High-Fidelity Patient Simulation

IN NURSING EDUCATION

Edited by

Wendy M. Nehring, PhD,

Dean and Professor
College of Nursing
East Tennessee State University
Johnson City, Tennessee

Felissa R. Lashley, PhD, RN, FACMG, FAAN

Professor and Past Dean
College of Nursing
Rutgers, The State University of New Jersey
Newark, New Jersey

Dean Emerita
School of Nursing
Southern Illinois University Edwardsville
Edwardsville, Illinois

JONES AND BARTLETT PUBLISHERS

Sudbury, Massachusetts

BOSTON   TORONTO   LONDON   SINGAPORE

World Headquarters

Jones and Bartlett Publishers
40 Tall Pine Drive
Sudbury, MA 01776
978-443-5000
info@jbpub.com
www.jbpub.com

Jones and Bartlett Publishers
Canada
6339 Ormindale Way
Mississauga, Ontario L5V 1J2
Canada

Jones and Bartlett Publishers
International
Barb House, Barb Mews
London W6 7PA
United Kingdom

Jones and Bartlett's books and products are available through most bookstores and online booksellers. To contact Jones and Bartlett Publishers directly, call 800-832-0034, fax 978-443-8000, or visit our website www.jbpub.com.

Substantial discounts on bulk quantities of Jones and Bartlett's publications are available to corporations, professional associations, and other qualified organizations. For details and specific discount information, contact the special sales department at Jones and Bartlett via the above contact information or send an email to specialsales@jbpub.com.

The authors, editor, and publisher have made every effort to provide accurate information. However, they are not responsible for errors, omissions, or for any outcomes related to the use of the contents of this book and take no responsibility for the use of the products and procedures described. Treatments and side effects described in this book may not be applicable to all people; likewise, some people may require a dose or experience a side effect that is not described herein. Drugs and medical devices are discussed that may have limited availability controlled by the Food and Drug Administration (FDA) for use only in a research study or clinical trial. Research, clinical practice, and government regulations often change the accepted standard in this field. When consideration is being given to use of any drug in the clinical setting, the health care provider or reader is responsible for determining FDA status of the drug, reading the package insert, and reviewing prescribing information for the most up-to-date recommendations on dose, precautions, and contraindications, and determining the appropriate usage for the product. This is especially important in the case of drugs that are new or seldom used.

Production Credits

Publisher: Kevin Sullivan
Acquisitions Editor: Emily Ekle
Acquisitions Editor: Amy Sibley
Associate Editor: Patricia Donnelly
Editorial Assistant: Rachel Shuster
Senior Production Editor: Carolyn F. Rogers
Production Assistant: Roya Millard
Senior Marketing Manager: Barb Bartoszek

V.P., Manufacturing and Inventory Control: Therese Connell
Composition: Spearhead, Inc.
Cover Design: Scott Moden
Cover Image: © Pixac/Dreamstime.com
Printing and Binding: Malloy, Inc.
Cover Printing: Malloy, Inc.

Library of Congress Cataloging-in-Publication Data
Nehring, Wendy M., 1957-
  High-fidelity patient simulation in nursing education / Wendy Nehring
and Felissa Lashley.
       p. ; cm.
    Includes bibliographical references and index.
    ISBN-13: 978-0-7637-5651-2 (pbk.)
    ISBN-10: 0-7637-5651-2 (pbk.)
  1. Nursing—Study and teaching. 2. Simulated patients. I. Lashley,
    Felissa R., 1941- II. Title.
    [DNLM: 1. Education, Nursing—methods—United States. 2. Patient Simulation—United States.
    3. Nursing Education Research—methods—United States. WY 18 N396h 2010]
    RT73.5.N44 2010
    610.73076—dc22
                                    2008050242

6048

Printed in the United States of America
13 12 11 10 09   10 9 8 7 6 5 4 3 2 1

In loving memory of my parents, Virgil
and Allene Nehring

Wendy M. Nehring

Special love to my special family—Neal, Anne,
Jacob, and Grace; Heather; Pete,
Julie, Ben, Hannah, and Lydia

Felissa R. Lashley

Contents

**Chapter 8—An Interdisciplinary Simulation Training and
       Education Program for an All-Hazards Response . 149**
Joy Spellman

Chapter 9—Hospital-Based Competency Development 167
Linda J. von Reyn

UNIT III: DEVELOPING AND IMPLEMENTING SCENARIOS . . . 187

Chapter 10—Baccalaureate Nursing Education 189
*Deatrah Dubose, Laurie D. Sellinger-Karmel, and
Robert L. Scoloveno*

Kathy Carver and Penny L. Marshall

Karen S. Kesten, Helen F. Brown,
Stephen Hurst, and Linda A. Briggs

Preface

Recent national trends related both to the healthcare delivery system and to higher education have created an environment of change for nursing education, especially for pre-licensure students. Driven by the need to address patient safety concerns and improve quality of care, a nursing faculty shortage, increased technology with which to deliver health care, higher patient acuity, decreased length of hospital stays, decreased availability of clinical sites, and, in some cases, less funding for clinical sites, nursing deans and directors must determine alternative and creative ways to teach future nurses. Likewise, agency-based nurse educators and administrators face a number of challenges, such as a nursing shortage, increased patient acuity, introduction of more complicated technology with which to deliver health care, limitations on orientation times, a need to address concerns related to patient safety and quality of care, and a need for improved interdisciplinary team performance—all of which require new and creative solutions. Increasing numbers of state boards of nursing are also requiring nurses to obtain a specific number of continued education units for relicensure, resulting in new opportunities for continuing education programs.

One solution to the growing concerns linked to these trends is the advent of high-fidelity patient simulators in nursing programs and in hospitals. These simulators, which serve as adjuncts to didactic learning, represent the closest possible technology to real patients and allow for repetitive "hands-on" learning in a safe environment where mistakes can be safely made. In turn, the nurse or nursing student who participates in simulation gains experience and confidence in his or her ability to make critical clinical decisions in acute care situations, where time and skill often have critical consequences. Hospitals have used high-fidelity patient simulators to address, for example, patient conditions and their intervention, competency assessments, hospital protocols, and organizational goals.

High-fidelity full-body patient simulators first appeared in the 1970s as a tool for anesthesiology education. Their development for this application was inspired by the successful use of simulation primarily in aviation training. Nevertheless, such simulators were not widely used by nurses until the 1990s. Thus such technology for nursing education has essentially been available—albeit not widely—for approximately 10 years. In that time, nurses have written several articles on the use of simulation in nursing programs, though the nurse-generated literature does not match the volume of articles written by physicians and anesthesiologists on use of simulators. Less research has also been done by nurses in this area. Increasing numbers of nursing programs are now acquiring high-fidelity patient simulators, however, and this book both provides a necessary primer for nursing programs starting out and stands as a state-of-the-science review for nurses interested in nursing's achievements in this field.

In 2008, Wendy Nehring conducted a survey of boards of nursing in each U.S. state, the District of Columbia, and Puerto Rico. She found that the boards of nursing were well aware of the national trends and concerns noted earlier in this preface and were very interested in how the use of high-fidelity patient simulation might address these concerns and enhance the practice of graduating nurses. In some cases, states allowed for the use of high-fidelity patient simulation to replace clinical hours and had written this approval into their regulations.

Given that high-fidelity patient simulation is gaining a well-respected place in nursing education and practice, it is important that nurse educators be familiar with what the technology can do and how to optimally use it. As a result, we organized this book into four units.

The first unit provides background information on high-fidelity patient simulation. Chapter 1 offers a detailed history of simulation in nursing education and practice. An overview of the use of models, computer-assisted instruction, role-playing, standardized patients, virtual reality, and mannequins with different levels of fidelity across time is given here. Chapter 2 covers the use of theoretical frameworks in structuring high-fidelity patient simulation experiences, and discusses the current body of nursing research using high-fidelity patient simulation. Recommendations for future nursing research are provided as well.

The second unit covers the development and implementation of nursing simulation programs in a variety of settings, including associate, baccalaureate, and graduate nursing education programs; a statewide nursing simulation program; an interdisciplinary simulation center; a focused bioterrorism interdisciplinary simulation program; and a hospital. The authors discuss planning, personnel decisions, faculty education, space concerns, equipment decisions, lessons learned, and future plans as they relate to simulation. This unit provides very helpful advice for anyone who is thinking about or just beginning to implement such a program.

The third unit will benefit any nurse educator who is currently working with high-fidelity patient simulators, as it addresses the development and implementation of scenarios. The authors of these chapters describe how they identify the topic of the scenario, who develops the scenario, and how the scenario is developed; they also outline the implementation process, the successes and challenges inherent in simulation development, use of simulation with different fidelity to complete the scenario, and future changes. The chapters in this unit were contributed from faculty members in associate, baccalaureate, and graduate nursing programs; a regional nursing simulation program; an interdisciplinary simulation center; an international interdisciplinary simulation center; and a hospital. Additional chapters in this unit include information on debriefing, a curriculum for pre-licensure nursing education programs, and evaluation. Again, helpful advice from these experienced users is shared to benefit the reader.

The fourth unit completes the book by speculating on the future of simulation in nursing education and practice. As we reflect on the use of simulation in nursing education and practice as it stands now (as is the first chapter) and on the future of this technology for the future education of nurses and nursing students (in the last chapter), it becomes clear how the use of simulation, in its many forms, has advanced the art and science of nursing.

We would like to thank Rachel Shuster and Amy Sibley of Jones and Bartlett Publishers for their assistance throughout the process of publishing this book. We would also like to thank all of the nursing pioneers in simulation who have dared to be innovative. We hope that this book will be beneficial to any nurse educator, in any setting, who wishes to implement high-fidelity patient simulation in his or her teaching.

Wendy M. Nehring and Felissa R. Lashley

Contributors

Wendy M. Nehring, PhD, RN, FAAN, FAAIDD
Editor
Dean and Professor
College of Nursing
East Tennessee State University
Johnson City, TN
(Chapter 1, Chapter 2)

Felissa R. Lashley, PhD, RN, FACMG, FAAN
Editor
Professor and Past Dean
College of Nursing
Rutgers, The State University of New Jersey
Newark, NJ
Dean Emerita
School of Nursing
Southern Illinois University Edwardsville
Edwardsville, IL
(Chapter 20)

Catherine Bailey, RN, PhD
Associate Professor
College of Nursing
Texas Woman's University
Dallas, TX
(Chapter 17)

Marcy Beck, RN, MSN
Co-director, Regional Simulation Center
Midwestern State University
Wichita Falls, TX
(Chapter 13)

Jana F. Berryman
Project Coordinator
Colorado Center for Nursing Excellence
Aurora, CO
(Chapter 6)

Linda A. Briggs, MSN, ACNP-BC, ANP-BC
Clinical Assistant Professor
School of Nursing and Health Studies
Georgetown University
Washington, DC
(Chapter 12)

Helen F. Brown, MS, BC-ACNP, BC-FNP
Doctors Emergency Service, PA
Anne Arundel Medical Center, Emergency Department
Annapolis, MD
(Chapter 12)

Kathy Carver, RN, MN
Nursing Professor
Johnson County Community College
Overland Park, KS
(Chapter 11)

Thomas J. Doyle, RN, MSN
Vice President and Chief Learning Officer
Medical Education Technologies, Inc.
Sarasota, FL
(Chapter 18)

Deatrah Dubose, RN, MSN, APN-C
Clinical Instructor
Rutgers, The State University of New Jersey
Newark, NJ
(Chapter 10)

Margaret Faut-Callahan, PhD, CRNA, FAAN
Dean and Professor
College of Nursing
Marquette University
Milwaukee, WI
(Chapter 5)

Paula Gubrud, RN, EdD
Statewide Director of Simulation
Oregon Health & Sciences School of Nursing
Portland, OR
(Chapter 14)

Stephen Hurst, BEng
Director of Medical Technologies
School of Nursing and Health Sciences
Georgetown University
Washington, DC
(Chapter 12)

Pamela R. Jeffries, RN, DNS, FAAN, ANEF
Associate Dean for Academic Affairs
Johns Hopkins University
Baltimore, MD
(Chapter 19)

Judy Johnson-Russell, RN, EdD
Clinical Educator
Education and Training Services
Medical Education Technologies, Inc.
Sarasota, FL
(Chapter 17)

Robert L. Kerner, Jr., JD, RN, CEN
Clinical Education Specialist
Patient Safety Institute
Lake Success, NY
(Chapter 7)

Karen S. Kesten, MSN, APRN, CCNS
Assistant Professor and Program Director of Acute Care Nursing
Practitioner and Acute and Critical Care Clinical Nurse Specialist Programs
School of Nursing and Health Sciences
Georgetown University
Washington, DC
(Chapter 12)

**Tan Khoon Kiat, MEd, BSc (Hons) Nursing Studies,
PG Cert Public Health**
Senior Technologist
School of Applied & Health Sciences (Nursing)
ITE College East
Singapore
(Chapter 15)

Beth Kuzminsky, RN, MSN
Curriculum Development Manager
Winter Institute for Simulation, Education, and Research
Pittsburgh, PA
(Chapter 16)

**Yvonne Lau, Master's Degree in Health Sciences (Education),
Bachelor's Degree in Health Science (Nursing), Diploma in Nursing**
Lecturer
School of Applied and Health Sciences (Nursing)
ITE College East
Singapore
(Chapter 15)

Kim Leighton, RN, PhD, CNE
Dean of Instructional Technology
Bryan LGH College of Health Sciences
Lincoln, NE
(Chapter 18)

Keith Marino, MSN, CRNA
Instructor
Nurse Anesthesia Program
Rush University
Chicago, IL
(Chapter 5)

Penny L. Marshall, RN, PhD
Nursing Professor
Johnson County Community College
Overland Park, KS
(Chapter 11)

Karen Mayes, RN, MSN
Professor and Acting Director of Nursing Education
St. Louis Community College
St. Louis, MO
(Chapter 4)

Marilyn McGuire-Sessions, RN, MSN
Nursing Program Director
Portland Community College
Portland, OR
(Chapter 14)

Angela M. McNelis, RN, PhD
Associate Professor
Indiana University School of Nursing
Indianapolis, IN
(Chapter 19)

Suppiah Nagammal, RN, BHSN, Cert Ed
ITE College East
Singapore
(Chapter 15)

John M. O'Donnell, CRNA, MSN, DrPh(c)
Director, University of Pittsburgh Nurse Anesthesia Program
Associate Director, Winter Institute for Simulation, Education, and Research
Pittsburgh, PA
(Chapter 16)

Patricia Ravert, RN, PhD
Associate Professor and Associate Dean of Undergraduate Affairs
College of Nursing
Brigham Young University
Provo, UT
(Chapter 3)

Robert L. Scoloveno, RN, MS, CCRN
Clinical Instructor
Rutgers, The State University of New Jersey
Newark, NJ
(Chapter 10)

Laurie D. Sellinger-Karmel, RN, MSN
Clinical Instructor
Rutgers, The State University of New Jersey
Newark, NJ
(Chapter 10)

Joy Spellman, RN, MSN
Director, Center for Public Health Preparedness
Burlington County College
Mt. Laurel, NJ
(Chapter 8)

Susan Sportsman, RN, PhD
Dean
College of Health Sciences and Human Services
Midwestern State University
Wichita Falls, TX
(Chapter 13)

Linda J. von Reyn, RN, PhD
Dartmouth-Hitchcock Medical Center
Acting Chief Nursing Officer
Lebanon, NH
(Chapter 9)

Judith Wiley, CRNA, DNP
Instructor and Associate Director
Nurse Anesthesia Program
Rush University
Chicago, IL
(Chapter 5)

Unit 1

Foundations

CHAPTER 1

History of Simulation in Nursing

Wendy M. Nehring

Simulation, in its many forms, has been a beneficial adjunct to teaching nursing since the beginning of formalized nursing education. The purpose of simulation is "to replicate some or nearly all of the essential aspects of a clinical situation so that the situation may be more readily understood and managed when it occurs for real in clinical practice" (Morton, 1995, p. 76). Today, advances in technology both in the educational and healthcare settings provide many opportunities to enhance the learning of the nursing student. Prensky (2001), however, emphasized that the way in which today's students learn is not compatible with the current educational system. Today's students have had access to various forms of technology and ways of thinking that significantly differ from those experiences of most faculty.

This chapter reviews the history of simulation in nursing. Specific attention is paid to factors influencing the use of simulation in nursing education and the identification and discussion of the continuum of simulation in nursing education.

FACTORS INFLUENCING THE USE OF SIMULATION

As nursing education has evolved across time, various factors have influenced those changes. Today's influences are not novel; indeed, most likely played a role in the past. Today's primary influences are (1) societal demands for safety and quality, (2) a need to recreate health professions education, (3) ethical considerations, (4) technological advances, (5) professional shortages, and (6) a changing landscape for the delivery of patient care. Each of these factors, which frequently overlap, is discussed in more detail in the following subsections.

Safety and Quality

One cannot read a newspaper today without seeing an article about an incident of patient care that resulted in an unfavorable outcome. To address this issue, many federal agencies and private organizations have responded. Each year the Joint Commission releases its annual national patient safety goals (Joint Commission, 2009), which healthcare agencies must in turn address in their annual reports. In 2006, the Agency for Healthcare Research and Quality (AHRQ) published *AHRQ Quality Indicators: Guide to Patient Safety Indicators*, which serve as a further check on healthcare professional practice and agency outcomes. Several Institute of Medicine (IOM) reports over the past decade have also focused on this reality and addressed the need for reform in the practice and education of healthcare professionals (e.g., Aspden, Corrigan, Wolcott, & Erickson, 2004; Committee on Quality of Health Care in America, Institute of Medicine, 2001; Kohn, Corrigan, & Donaldson, 2000).

The IOM concluded that there are five areas of competence in health professions education that needed to be included in the curriculum: patient-centered care, interdisciplinary teams, evidence-based practice, quality improvement, and informatics (Greiner & Knebel, 2003). It is likely that nursing schools will need to document how these competencies are included in the undergraduate and graduate curricula in the future as measurements of their won quality and competence for accreditation purposes. Nursing, to date, has measured competence for the pre-licensure nursing student only by means of the passing of a multiple-choice test (i.e., NCLEX-RN).

Kane (1992) defined competence as the "degree to which the individual can use the knowledge, skills, and judgment associated with the profession to perform effectively in the domain of possible encounters defining scope of professional practice" (p. 166). del Bueno and her colleagues (1987) discussed competency development as being multidimensional and judged on knowledge, skills, and critical thinking. The National Council of State Boards of Nursing (NCSBN) has discussed the issue of competency in nursing for a number of years (1996, 2005) and found that "one of the greatest challenges to all health care practitioners is the attainment, maintenance, and advancement of professional competence (2005, p. 1). This organization continues to debate what the best measurements of competence should be. In its 2007 publication, *Position Statement on Competence and Competency*, the American Nurses Association stated that the measurement criteria found under the standards of nursing practice and standards of professional performance in each of the individual scope and standards of practice documents they publish serve as competency statements. Furthermore, as the *Essentials of Baccalaureate Nursing Education* document is revised, the American Association of

Colleges of Nursing (AACN, 2007) has stated that this document will serve as recommendations for the competencies needed for entry into professional practice and will include essential knowledge, skills, and attitudes.

In 1989, the NCSBN received funding from the Kellogg Foundation to develop a computerized clinical-decision-making assessment exam using clinical simulations. This exam was proposed as a second measure of competence, along with the NCLEX-RN, which was a paper-and-pencil exam at that point in time, for individuals seeking licensure as a registered nurse. This new assessment test would involve written answers to interactive case studies. In 1999, the NCSBN Delegate Assembly voted down the use of this test (Bersky & Krawczak, 1995; Bersky, Krawczak, & Kumar, 1998; Bremner & Brannan, 2000; Forker & McDonald, 1996).

It is again time for nursing to consider expanding the measurement of competence to include an assessment of skills. Obviously, the practice of nursing involves the successful completion of psychomotor skills (e.g., inserting a catheter, inserting a needle for intravenous fluids) in a timely manner.

In other healthcare fields, such as medicine, the national licensure exam already includes both multiple-choice written examinations and skills assessment, with and without the use of standardized patients (Tetzlaff, 2007). Specific medical organizations have also embraced the use of simulation in education and certification. The American College of Surgeons (2007) will accredit skill centers that include simulation. The Accreditation Council for Graduate Medical Education (ACGME) (2007) has mandated training using simulation. The American Society of Anesthesiologists' Committee on Outreach Education (2006) will evaluate and give approval for simulation programs. Finally, beginning in 2007, the American Board of Anesthesiologists will include simulation as a component of recertification for those graduating from their initial anesthesiology program from that year on (Gaba & Raemer, 2007).

Changes in Nursing Education

New knowledge and technology, which are currently proliferating at an exponential rate, as well as changes in the delivery of health care should be integrated into nursing education in a timely manner. Active learning techniques and interprofessional learning opportunities have been emphasized as essential to healthcare professional education in the twenty-first century (Greiner & Knebel, 2003).

Tanner (2006) called for a transformation of clinical education based on increased patient acuity, decreased numbers of clinical sites, costs of clinical sites in some locations, inefficiency of student time while at the clinical site, and the faculty shortage, among other factors. She advocated for new ways of meeting learning outcomes including simulation. AACN (2007) has concurred with this position, stating that the new *Essentials* document for baccalaureate nursing education should include a set of quality indicators for clinical learning. In the revision of the *Essentials of Baccalaureate Nursing Education* (AACN, 2008), the sixth essential—"Interprofessional communication and collaboration for improving patient health outcomes"—specifically addresses the use of simulation. NCSBN (2006) has also stated that research needs to be conducted to ascertain best practices for developing clinical competency, although this organization does state that innovative teaching strategies, such as simulation, are beneficial for this purpose. The Health Resources and Services Administration (HRSA, 2002) has recommended the use of simulation in clinical settings and suggested that faculty should develop skills on the use of simulation. According to Boller and Jones (2008), nursing curricula need to be revised to include the use of simulation and the appropriate infrastructure needs to be supported and developed. This perspective has been supported by state nursing workforce reports issued in the past several years by 15 states (e.g., Bristol, 2006; Oregon Nursing Leadership Council, 2005; Waneka, 2008) as a means of increasing the numbers of nursing students and remaining cost-effective in the use of faculty resources.

Patel and Gould (2006) have identified several problems in the mentor–apprenticeship model currently used in health professional education, including nursing. They list five notable problems: practicing on patients, timing for advancement, finding consistency in clinical sites, educating expenses, and increasing time issues. Practicing skills and procedures on patients carries increased risk and brings up ethical considerations (discussed in the next section). Students learn and reach competence at different rates, so competency-based advancement may be more efficient than time-based advancement. In addition, not only are clinical sites decreasing, but the quality of the available sites is also variable, although it is hoped that nursing students obtain comparable clinical experiences. Furthermore, whether or not a clinical site charges for a nursing program, it is costly for a hospital to have students present. The student–faculty ratio on the unit also influences the amount of time that the faculty member or staff nurse has to spend with a particular student. The use of simulation can help to counteract these problems in nursing education.

Ethical Considerations

Given the well-known trends toward higher patient acuity and shorter hospital stays, Decker (2007) has wondered whether there would come a time when nursing students would need to tell patients that they have never performed a particular skill or procedure on a patient before and this would be their first time. Patel and Gould (2006) state that the goal of simulation is "to eliminate the initial learning curve in the clinical setting so first attempts are optimal" (p. S166). This is an important consideration as nursing faculty review curricular changes.

Technological Advances

Technology and its applications to assessment, diagnosis, intervention, and evaluation require the implementation of nursing curricular changes at a constant rate. For example, computer modeling allows students to visualize the body in greater detail and depth than ever before. With this technology, students can study the internal structures of the body at any time with the use of the computer. We can also treat an individual thousands of miles away as a result of advances in telemedicine and informatics. Yet even with the use of this technology, we are reminded of the influence of human factors for a successful patient outcome and the need to provide hands-on patient care.

Professional Shortages

The nursing shortage and the need to increase the numbers of nursing students, coupled with the faculty shortage, have further contributed to the need for a paradigm shift in nursing education, which should include simulation (Seropian, Brown, Gavilanes, & Driggers, 2004). After conducting an integrative review of the literature, Goodin (2003) stated that the current nursing shortage is a result of aging nurses in the workforce, fewer nursing graduates in relation to retiring nurses, a changing work environment with challenges including sicker patients staying in healthcare settings for shorter periods of time, and a poor image of nursing. According to this author, solutions to this problem might include revising recruitment and retention strategies, improving the image of nursing, and supporting the development of legislation to positively alter the impediments to reverse the shortage. Elgie (2007) has emphasized that the most viable solution would be to alter the wages and benefits of nurses so as to recruit and retain nurses over the long term.

Similarly, the nursing faculty shortage has been influenced by an aging workforce, decreased interest in academia by younger nurses largely due to its relatively low salaries, the costs of higher education for achieving graduate degrees to meet criteria for faculty positions, the decreased numbers of graduates from nursing graduate programs in proportion to faculty leaving their positions for retirement and other reasons, faculty workloads, and age of graduates of nursing doctoral programs (AACN, 2005). Innovative solutions have included forming partnerships with clinical agencies to provide clinical faculty, use of retired faculty to teach part-time in didactic courses, and simulation to augment clinical education. These shortages in the nursing and nursing faculty workforces will persist for a number of years, so it is imperative that nursing schools take a proactive stance in addressing these challenges for their specific geographic area.

Changes in the Delivery of Health Care

The delivery of health care in our society today has been evaluated on cost, quality, and access. Nursing care, by comparison, can best be judged by the quality. Nurses today must be competent in critical thinking, problem solving, clinical judgment, evidence-based best practices, and performance of skills to achieve optimal patient outcomes, and they must be able to evolve from novice to expert in as little time as possible (Boller & Jones, 2008). To prepare pre-licensure nursing students to achieve these competencies, changes must be made to our current system of providing nursing education. Several states have developed regional or state simulation centers to facilitate such competencies in both nursing students and practicing nurses, including Colorado (Colorado Center for Nursing Excellence, 2007), North Carolina (Metcalfe, Hall, & Carpenter, 2007), and Oregon (Krautscheid & Burton, 2003). In addition, a growing number of nursing programs have purchased high-fidelity patient simulators in an effort to enhance clinical experiences by decreasing the number of clinical sites, patient selection and acuity, and ability for students to perform all essential nursing tasks (Tanner, 2006).

A historical overview of the continuum of simulation is presented in the next section. It illustrates how the traditional lecture method must now be supplemented with simulation for optimal learning.

THE CONTINUUM OF SIMULATION

The continuum of simulation involves seven components:

- Partial and complex task trainers
- Role-play
- Games
- Computer-assisted instruction
- Standardized patients
- Virtual reality and haptic systems
- Integrated simulators: low- through high-fidelity simulators (instructor-driven and model-driven)

Case studies will not be discussed here as a category because each of the preceding components, with the possible exception of partial and complex task trainers, involves the use of a case study. The personnel, equipment, and costs of each component vary and, as the technology has evolved, many of these categories have converged.

In the past, the educational question in the nursing literature for each category has primarily been the same: Does the use of this technology enhance the learning of the student? In addition, the advantages and disadvantages listed for each category in the nursing literature are also similar; they are summarized here. The advantages of the use of simulation in the nursing literature include these points:

- Simulation involves active learning (Clark, 1976; Corbett & Beveridge, 1982; Davidhizar, 1977; Greenblatt & Duke, 1975).
- Simulation increases knowledge, communication skills, motivation, confidence, and affective learning (Corbett & Beveridge, 1982; Davidhizar, 1977; de Tornyay & Thompson, 1982; Dooling, 1986; Greenblatt & Duke, 1975; Krautscheid & Burton, 2003; Kuipers & Clemens, 1998; Taylor, 1980; Theroux & Pearce, 2006; Thomas, O'Connor, Albert, Boutain, & Brandt, 2001).
- Simulation improves critical thinking (Monti, Wren, Haas, & Lupine, 1998; Nehring, Ellis, & Lashley, 2001; O'Donnell, Fletcher, Dixon, & Palmer, 1998; Thomas et al., 2001).
- Simulation decreases anxiety (Blau, 1983; Davidhizar, 1977; Theroux & Pearce, 2006).
- Simulation allows for the application of knowledge and skills and the ability to make mistakes in a safe environment (Clark, 1976; Davidhizar, 1977; Dooling, 1987; Howard, 1987; Monti et al., 1998; Nehring et al., 2001; O'Donnell et al., 1998).
- Scenarios may be developed based on course objectives (Bosek, Li, & Hicks, 2007; Vessey & Huss, 2002).
- Standardized experiences can be offered to all students, including those not commonly found in the clinical setting (Dooling, 1987; Grobe, 1984; Krautscheid & Burton, 2003; Lasater, 2007b; Sweeney, O'Malley, & Freeman, 1982; Thomas et al., 2001).
- Simulation provides instant feedback (de Tornyay & Thompson, 1982; Feingold, Calaluce, & Kallen, 2004; Taylor, 1980; Theroux & Pearce, 2006; Vessey & Huss, 2002).
- Simulation increases teamwork skills (Krautscheid & Burton, 2003; Lasater, 2007b).

Disadvantages include the following issues:

- Simulation is time-consuming to develop and implement (Clark, 1977; Dooling, 1987; Monti et al., 1998; Nehring et al., 2001).

- For many instructors, simulation is an unfamiliar mode of teaching at first (Clark, 1977).
- Simulation is expensive (Colliver & Swartz, 1997; Ebbert & Connors, 2004; King, Perkowski-Rodgers, & Pohl, 1994; Monti et al., 1998; Nehring et al., 2001).
- Limited numbers of students can be actively involved at one time (Henrichs, Rule, Grady, & Ellis, 2002; Monti et al., 1998; Nehring et al., 2001; O'Donnell et al., 1998).

Nursing research for most forms of simulation has resulted in mixed results, with some studies finding statistical significance and others finding none (see Nehring & Lashley, in press). Nursing research specific to the use of high-fidelity patient simulation is discussed in Chapter 2. Students have consistently noted that they feel that they learn more with simulation, so further research is needed to prove the efficacy of simulation in nursing education. A review of each category of simulation in nursing education follows.

Partial and Complex Task Trainers

In 1874, Lees wrote that every nursing school should have "a mechanical dummy, models of legs and arms to learn bandaging, a jointed skeleton, a black drawing board, and drawings, books, and models" (p. 34). The first "mechanical dummy" to be produced for the purpose of nursing education in the United States came in 1911 in the form of Mrs. Chase, a life-size mannequin (see Figure 1-1). Manufactured by the M. J. Chase Company of Pawtucket, Rhode Island (a doll company), Mrs. Chase came with jointed hips, elbows, and knees. She was originally conceived by Lauder Sutherland, who was the principal of the Hartford Hospital Training School in Hartford, Connecticut, between 1905 and 1918. Sutherland believed that this doll could help with classroom demonstrations and allow nursing students the opportunity to practice their skills without causing possible discomfort to patients. Improvements in Mrs. Chase occurred over the years allowing for procedures involving the urethra, vagina, and rectum, as well as an injection site in her arm. Baby and male versions were produced later, with production of the Chase mannequins continuing until the 1970s (Herrmann, 1981, 2008). Interestingly, Mrs. Chase is mentioned in the first Cherry Ames book (Wells, 1944).

In 1919, the Committee on Education of the National League of Nursing Education (now the National League for Nursing) published its first standard curriculum. In this document, the authors listed the equipment and supplementary materials needed to enhance the lectures for each area. For example, in a lecture on infant feeding, the suggested equipment and illustrative materials included "charts, models, pictures, utensil and materials for infant feeding,

Figure 1-1   Mrs. Chase

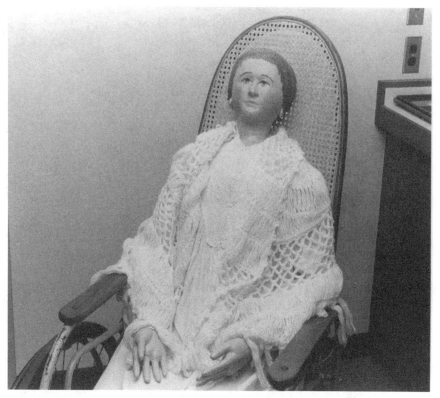

Source: Courtesy of the Hamilton Archives at Hartford Hospital (Hartford, CT).

food-charts, etc." (Committee on Education of the National League of Nursing Education, 1919, p. 100).

Today, task trainers range from simple to complex (see Figure 1-2). Early two-dimensional charts have been replaced with three-dimensional computer modeling (e.g., A.D.A.M. interactive anatomy). Specific body parts and full-size static mannequins can also be purchased to represent different ethnic groups. Task trainers represent the most common form of simulation (Gaba, Fish, & Howard, 1994).

Role-Play

Role-playing has been used with nursing students for many years, primarily to allow students time to practice their communication skills and learn

Figure 1-2   Examples of Task Trainers

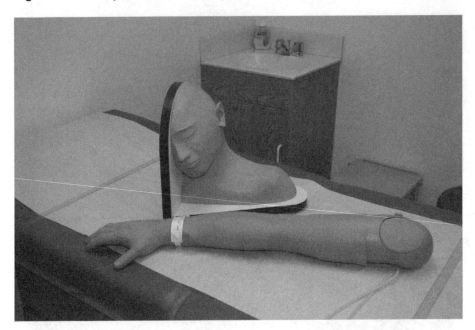

empathy for their patients (Jenkins & Turick-Gibson, 1999; Schoenly, 1994). During a role-playing experience, nursing students are assigned different roles, such as the nurse, patient, or family member. After the role-playing experience is over, the students and their faculty member participate in a debriefing period (Jenkins & Turick-Gibson, 1999; Newcomb & Riddlesperger, 2007; Schoenly, 1994). A videotaped, role-playing experience involving several students, faculty, and props was described by Johnson, Zerwic, and Theis (1999). Swart (1992) suggested that role-playing might replace time in a clinical setting under certain circumstances.

Although role-playing experiences with students and faculty continue to be used in nursing education today, more sophisticated formats, such as standardized patients, computerized games and Internet sites, and high-fidelity patient simulation are more commonly used.

Games

Nursing educators have developed a variety of games in an attempt to teach nursing students decision-making skills. Specific games incorporate the educators' knowledge on a particular client population (e.g., the elderly) (Chaisson, 1977; Marte, 1988) or nursing specialization (e.g., psychiatric care) (Cosgray, Davidhizar, Grostefon, Powell, & Wringer, 1990; Davidhizar, 1977). Ulione (1983) felt that games differed from role-playing because they had more structure and were based on a theoretical framework.

Today, games that involve educational goals are called "serious gaming." Skiba (2008) has reported on several game-oriented initiatives related to the promotion of physical activity and rehabilitation and therapy. She described a nursing research study by Dr. Glenna Dowling at the University of California at San Francisco, who is using the Wii platform to assist patients with Parkinson's disease to improve their ambulation and balance. As serious gaming advances, the lines between games, computer-assisted instruction, and virtual reality will continue to blur.

Computer-Assisted Instruction

Computer-assisted instruction (CAI) first appeared in the late 1970s, although the first nursing literature on the topic was published in the early 1980s (e.g., Lange, 1982; Sweeney et al., 1982). The American Nurses Association's Council on Computer Applications in Nursing (1986) found that nursing students can learn the same material in half the time through the use of CAI. As nursing educators saw this benefit, CAI was developed for a variety of learning needs, including health assessment (Bradburn, Zeleznikow, & Adams, 1993; Sweeney et al., 1982), decision making (Grossman & Hudson, 2001; Wong, Wong, & Richard, 1992), and obstetrical nursing skills (Weiner, Gordon, & Gilman, 1993). More recently, Giddens (2007), working at the University of New Mexico College of Nursing, developed a virtual neighborhood in which 30 characters interact and experience health problems that require nursing assessment and intervention across the undergraduate curriculum.

Online instruction for nursing courses is now commonplace. New evolutions of online course platforms allow for increased interactivity and virtual reality experiences. An example is the Croquet Project (2007), which is an open-source online platform that allows for interactive, multiuser, multiformat applications.

Another example is Pulse!! The Virtual Clinical Learning Lab (http://www.sp.tamucc.edu/pulse/home.asp), which allows students from various health professions to work together in their distinctive roles to solve a critical incident in a patient as part of a team. Skiba (2007) has discussed the development of virtual worlds, also called live-action role-playing games (LARPs), in which players can interact in different levels of a three-dimensional (3-D) virtual world. To participate in a LARP, each player develops an avatar that represents the individual. An example that has been used in many university courses is Second Life, although its use in a nursing course has not been detailed in the literature.

Standardized Patients

Traditionally, standardized patients involve people who may or may not be professional actors who are instructed on how to act as if they have a particular disease or condition in a given patient situation in a given healthcare setting. The first standardized patient was introduced in the United States in the School of Medicine at the University of Southern California by Dr. Howard Barrows (Jenkins & Schaivone, 2007). Encounters with such patients soon became an essential standard of medical education and later became part of the medical licensing examination.

Traditionally, standardized patients are used to teach and evaluate assessment, communication, and interviewing skills (Ebbert & Connors, 2004; Kruijver, Kerkstra, Kerssens, Hoitkamp, Bensing, & van de Wiel, 2001). They are used alone or as an element of a multistation evaluation exercise, called an objective structured clinical experience (OSCE) (Vessey & Huss, 2002). The documentation of the use of standardized patients in undergraduate nursing programs has been less frequent (e.g., Johnsson, Kjellberg, & Lagerstrom, 2006; Wilson et al., 2006; Yoo & Yoo, 2003) than in graduate nursing education (e.g., Ebbert & Connors, 2004; Gibbons et al., 2002; McDowell, Nardini, Negley, & White, 1984; Miller, Wilbur, Dedhiya, Talashek, & Mrtek, 1999; O'Connor, Albert, & Thomas, 1999; Ross et al., 1988; Rutledge, Garzon, Scott, & Karlowicz, 2004; Theroux & Pearce, 2006; Vessey & Huss, 2002).

Virtual Reality and Haptic Systems

Virtual reality allows the user to interact with a computer-based world and often involves haptics (i.e., tactile simulation). The first mention of the use of virtual reality in nursing education was by Phillips (1993). Many virtual reality systems are available for surgeons to practice their surgical skills, but at present the only virtual reality system using haptics that is available for nursing education is the Laerdal Virtual IV System for learning intravenous catheterization. This product was originally a prototype developed as a collaboration between a university and a technology corporation (Merril & Barker, 1996).

In the near future, Internet virtual worlds will be used by nursing educators to teach and evaluate a variety of skills in their nursing students. The classroom will be virtual without university borders (Skiba, 2007). (See Chapter 20.)

Recently, physicians have collaborated with computer specialists to develop two-dimensional, life-size virtual patients to replace simulated patients for medical education (Stevens et al., 2006). The virtual patient is projected on an exam room wall and the student, after reviewing the patient information, is instructed to take a health history from the virtual patient. The student wears a device on his or her head that allows the faculty member to see where the student looked while conversing with the virtual patient. Advantages of this system over the use of standardized patients include (1) no training is needed for the virtual patient, (2) there is a potential limitless repertoire of patient scenarios, (3) faculty can log students' achievement of performance indicators in real time, (4) scenarios may be tailored to meet individual student needs, and (5) the simulator provides a safe environment in which to practice. This technology will be of benefit to both undergraduate and graduate nursing education.

Integrated Simulators

Integrated simulators range from low- to high-fidelity models. The fidelity of a simulator is related to "how closely it replicates the selected domain and is determined by the number of elements that are replicated as well as the error between each element and the real world" (Gaba, 2004, p. 8).

Low-fidelity simulators usually provide for simple, gross movements without joint movement and are best used for the instruction of psychomotor skills. This type of simulator was described in the section on task trainers.

Moderate-fidelity simulators allow the student to listen for breath and heart sounds and to feel for some pulses, but lack the ability to show chest movements when breathing or eyes that blink or pupils that dilate, for example. VitalSim by Laerdal is an example of a moderate-fidelity simulator (Gaba et al., 1994). (See Figure 1-3.)

A *high-fidelity* patient simulator "is a computerized full-body mannequin that is able to provide real-time physiological and pharmacological parameters of persons of both genders, varying ages, and with different health conditions" (Nehring et al., 2001, p. 195). (See Figure 1-4.) High-fidelity patient simulators can be instructor-driven (more faculty time required to run scenario) or model-driven (less faculty time after physiological parameters are set for running of scenario). Leading manufacturers of high-fidelity

Figure 1-3   Example of a Moderate-Fidelity Patient Simulator

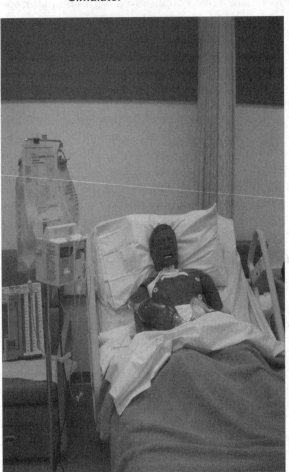

patient simulators are Gaumard, Laerdal, and Medical Education Technologies, Inc. (METI).

Integrated simulators first appeared with the development of SimOne, a partial body anesthesiology model that was introduced in the late 1960s (Denson & Abrahamson, 1969), and Harvey, a partial body mannequin that simulated 40 cardiovascular disease states (Gordon, 1974; Gordon et al., 1980) and was introduced in the 1970s. These prototypes were influenced by the cardiac resuscitation models introduced in the 1950s by Peter Safar and manufactured by Asmund Laerdal, a company that was originally a toy maker (Sinz, 2007).

Figure 1-4   Example of a High-Fidelity Patient Simulator

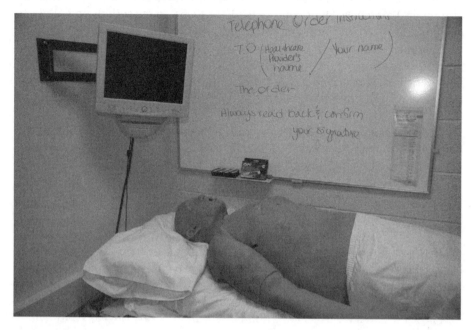

The high-fidelity patient simulators used today were modeled after the Comprehensive Anesthesia Simulation Environment (CASE) (Gaba & DeAnda, 1988) developed at Stanford and the Gainesville Anesthesia Simulator (GAS) (Good et al., 1988) developed at the University of Florida (Cooper & Taqueti, 2004). Although originally designed for the practice of anesthesia, nurses have provided input that influenced the evolution of these models over the past decade.

Use in Nursing Education

High-fidelity patient simulators have been used in nursing education for roughly a decade. The use of high-fidelity patient simulation in nursing education has been described for specific fields of practice, including critical care (Rauen, 2004), community health (Brady, Molzen, Graham, & O'Neill, 2006), pediatrics (Lambton, 2008), and nurse anesthesia (Fletcher, 1998; Monti et al., 1998; O'Donnell et al., 1998). Rauen (2001) emphasized this technology's ability to enhance critical thinking skills in nursing students through the use of high-fidelity patient simulation; Lasater (2007a, 2007b) discussed how high-fidelity patient simulation helped to increase clinical judgment among nursing students; and Bremner and colleagues (2006) described the use of high-fidelity patient simulation with nursing students prior to their first clinical experience. Moreover, Worzala, Glaser, and McGinley (2006) discussed a curriculum to teach mock codes for third- and fourth-year medical students and senior nursing students. Kappus and associates (2006) described a continuing education program in critical care using high-fidelity patient simulation. More recently, Lambton (2008) described a plan to substitute 25% of the pediatric clinical experience in a nursing program with a structured high-fidelity patient simulation experience.

The use of debriefing (see Chapter 17) and evaluation (see Chapter 19) will be covered elsewhere in this book. Nevertheless, it is clear that these important aspects of high-fidelity patient simulation have been discussed by nurse-authors. In addition, the first book on the use of simulation in nursing education was edited by Jeffries (2007).

Use in Nursing Practice

In the past few years the use of high-fidelity patient simulation in healthcare settings has taken off. The increased use of high-fidelity patient simulators and other forms of simulation has been accompanied by a corresponding decrease in time and expense for orientation or residency programs for new nursing graduates (Ackermann, Kenny, & Walker, 2007; Beyea, von Reyn, & Slattery, 2007; Zekonis & Gantt, 2007). Beyea and associates (2007) focused on the development of skills, critical thinking, patient safety, and human factors engineering in conjunction with this technology. Patient safety and the development of safer patient and nurse environments was the focus of articles by Nelson (2003) and Paparella, Mariani, Layton, and Carpenter (2004). Another area of focus has been competency testing of skills using high-fidelity patient simulation and other forms of simulation (Landry, Oberleitner, Landry, & Borazjani, 2006; Winslow, Dunn, & Rowlands, 2005). Other nurse-authors have discussed the use of high-fidelity patient simulation in the development of effective healthcare teams (Cole & Crichton, 2006; Johannsson, Ayida, & Sadler, 2005). Comprehensive educational models for the development of the graduate nurse from novice to expert have also been outlined for a hospital setting using a variety of simulations (Ferguson, Beeman, Eichorn, Jaramillo, & Wright, 2004), and assessment for a nurse internship for nurses joining the Air Force has used high-fidelity patient simulation (Eaves & Flagg, 2001).

Nursing Conceptual Models

Two conceptual models involving the use of high-fidelity patient simulation have been introduced by nurse-authors.

The first model is *critical incident nursing management* (CINM), which was introduced by Nehring, Lashley, and Ellis (2002). It follows in the footsteps of the anesthesiology model of *anesthesia crisis resource management* (ACRM) developed by Gaba, Fish, and Howard (1994). The CINM focuses on the nurse's response to a patient's critical incident based on characteristics of the nurse, characteristics of the patient, other members of the healthcare team, and the environment (Nehring & Lashley, 2004).

The second model is the *Nursing Education Simulation Framework* introduced by Jeffries (2005). Jeffries's framework takes into account characteristics of both teacher and student, educational practices, design characteristics of the simulation, and identification of outcomes. Further discussion of both this framework and the CINM model appears in Chapter 2.

Simulated Environments

Simulated environments rely on the ability of the environment to mimic the real world. Nursing faculty need to determine the setup of the simulation environment, which varies based on the number of beds, rooms, type of units, access from room to room, presence or absence of a "control" room, types of equipment and props, and use of audiovisual equipment for documentation. Wallpaper can be obtained to represent a specific real location or to represent a specific site such as an emergency department. Further study is required to identify how much realism is needed to adequately represent the real world for learning to take place.

CONCLUSION

It is obvious that the forms of simulation across this continuum arose at distinct points in time based on the level of technology present at that time. As time has advanced, the different forms of simulation have converged. More than likely, the simulation techniques employed in the next 10 years will differ radically from those in use today.

Jeffries (2005) has stressed that the nursing discipline should formulate guidelines to frame simulation development, best practices for implementation, and research to evaluate its efficacy for nursing education. Across time, nurse educators have recognized the significance of the supplementation of simulation in its various forms in nursing education. Today, more effort is needed to integrate high-fidelity patient simulators into the undergraduate and graduate nursing curricula as learning tools and as means to measure clinical competence. Moreover, a concerted effort is needed by nursing faculty and nursing administrators to identify a program of nursing research that will provide definitive proof that simulation—and especially the use of high-fidelity patient simulators—is efficacious and can be used to provide for the initial, advanced, and continuing education of competent nurses for years to come. Nurses must keep in line with the other health professions in the use of technology in their education and practice.

References

Accreditation Council for Graduate Medical Education (ACGME). (2007). *ACGME program requirements for graduate medical education in surgery.* Retrieved September 26, 2007, from: http://www.acgme.org/acWebsite/downloads/RRC.progReq/440generalsurgery01012008.pdf

Ackermann, A. D., Kenny, G., & Walker, C. (2007). Simulator programs for new nurses' orientation: A retention strategy. *Journal for Nurses in Staff Development, 23,* 136–139.

American Association of Colleges of Nursing. (2005). *Faculty shortages in baccalaureate and graduate nursing programs: Scope of the problem and strategies for expanding the supply.* Washington, DC: Author.

American Association of Colleges of Nursing. (2007). *Joint Commission Nursing Advisory Council report on the revision of "The Essentials of Baccalaureate Nursing Education."* Washington, DC: Author.

American Association of Colleges of Nursing. (2008). *The essentials of baccalaureate nursing education.* Washington, DC: Author.

American College of Surgeons, Division of Education Accredited Education Institutes. (2007). *Welcome to the American College of Surgeons Division of Education Accredited Education Institutes.* Retrieved May 15, 2007, from: http://www.facs.org/education/accreditationprogram/index.html

American Nurses Association, Council on Computer Applications in Nursing. (1986). *Computers and CAI in nursing education.* Kansas City, MO: American Nurses Association.

American Society of Anesthesiologists, Committee on Outreach Education. (2006). *ASA approval of anesthesiology simulation programs.* Park Ridge, IL: American Society of Anesthesiologists.

Aspden, P., Corrigan, J. M., Wolcott, J., & Erickson, S. M. (Eds.). (2004). *Patient safety: Achieving a new standard of care.* Washington, DC: National Academies Press.

Bersky, A., & Krawczak, A. (1995). Computerized Clinical Simulation Testing (CST) update. *Issues, 16*(1), 6–7.

Bersky, A., Krawczak, A., & Kumar, T. D. (1998). Computerized clinical simulation testing. A new look for the NCLEX-RN examination? *Nurse Educator, 23*(1), 20–25.

Beyea, S. C., von Reyn, L., & Slattery, M. J. (2007). A nurse residency program for competency development using human patient simulation. *Journal for Nurses in Staff Development, 23,* 77–82.

Blau, S. (1983). Role-playing, an effective way of dealing with anxiety prior to psychiatric nursing rotation. *Free Association: A Newsletter for Psychiatric Nurses, 10*(3), 10.

Boller, J., & Jones, D. (2008). *Nursing education redesign for California: White paper and strategic action plan recommendations.* Berkeley, CA: California Institute for Nursing and Health Care.

Bosek, M. S., Li, S., & Hicks, F. D. (2007). Working with standardized patients: A primer. *International Journal of Nursing Education Scholarship, 4*(1), Article 16.

Bradburn, C., Zeleznikow, J., & Adams, A. (1993). FLORENCE: Synthesis of case-based and model-based reasoning in a nursing care planning system. *Computers in Nursing, 11,* 20–24.

Brady, D., Molzen, S., Graham, S., & O'Neill, V. (2006). Using the synergy of online education and simulation to inspire a new model for a community critical care course. *Critical Care Nursing Quarterly, 29*, 231–236.

Bremner, M. N., Aduddell, K., Bennett, D. N., & VanGeest, J. B. (2006). The use of human patient simulators: Best practices with novice nursing students. *Nurse Educator, 31*, 170–174.

Bremner, M. N., & Brannan, J. D. (2000). A computer simulation for the entry-level RN: Enhancing clinical decision making. *Journal for Nurses in Staff Development, 16*(1), 5–9.

Bristol, T. J. (2006). *Evidence-based e-learning for nursing educators.* Iowa City, IA: Center for Health Workforce Planning, Bureau of Health Care Access, Iowa Department of Public Health.

Chaisson, M. G. (1977). Life cycle: Simulating the problems of the aging and the aged. *Health Education Monographs, 5*(suppl 1), 28.

Clark, C. C. (1976). Simulation gaming: A new teaching strategy in nursing education. *Nurse Educator, 1*, 4–9.

Clark, C. C. (1977). Learning outcomes in a simulation game for associate degree nursing students. *Health Education Monographs, 5*(suppl 1), 25.

Cole, E., & Crichton, N. (2006). The culture of a trauma team in relation to human factors. *Journal of Clinical Nursing, 15*, 1257–1266.

Colliver, J. A., & Swartz, M. H. (1997). Assessing clinical performance with standardized patients. *Journal of the American Medical Association, 278*, 790–791.

Colorado Center for Nursing Excellence. (2007). *Work, Education and Lifelong Learning Simulation (WELLS) Center.* Retrieved March 31, 2007, from: http://www.coloradonurisngcenter.org/CurrentProjects/WellsCenter.html

Committee on Education, National League of Nursing Education. (1919). *Standard curriculum for schools of nursing.* New York: National Nursing Association.

Committee on Quality of Health Care in America, Institute of Medicine. (2001). *Crossing the quality chasm: A new health system for the 21st century.* Washington, DC: National Academies Press.

Cooper, J. B., & Taqueti, V. R. (2004). A brief history of the development of mannequin simulators for clinical education and training. *Quality and Safety in Health Care, 13*(suppl 1), i11–i18.

Corbett, N. A., & Beveridge, P. (1982). Simulation as a tool for learning. *Topics in Clinical Nursing, 4*(3), 58–67.

Cosgray, R. E., Davidhizar, R. E., Grostefon, J. D., Powell, M., & Wringer, P. H. (1990). A day in the life of an inpatient: An experiential game to promote empathy for individuals in a psychiatric hospital. *Archives of Psychiatric Nursing, 4*, 354–359.

Croquet project. (2007). Retrieved April 1, 2008, from: http://www.croquetconsortium.org

Davidhizar, R. E. (1977). Use of simulation games in teaching psychiatric nursing. *Journal of Nursing Education, 16*, 9–12.

del Bueno, D. J., Weeks, L., & Brown-Stewart, P. (1987). Clinical assessment centers: A cost-effective alternative for competency development. *Nursing Economics, 5*(1), 21–26.

Denson, J. S., & Abrahamson, S. (1969). A computer-controlled patient simulator. *Journal of the American Medical Association, 208*, 504–508.

de Tornyay, R., & Thompson, M. (1982). *Strategies for teaching nursing* (2nd ed.). New York: Wiley.

Decker, S. (2007). Integrating guided reflection into simulated learning experiences. In P. R. Jeffries (Ed.), *Simulation in nursing education: From conceptualization to evaluation* (pp. 73–85). New York: National League for Nursing.

Dooling, S. L. (1986). Designing computer simulations for staff nurse education. *Journal of Medical Systems, 10*, 139–149.

Dooling, S. L. (1987). Designing computer simulations. *Computers in Nursing, 5*, 219–224.

Eaves, R. H., & Flagg, A. J. (2001). The U. S. Air Force pilot simulated medical unit: A teaching strategy with multiple applications. *Journal of Nursing Education, 40*, 110–115.

Ebbert, D. W., & Connors, H. (2004). Standardized patient experiences: Evaluation of clinical performance and nurse practitioner student satisfaction. *Nursing Education Perspectives, 25*, 12–15.

Elgie, R. (2007). Politics, economics, and nursing shortages: A critical look at United States government policies. *Nursing Economics, 25*, 285–292.

Feingold, C. E., Calaluce, M., & Kallen, M. A. (2004). Computerized patient model and simulated clinical experiences: Evaluation with baccalaureate nursing students. *Journal of Nursing Education, 43*, 156–163.

Ferguson, S., Beeman, L., Eichorn, M., Jaramillo, Y., & Wright, M. (2004). High-fidelity simulation across clinical settings and educational levels. In G. E. Loyd, C. L. Lake, & R. B. Greenberg (Eds.), *Practical health care simulations* (pp. 184–203). Philadelphia: Elsevier.

Fletcher, J. L. (1998). AANA journal course: Update for nurse anesthetists: ERR WATCH: Anesthesia crisis resource management from the nurse anesthetist's perspective. *Journal of the American Association of Nurse Anesthetists, 66*, 595–602.

Forker, J. E., & McDonald, M. E. (1996). Methodologic trends in the healthcare professions: Computer adaptive and computer simulation testing. *Nurse Educator, 21*(4), 13–14.

Gaba, D. M. (2004). A brief history of mannequin-based simulation and application. In W. F. Dunn (Ed.). *Simulations in critical care and beyond* (pp. 7–14). Des Plaines, IL: Society of Critical Care Medicine.

Gaba, D. M., & DeAnda, A. (1988). A comprehensive anesthesia simulator environment: Re-creating the operating room for research and training. *Anesthesiology, 69*, 387–394.

Gaba, D. M., Fish, K. J., & Howard, S. K. (1994). *Crisis management in anesthesiology.* New York: Churchill Livingston.

Gaba, D. M., & Raemer, D. (2007). The tide is turning: Organizational structures to embed simulation in the fabric of healthcare. *Simulation in Healthcare, 2*(1), 1–3.

Gibbons, S. W., Adamo, G., Padden, D., et al. (2002). Clinical evaluation in advanced practice nursing education: Using standardized patients in health assessment. *Journal of Nursing Education, 41*, 215–221.

Giddens, J. F. (2007). The neighborhood: A web-based platform to support conceptual teaching and learning. *Nursing Education Perspectives, 28*, 251–256.

Good, M., Lampotang, S., & Gibby, G. (1988). Critical events simulation for training in anesthesiology. *Journal of Clinical Monitoring and Computing, 4*, 140.

Goodin, H. J. (2003). The nursing shortage in the United States of America: An integrative review of the literature. *Journal of Advanced Nursing, 43*, 335–343.

Gordon, M. S. (1974). Cardiology patient simulator: Development of an animated manikin to teach cardiovascular disease. *American Journal of Cardiology, 34*, 350–355.

Gordon, M. S., Ewy, G. A., DeLeon, A. C. Jr., Waugh, R. A., Felner, J. M., Forker, A. D. et al. (1980). "Harvey," the cardiology patient simulator: Pilot studies on teaching effectiveness. *American Journal of Cardiology, 45*, 791–796.

Greenblatt, C. S., & Duke, R. D. (1975). *Gaming-simulation: Rationale, design and application.* New York: John Wiley and Sons.

Greiner, A. C., & Knebel, E. (Eds.). (2003). *Health professions education: A bridge to quality.* Washington, DC: National Academies Press.

Grobe, S. (1984). Computer assisted instruction: An alternative. *Computers in Nursing, 2*(3), 92–97.

Grossman, C. C., & Hudson, D. B. (2001). Rating students' technology generated clinical decision making scores. *Nurse Educator, 26,* 5–6.

Health Resources and Services Administration. (2002). *National Advisory Council on Nurse Education and Practice: Second report to the Secretary of Health and Human Services and Congress.* Rockville, MD: Author.

Henrichs, B., Rule, A., Grady, M., & Ellis, W. (2002). Nurse anesthesia students' perceptions of the anesthesia patient simulator: A qualitative study. *AANA Journal, 70,* 219–225.

Herrmann, E. K. (1981). Mrs. Chase: A noble and enduring figure. *American Journal of Nursing, 81,* 1836.

Herrmann, E. K. (2008). Remembering Mrs. Chase. *NSNA Imprint,* 52–55.

Howard, E. P. (1987). Use of a computer simulation for the continuing education of registered nurses. *Computers in Nursing, 5,* 208–213.

Jeffries, P. R. (2005). A framework for designing, implementing, and evaluating simulations used as teaching strategies in nursing. *Nursing Education Perspectives, 26,* 96–103.

Jeffries, P. R. (Ed.). (2007). *Simulation in nursing education: From conceptualization to evaluation.* New York: National League for Nursing.

Jenkins, L. S., & Schaivone, K. (2007). Standardized patients in nursing education. *Annual Review of Nurisng Education, 5,* 3–23.

Jenkins, P., & Turick-Gibson, T. (1999). An exercise in critical thinking using role playing. *Nurse Educator, 24*(6), 11–14.

Johannsson, H., Ayida, G., & Sadler, C. (2005). Faking it? Simulation in the training of obstetricians and gynaecologists. *Current Opinion in Obstetrics and Gynecology, 17,* 557–561.

Johnson, J. H., Zerwic, J. J., & Theis, S. L. (1999). Clinical simulation laboratory: An adjunct to clinical teaching. *Nurse Educator, 24*(5), 37–41.

Johnsson, A. C., Kjellberg, A., & Lagerstrom, M. I. (2006). Evaluation of nursing students' work technique after proficiency training in patient transfer methods during undergraduate education. *Nursing Education Today, 26,* 322–331.

Joint Commission. (2009). *2009 national patient safety goals.* Retrieved January 19, 2009, from: http://www.jointcommission.org/PatientSafety/NationalPatientSafetyGoals/

Kane, M. T. (1992). The assessment of professional competence. *Evaluation & the Health Professions, 15,* 163–182.

Kappus, L., Leon, V., Lyons, A., Meehan, P., & Hamilton-Bruno, S. (2006). Simulation training: An innovative way to teach critical care nursing skills. *Critical Care Nurse, 26*(2), S15.

King, A. M., Perkowski-Rodgers, L. C., & Pohl, H. S. (1994). Planning standardized patient programs: Case development, patient training, and costs. *Teaching and Learning in Medicine, 6,* 6–14.

Kohn, L. T., Corrigan, J. M., & Donaldson, M. S. (Eds.). (2000). *To err is human: Building a safer health system.* Washington, DC: National Academies Press.

Krautscheid, L., & Burton, D. (2003). *Technology in nursing education: Oregon education-based technology needs assessment: Expanding nursing education capacity.* Portland, OR: Oregon Nursing Center.

Kruijver, I. P., Kerkstra, A., Kerssens, J. J., Hoitkamp, C. C., Bensing, J. M., & van de Wiel, H. B. (2001). Communication between nurses and simulated patients with cancer: Evaluation of a communication training programme. *European Journal of Oncology Nursing, 5,* 140–150.

Kuipers, J. C., & Clemens, D. L. (1998). Do I dare? Using role-play as a teaching strategy. *Journal of Psychosocial Nursing & Mental Health Services, 36*(7), 12–17, 42–43.

Lambton, J. (2008). Integrating simulation into a pediatric nursing curriculum: A 25% solution. *Simulation in Healthcare, 3,* 53–57.

Landry, M., Oberleitner, M. G., Landry, H., & Borazjani, J. G. (2006). Using simulation and virtual reality technology to assess continuing nurse competency in the long-term acute care setting. *Journal for Nurses in Staff Development, 22,* 163–169.

Lange, C. M. (1982). Creation of self-learning centers. *Topics in Clinical Nursing, 4,* 20–28.

Lasater, K. (2007a). Clinical judgment development: Using simulation to create an assessment rubric. *Journal of Nursing Education, 46,* 496–503.

Lasater, K. (2007b). High-fidelity simulation and the development of clinical judgment: Students' experiences. *Journal of Nursing Education, 46,* 269–280.

Lees, F. (1874). *Handbook for hospital sisters.* London: W. Ibister & Co.

Marte, A. L. (1988). How does it feel to be old? Simulation game provides "into aging" experience. *Journal of Continuing Education in Nursing, 19,* 166–168.

McDowell, B. J., Nardini, D. L., Negley, S. A., & White, J. E. (1984). Evaluating clinical performance using simulated patients with student nurse practitioners. *Journal of Nursing Education, 23*(1), 37–39.

Merril, G. L., & Barker, V. L. (1996). Virtual reality debuts in the teaching laboratory in nursing. *Nurse Educator, 19,* 182–187.

Metcalfe, S. E., Hall, V. P., & Carpenter, A. (2007). Promoting collaboration in nursing education: The development of a regional simulation laboratory. *Journal of Professional Nursing, 23,* 180–183.

Miller, A. M., Wilbur, J., Dedhiya, S., Talashek, M. L., & Mrtek, R. (1999). Interpersonal styles of nurse practitioner students during simulated patient encounters. *Clinical Excellence for Nurse Practitioners, 2,* 166–171.

Miller, A. M., Wilbur, J., Montgomery, A. C., & Talashek, M. L. (1998). Standardized faculty evaluation of nurse practitioner students by using simulated patients. *Clinical Excellence for Nurse Practitioners, 2,* 102–109.

Monti, E. J., Wren, K., Haas, R., & Lupien, A. E. (1998). The use of an anesthesia simulator in graduate and undergraduate education. *CRNA: The Clinical Forum for Nurse Anesthetists, 9,* 59–66.

Morton, P. G. (1995). Creating a laboratory that simulates the critical care environment. *Critical Care Nurse, 16*(6), 76–81.

National Council of State Boards of Nursing (NCSBN). (1996). *Assuring competence: A regulatory responsibility.* Chicago: Author.

National Council of State Boards of Nursing (NCSBN). (2005). *Meeting the ongoing challenge of continued competence.* Chicago: Author.

Nehring, W. M., Ellis, W. E., & Lashley, F. R. (2001). Human patient simulators in nursing education: An overview. *Simulation & Gaming, 32,* 194–204.

Nehring, W. M., & Lashley, F. R. (2004). Using the Human Patient Simulator in nursing education. *Annual Review of Nursing Education, 2,* 163–181.

Nehring, W. M., & Lashley, F. R. (in press). Nursing simulation: A review of the past 40 years. *Simulation & Gaming*.

Nehring, W. M., Lashley, F. R., & Ellis, W. E. (2002). Critical incident nursing management using human patient simulators. *Nursing Education Perspectives, 23*, 128–132.

Nelson, A. (2003). Using simulation to design and integrate technology for safer and more efficient practice environments. *Nursing Outlook, 51*, S27–S29.

Newcomb, P., & Riddlesperger, K. (2007). Using improvisational theater to teach genetics concepts. *Nurse Educator, 32*, 227–230.

O'Connor, F. W., Albert, M. L., & Thomas, M. D. (1999). Incorporating standardized patients into a psychosocial nurse practitioner program. *Archives of Psychiatric Nursing, 13*, 240–247.

O'Donnell, J., Fletcher, J., Dixon, B., & Palmer, L. (1998). Planning and implementing an anesthesia crisis resource management course for student nurse anesthetists. *CRNA: The Clinical Forum for Nurse Anesthetists, 9*, 50–58.

Oregon Nursing Leadership Council. (2005). *Oregon Nursing Leadership Council strategic plan: Solutions to Oregon's nursing shortage 2005–2008*. Portland, OR: Author.

Paparella, S. F., Mariani, B. A., Layton, K., & Carpenter, A. M. (2004). Patient safety simulation: Learning about safety never seemed more fun. *Journal for Nurses in Staff Development, 20*, 247–252.

Patel, A. A., & Gould, D. A. (2006). Simulators in interventional radiology training and evaluation: A paradigm shift is on the horizon. *Journal of Vascular Interventional Radiology, 17*, S163–S173.

Phillips, J. R. (1993). Virtual reality: A new vista for nurse researchers? *Nursing Science Quarterly, 6*(1), 5–7.

Practice Education & Regulation Committee, National Council of State Boards of Nursing (NCSBN). (2006). *Report of the invitational forum: January 26, 2006*. Chicago, IL: Author.

Prensky, M. (2001). Digital natives, digital immigrants. *On the Horizon, 9*(5), 1–6.

Rauen, C. A. (2001). Using simulation to teach critical thinking skills: You can't just throw the book at them. *Critical Care Nursing Clinics of North America, 13*(1), 93–103.

Rauen, C. A. (2004). Simulation as a teaching strategy for nursing education and orientation in cardiac surgery. *Critical Care Nurse, 24*(3), 46–51.

Ross, M., Carroll, G., Knight, J., Chamberlain, M., Fothergill-Bourbonnais, F., & Lindon, J. (1988). Using the OSCE to measure clinical skills performance in nursing. *Journal of Advanced Nursing, 19*(1), 45–56.

Rutledge, C. M., Garzon, L., Scott, M., & Karlowicz, K. (2004). Using standardized patients to teach and evaluate nurse practitioner students on cultural competency. *International Journal of Nursing Education Scholarship, 1*(1), Article 17.

Schoenly, L. (1994). Teaching in the affective domain. *Journal of Continuing Education in Nursing, 25*, 209–212.

Seropian, M. A., Brown, K., Gavilanes, J. S., & Driggers, B. (2004). Simulation: Not just a manikin. *Journal of Nursing Education, 43*, 164–169.

Sinz, E. H. (2007). Anesthesia national CME program and ASA activities in simulation. *Anesthesiology Clinics, 25*, 209–223.

Skiba, D. J. (2008). Games for health. *Nursing Education Perspectives, 29*, 230–232.

Skiba, D. (2007). Nursing education 2.0: Second life. *Nursing Education Perspectives, 28*, 156–157.

Stevens, A., Hernandez, J., Johsen, K., Dickerson, R., Raij, A., Harrison, C., et al. (2006). The use of virtual patients to teach medical students history taking and communication skills. *The American Journal of Surgery, 191*, 806–811.

Swart, J. (1992). Can simulation replace practica? *Nursing RSA Verpleging, 7*(4), 35–38.

Sweeney, M. A., O'Malley, M., & Freeman, E. (1982). Development of a computer simulation to evaluate the clinical performance of nursing students. *Journal of Nursing Education, 21*(9), 28–38.

Tanner, C. A. (2006). The next transformation: Clinical education. *Journal of Nursing Education, 45*, 99–100.

Taylor, A. P. (1980). Clinical simulations in nursing. *Nursing Times, 76*(26), 1217–1218.

Tetzlaff, J. E. (2007). Assessment of competency in anesthesiology. *Anesthesiology, 106*(4), 812–825.

Theroux, R., & Pearce, C. (2006). Graduate students' experiences with standardized patients as adjuncts for teaching pelvic examinations. *Journal of the American Academy of Nurse Practitioners, 18*, 429–435.

Thomas, M. D., O'Connor, F. W., Albert, M. L., Boutain, D., & Brandt, P. A. (2001). Case-based teaching and learning experiences. *Issues in Mental Health Nursing, 22*, 517–531.

Ulione, M. S. (1983). Simulation gaming in nursing education. *Journal of Nursing Education, 22*, 349–351.

Vessey, J. A., & Huss, K. (2002). Using standardized patients in advanced practice nursing education. *Journal of Professional Nursing, 18*, 29–35.

Waneka, R. (2008). *California Board of Registered Nursing 2006–2007 annual school report: Pre-licensure nursing programs data summary.* San Francisco: Center for the Health Professions.

Weiner, E. E., Gordon, J. S., & Gilman, B. R. (1993). Evaluation of a labor and delivery videodisc simulation. *Computers in Nursing, 11*, 191–196.

Wells, H. (1944). *Cherry Ames: Student nurse.* New York: Grosset & Dunlap.

Wilson, L., Gordon, M. G., Cornelius, F., Glascow, M. E. S., Suplee, P. D., Vasso, M., et al. (2006). The standardized patient experience in undergraduate nursing education. *Studies in Health Technology & Informatics, 122*, 830.

Winslow, S., Dunn, P., & Rowlands, A. (2005). Establishment of a hospital-based simulation skills laboratory. *Journal for Nurses in Staff Development, 21*, 62–65.

Wong, J., Wong, S., & Richard, J. (1992). Implementing computer simulations as a strategy for evaluating decision-making skills of nursing students. *Computers in Nursing, 10*, 264–269.

Worzala, K. T., Glaser, K. M., & McGinley, A. (2006). A collaborative curriculum for medical and nursing students. *Medical Education, 40*, 478.

Yoo, M. S., & Yoo, I. Y. (2003). The effectiveness of standardized patients as a teaching method for nursing fundamentals. *Journal of Nursing Education, 42*, 444–448.

Zekonis, D., & Gantt, L. T. (2007). New graduate nurse orientation in the emergency department: Use of a simulation scenario for teaching and learning. *Journal of Emergency Nursing, 33*, 283–285.

CHAPTER 2

A Synthesis of Theory and Nursing Research Using High-Fidelity Patient Simulation

Wendy M. Nehring

Nursing educators have used simulation as an adjunct to enhance their teaching in a variety of forms for more than a century. High-fidelity patient simulation has been used by nursing educators for about a decade. (This history was detailed in Chapter 1.) The popularity of this technology largely reflects the need to assure the public that nursing students are safe and competent to practice upon graduation. There is no question that part of the nursing educational experience needs to involve time in the healthcare setting. Yet, this setting cannot be standardized. Nursing students inevitably receive varied experiences in which the patient load and acuity prevent them from consistent opportunities to practice their psychomotor and psychosocial skills ensuring competency in all areas. High-fidelity patient simulation provides standardized experiences to assist in the progression to competency, as evidenced by graduation from the nursing program.

As this technology is integrated in the nursing curriculum, nursing educators have begun to use theoretical frameworks to organize these teaching and learning experiences. This chapter takes an in-depth look at these theoretical frameworks used by nursing educators, which derive from the literature. Additional theoretical frameworks that have been used in medicine will also be mentioned. Moreover, nursing educators have conducted research studies using high-fidelity patient simulators in the past several years; the results of these studies will be detailed in the second section of this chapter. Finally, recommendations for further research will be given.

THEORETICAL FRAMEWORKS USED IN NURSING SIMULATION

The curriculum of a nursing program is the foundation of learning. As Leddy (2008) states, the "curriculum is the totality of formal and informal content that imparts the skills, attitudes, and values considered important in achieving specific educational goals" (p. 68). These goals are often listed as

27

program objectives and are further broken down into level and course objectives. As simulation becomes an important component of every nursing program curriculum, it is important to include this technology in a description of how nursing students will meet the objectives at each level. To organize the curriculum, faculty often develop curriculum frameworks. In recent years, nursing educators using high-fidelity patient simulation have identified a variety of theoretical frameworks to explain how simulation is being used to meet the educational goals of the program. These frameworks often involve an aspect of the overall curriculum framework, making it important to note whether these theoretical frameworks will become part of the overall curriculum frameworks of most nursing programs in the coming years.

Patricia Benner (1984) developed a theory of skill acquisition for nurses that describes levels of competence as ranging from novice to expert. This theory was originally proposed for the nurse in practice and has become a popular theory to be used in conjunction with high-fidelity patient simulation. Ferguson and colleagues (2004) described a nursing staff development model for use in their hospital that incorporated Benner's model and simulation, including high-fidelity patient simulation. Long (2005) discussed the use of Benner's model using high-fidelity patient simulation to teach resuscitation skills. Larew et al. (2006) described how Benner's theory could be applied in nursing education using high-fidelity patient simulation. Waldner and Olson (2007) combined Benner's first three stages with Kolb's (1984) theory of experiential learning to provide the framework for using high-fidelity patient simulation in the nursing curriculum.

Additional theoretical frameworks used by nursing educators with high-fidelity patient simulation include Schon's (1983) theory of reflective thinking (Decker, 2007), Pesut and Herman's (1999) model of clinical reasoning (Kuiper, Heinrich, Mattias, Graham, & Bell-Kotwall, 2008), and Tanner's (2006) theory of clinical judgment (Lasater, 2007a). These theoretical frameworks are similar to those being used in medicine. Bradley and Postlethwaite (2003) outlined a variety of theories, both traditional and contemporary, that have been used by medicine in framing their use of high-fidelity patient simulation in the medical curriculum and in practice. These theoretical frameworks include behaviorism, constructivism, social constructivism, reflective practice, situated learning, and mastery learning. Each of these theoretical frameworks to some degree involves repetitive practice, feedback, personal and group reflection on role-play, a safe environment, and movement from dependent to independent learning; all offer advantages when used with high-fidelity patient simulation (Issenberg, McGaghie, Petrusa, Gordon, & Scalese, 2005).

A recent theoretical framework by Jeffries and Rogers (2007), called *Nursing Education Simulation Framework*, was designed specifically for the use of simulation in nursing education (see Chapter 19) and is being used by many nursing programs across the United States. This framework comprises three spheres. Faculty and student characteristics together with educational practices make up one sphere, which in turn influences student outcomes (second sphere) and the simulation design characteristics (third sphere). In other words, the nature of the simulation must be determined by the learning needs of the student. Availability of technology and faculty expertise, for example, will influence the type of simulation that can be done. Evaluation of the outcomes can also take place based on this framework.

Nehring and Lashley (2004b) developed *critical incident nursing management* (CINM), a nursing practice model that was adopted from the anesthesia crisis management model developed by Gaba, Fish, and Howard (1994). The CINM model includes both internal and external factors that may influence the nurse's performance in the work setting. For example, given a critical incident in a patient, such as a myocardial infarction, the nurse's actions are influenced by the antecedents and consequences of the critical incident, the members of the healthcare team, and the environment, in addition to the nurse's characteristics, such as fatigue (Nehring & Lashley, 2004b; Nehring, Lashley, & Ellis, 2002).

In the coming years it will be important for nurse researchers to continue to test all of these theoretical frameworks so that they can better understand how nursing education and practice can be improved.

NURSING RESEARCH INVOLVING HIGH-FIDELITY PATIENT SIMULATION

Nurse researchers have examined the use of high-fidelity patient simulation in nursing education and practice for less than a decade. In a review of published nursing research articles involving high-fidelity patient simulation, only 26 articles were found. Published abstracts and dissertations were not included. Twenty-two of these articles involved nursing education, either in nursing programs or in practice, and four articles involved team management. Table 2-1 provides further details on each of these nursing research articles.

Nursing Education Research Studies

The 22 nursing education articles can be divided into four categories based on the use of high-fidelity patient simulation: an adjunct to traditional teaching, as a means of assessing competence, as a substitute for clinical judgment, and as a method of teaching.

Table 2-1 Characteristics of Existing Nursing Research Studies Using High-Fidelity Patient Simulators ($n = 26$)

Study	Purpose	Participants	Design and Interventions	Outcome Measures	Outcomes
Nursing Education					
Alinier, G., Hunt, W. G., & Gordon, R. (2004). Determining the value of simulation in nurse education: Study design and initial results. *Nurse Education in Practice, 4*, 200–207.	"To determine the effect of realistic scenario-based simulation on nursing students' competence and confidence" (p. 200).	Conducted in United Kingdom (UK) 67 nursing students in fifth semester of 3-year program who have taken part in this study (more are being enrolled)	Study consists of three phases: phase one is an OSCE (Objective Structured Clinical Examination) session of which all participate, then group is randomly divided into control and experimental group with the experimental group receiving two simulation sessions (one as observer and the other as participant), then all complete a confidence questionnaire and participate in a second OSCE session.	Comparison of scores on the two OSCE sessions, as well as confidence questionnaire results between two groups. Time to complete all components of study is 5–6 months.	• Similar scores on first OSCE between groups. • Scores were improved on second OSCE with experimental group doing better (6.76% vs 13.43%, p < 0.05). • Control group was older and had more healthcare experience.
Alinier, G., Hunt, B., Gordon, R., & Harwood, C. (2006). Effectiveness of intermediate-fidelity simulation training technology in undergraduate nursing education.	"To determine the effect of scenario-based simulation training on nursing students' clinical skills and	Conducted in UK 99 nursing students in second year of 3-year program	Pre-test, post-test design. Used same design as above.	As above	• Scores were improved on second OSCE with experimental group doing better (7.18% vs 14.18%, p < 0.001).

30

Table 2-1 Characteristics of Existing Nursing Research Studies Using High-Fidelity Patient Simulators (n = 26) (continued)

Citation	Purpose	Sample / Setting	Intervention	Instrument	Findings
Journal of Advanced Nursing, 54, 359–369.	competence" (p. 359).	Continuation of above study			• No significant difference on confidence scale.
Bearnson, C. S., & Wiker, K. M. (2005). Human patient simulators: A new face in baccalaureate nursing education at Brigham Young University. *Journal of Nursing Education, 44,* 421–425.	"To explore the benefits and limitations of using an HPS as a patient substitute for one day of clinical for junior nursing students" (p. 421).	Conducted in United States (U.S.) Number of students not provided; all were junior nursing students.	Survey Students participated in a two-hour session that involved the care of three post-operative patients.	Students rated their agreement on a 4-point Likert scale (eg., 4 = strongly agree) to four statements regarding their experience with the simulators.	• Two knowledge questions both averaged over 3 (3.13 and 3.31). • One skill question also had an average of over 3 (3.06). • One confidence question had an average of 3.0.
Brenner, M. N., Aduddell, K., Bennett, D. N., & VanGeest, J. B. (2006). The use of human patient simulators: Best practices with novice nursing students. *Nurse Educator, 31,* 170–174.	"To determine the value of using human patient simulation (HPS) technology as an educational methodology from the perspective of the novice nursing student" (pp. 171–172).	Conducted in U.S. 41 novice undergraduate students	Survey Students assessed the simulator and were then asked by the instructor to assess the simulator again as they controlled changes in the simulator's status.	Students then completed the two-part questionnaire which consisted of questions answered on a Likert rating scale and any comments by the student.	• 95% agreed the experience was good to excellent • 68% felt it should be mandatory • 61% felt that they gained confidence • 42% felt such an experience helped to relieve stress for the first clinical day • General comments related to educational benefit, degree of realism, level of confidence, and limitations.

Table 2-1 Characteristics of Existing Nursing Research Studies Using High-Fidelity Patient Simulators (*n* = 26) (*continued*)

Study	Purpose	Participants	Design and Interventions	Outcome Measures	Outcomes
Nursing Education					
Childs, J. C., & Sepples, S. (2006). Clinical teaching by simulation: Lessons learned from a complex patient care scenario. *Nursing Education Perspectives, 27,* 154–158.	"To study the simulation development and implementation process and measure student satisfaction" (p. 154). This school participated in the first National League for Nursing (NLN)/Laerdal study.	Conducted in U.S. 55 senior generic and second-degree undergraduate nursing students	Survey Students participated in four stations that took a total of 2 hours to complete: identifying cardiac arrhythmias, identifying rhythm strips, discussing arrhythmia case studies, and participating in a mock code.	Students completed three Likert rating scale tools: *Educational Practice Scale for Simulation* (EPSS), *The Simulation Design Scale* (SDS), and a specific tool from the school that examined confidence level, degree of usefulness of the experience, and feelings related to the experience.	• Feedback and information from experience important followed by fidelity and complexity (SDS). • Each element of the EPSS was found to be important by the students (i.e., active learning, collaboration, diverse learning opportunities, and high expectations). • Students rated experience as positive. • Found mock code to be stressful but helpful. • Lessons learned provided by authors.

Table 2-1 Characteristics of Existing Nursing Research Studies Using High-Fidelity Patient Simulators (*n* = 26) *(continued)*

DeCarlo, D., Collingridge, D. S., Grant, C., & Ventre, K. M. (2008). Factors influencing nurses' attitudes toward simulation-based education. *Simulation in Healthcare, 3,* 90–96.	"To identify barriers to nurses' participation in simulation and to determine whether prior simulation exposure, professional experience, and practice location influence their tendency to perceive specific issues as barriers" (p. 90).	Conducted in U.S. 523 nurses employed in a children's hospital	Survey Surveys were distributed to staff and returned in drop boxes within the hospital.	"Staff completed a 54-item survey to gather data on professional demographics, simulation exposure, perceived barriers to participation in simulation, and training priorities" (p. 90).	• Lack of realism was noted most often by nurses with simulation experience, those with less experience, and those who practice in a nonacute unit in the hospital. • Higher level of stress and intimidation was found for those who did not work in acute care areas. • For those working in acute care units, simulation provided an opportunity to practice the care of patients with rare events.
Feingold, C. E., Calaluce, M., & Kallen, M. A. (2004). Computerized patient model and simulated clinical experiences: Evaluation with baccalaureate nursing students. *Journal of Nursing Education, 43,* 156–163.	"To evaluate student and faculty perceptions regarding the use of a computerized patient simulator in a simulated clinical scenario" (p. 156).	Conducted in U.S. 65 senior nursing students split between two semesters	Survey Students participated in two scenario experiences at the beginning and end of their first semester of their senior year in the Acute Care	Students completed a 20-item Likert style satisfaction survey that examined realism, transfer of skills to clinical setting, and value.	• The value subscale had the highest level of agreement (3.04 mean out of 4) and the transferability the lowest (2.52). • Technical skills (3.53) rated highest whereas competence improved as result of experience

Table 2-1 Characteristics of Existing Nursing Research Studies Using High-Fidelity Patient Simulators ($n = 26$) (continued)

Study	Purpose	Participants	Design and Interventions	Outcome Measures	Outcomes
Nursing Education					
			of the Adult course. Each experience allowed faculty to assess for skill level and decision-making abilities. The first experience assisted faculty to make clinical assignments.	Faculty completed a 17-item Likert style survey related to faculty support and necessary training needed to implement this technology.	with simulator rated lowest (2.50). • Students felt the experience provided appropriate realism (86.1%), tested clinical skills (83.0%) and decision-making (87.7%), was valuable to learning (76.5%), and provided adequate feedback (96.9%) (p. 160). • Less than half of the students felt that their confidence (46.9%) or competence (46.9%) increased. • Faculty felt that the experience was realistic and effective (100%).
Henrichs, B, Rule, A., Grady, M., & Ellis, W. (2002). Nurse anesthesia students' perceptions of	"To describe the perceptions of nurse anesthesia students	Conducted in U.S.	Qualitative Nurse anesthesia students partici-	The PI observed each of the sessions and made notes, a focus group with	• Advantages and disadvantages of the experience were identified by the students.

Table 2-1 Characteristics of Existing Nursing Research Studies Using High-Fidelity Patient Simulators ($n = 26$) (continued)

the anesthesia patient simulator: A qualitative study. *AANA Journal, 70,* 219–225.	who used a MedSim simulator" (p. 219).	12 first-year nurse anesthesia students	pated in four simulation sessions: (1) introduction to simulator, (2) performance of an anesthetic induction, (3) performance after a minor incident, and (4) performance after a major incident.	the students after the experience, and journal notes throughout the participation in the sessions.	• Anxiety was experienced. • All students felt that the simulator should be part of program. • Students did not feel that the simulator should be used for certification/ recertification.
Hoffmann, R. L., O'Donnell, J. M., & Kim, Y. (2007). The effects of human patient simulators on basic knowledge in critical care nursing with undergraduate senior baccalaureate nursing students. *Simulation in Healthcare, 2,* 110–114.	"To investigate whether participation in instruction involving human patient simulators, in conjunction with a traditional clinical experience, improves professional competence in critical care in senior nursing students" (p. 110).	Conducted in U.S. 29 senior baccalaureate nursing students in advanced medical-surgical nursing course	Pre- and post-test repeated measures design. Students completed seven weeks in the traditional clinical setting and the remaining seven weeks in a simulation experience.	The *Basic Knowledge Assessment Tool-6* (BKAT-6) was completed prior to the clinical experience and on the last day of the simulation experience.	• Significant differences were found between the results of the two BKAT-6 scores with improvement after simulation. • Only the subscales of endocrine and gastrointestinal were not significantly improved (note: these areas were not covered in the scenarios).

Table 2-1 Characteristics of Existing Nursing Research Studies Using High-Fidelity Patient Simulators ($n = 26$) (continued)

Study	Purpose	Participants	Design and Interventions	Outcome Measures	Outcomes
Nursing Education					
Jeffries, P. R., & Rizzolo, M. A. (2006). *Designing and implementing models for the innovative use of simulation to teach nursing care of ill adults and children: A national, multi-site, multi-method study.* New York: National League for Nursing.	"To: (1) develop and test models that nursing faculty can implement when using simulation to promote student learning, (2) develop a cadre of nursing faculty who can use simulation in innovative ways to enhance student learning, (3) contribute to the refinement of the body of knowledge related to the use of simulation in nursing education, and (4) demonstrate the value of collaboration between the corporate and not-for-profit worlds" (p. 1).	Conducted in U.S. 8 project sites 395 students participated in one part of the study as described in Childs & Sepples (2006). 403 students participated in a second part of the study. 110 students participated in the third part of the study.	Four phases of which the last two involved research: 1. Pre-test, post-test design 2. Pre-test, post-test, three group experimental design The EPSS and SDS were assessed and their scores evaluated (see Childs & Sepples, 2006). Students participated in 12-item pre- and post-test. Intervention consisted of 38-minute lecture and care of post-operative adult using a simulator by the faculty member. This procedure was repeated with three groups: paper and pencil case study,	SDS and EPSS scales *Student Satisfaction with Learning Scale* *Self-Confidence in Learning Using Simulations Scale* *Self-Perceived Judgment Performance Scale*	• In first study, there was a significant difference between the pre- and post-test results (p < .0001). • High expectations received the highest ratings on the EPSS. • In the second study, using the SDS, the students perceived the high-fidelity mannequin to be more real, feedback to be equal with both mannequins, and more problem-solving took place with both mannequins. • Using the EPSS, students felt that the high-fidelity mannequin provided more diverse ways of learning and active learning took place more with the mannequins.

Table 2-1 Characteristics of Existing Nursing Research Studies Using High-Fidelity Patient Simulators ($n = 26$) (continued)

			simulation with low-fidelity mannequin, and simulation with a high-fidelity mannequin. The third study divided the students in half and one half had the case study first and then simulation and the other half experienced the reverse order.	Pre- and post-test	• The pre- and post-test results were nonsignificant. • In the third study, students using the high-fidelity mannequin reported greater active learning and more diverse ways of learning and were more satisfied.
King, C. J., Moseley, S., Hindenlang, B., & Kuritz, P. (2008). Limited use of the human patient simulator by nurse faculty: An intervention program designed to increase use. *International Journal of Nursing Education Scholarship*, 5(1), article 12.	Two-phase study Phase 1 purpose: "To examine faculty member's attitudes, subjective norms, perceived behavioral control, and intent to use HPS" (p. 2). Phase 2 purpose: "To examine the effect of a HPS educational intervention on intent to use, attitudes, subjective norms, and perceived behavioral control. Second, to identify the most important factors in explaining intent to use the HPS" (p. 2).	Conducted in U.S. The participants in phase 1 were faculty from an Associate Degree in Nursing (AND) program in the southeastern United States. The participants in phase 2 were 15 faculty from the same program.	The first phase was a survey designed by the authors. The second phase consisted of a pre- and post-survey similar to phase 1 with an intervention which consisted of an education program for the 15 faculty on how to use the high-fidelity patient simulator.	In phase 1, the completion of the survey entitled, *The Faculty Attitudes and Intent to Use Related to the Human Patient Simulator.* In phase 2, the completion of the pre- and post-	In phase 1: • Issues raised were how the use of the high-fidelity patient simulator fit into the curriculum, confidence and competence of the faculty was low, pressure to use, amount of prep time, and lack of experience using the high-fidelity patient simulator. In phase 2: • After educational training on the high-fidelity patient simulator, faculty confidence, sense of competence, attitudes, and intent to use increased.

Table 2-1   Characteristics of Existing Nursing Research Studies Using High-Fidelity Patient Simulators ($n = 26$) (continued)

Study	Purpose	Participants	Design and Interventions	Outcome Measures	Outcomes
Nursing Education					
				surveys as well as participation in the educational intervention using the high-fidelity patient simulator.	
Kuiper, R., Heinrich, C., Matthias, A., Graham, M. J., & Bell-Kotwall, L. (2008). Debriefing with the OPT model of clinical reasoning during high fidelity patient simulation. *International Journal of Nursing Education Scholarship, 5*(1), article 17.	"To explore the impact of patient simulation technology on situated cognition of undergraduate nursing students with the long term goal of preparing a workforce of practitioners who effectively manage clinical issues" (p. 1).	Conducted in U.S. "44 undergraduate senior baccalaureate nursing student in an adult health medical/ surgical course" (p. 4).	Pre-test, post-test Completion of Outcome Present State-Test (OPT) worksheets after clinical experiences in the hospital and after simulation experiences.	Completion of OPT worksheets	• "No differences were found between the scores on the OPT worksheets after clinical in the hospital as compared to the simulation experiences. • Higher scores for simulation were found on listing interventions, recording laboratory data, making judgments regarding tests, and connecting present-outcome states and NANDA diagnoses" (p. 10).

Table 2-1 Characteristics of Existing Nursing Research Studies Using High-Fidelity Patient Simulators (n = 26) (continued)

| Lasater, K. (2007a). Clinical judgment development: Using simulation to create an assessment rubric. *Journal of Nursing Education, 46,* 496–503. | "To describe students' responses to simulated scenarios, within the framework of Tanner's Clinical Judgment Model, to develop a rubric that describes levels of performance in clinical judgment, and pilot test the rubric in scoring student's performance" (p. 496). | Conducted in U.S. 26 third-year students enrolled in the adult medical-surgical clinical course | "A cycle of theory-driven description-observation-revision-review method" (p. 498). "Students were used to develop and refine the Lasater Clinical Judgment Rubric through participation in simulation scenarios. In the pilot test, eight students were used to further test the rubric through participation in a focus group" (p. 498). | Participation in the simulation scenarios for all participants and further participation by a subset of the participants in a focus group. | • The rubric was developed.
 • Students discussed the strengths and limitations of the use of the simulator, feelings of anxiety, need for further feedback from faculty, the value of teamwork, and general comments. |
| Lasater, K. (2007b). High-fidelity simulation and the development of clinical judgment: Students' experiences. *Journal of Nursing Education, 46,* 269–276. | "To examine the clinical judgment of students in one nursing program's first term of using high-fidelity patient simulation" (p. 269). | Conducted in U.S. "48 junior undergraduate nursing students enrolled in the Nursing | Focus group Students participated in the focus group after their simulation experience which consisted of one clinical day per week for the course of the semester. | Participation in focus group | Five codes emerged:
 • "Strengths and limitations of high-fidelity patient simulation.
 • Paradoxical nature of simulation — provocation of anxious and stupid feelings to increased learning and awareness. |

Table 2-1 Characteristics of Existing Nursing Research Studies Using High-Fidelity Patient Simulators ($n = 26$) (continued)

Study	Purpose	Participants	Design and Interventions	Outcome Measures	Outcomes
Nursing Education					
		Care of the Acutely Ill Adult course" (p. 271).			• Intense desire for more direct feedback. • Value of students' connections with others. • General recommendations for facilitation and learning" (p. 272).
LeFlore, J. L., Anderson, M., Michael, J., Engle, W. D., & Anderson, J. (2007). Comparison of self-directed learning versus instructor-modeled learning during a simulated clinical experience. *Simulation in Healthcare, 2,* 170–177.	"To test the hypothesis that instructor-modeled learning is more effective compared with self-directed learning during a simulated clinical experience" (p. 170).	Conducted in U.S. 16 NP students were divided into three groups: control, self-directed learning, and instructor-modeled learning.	Descriptive pilot study The control group received a lecture and an orientation to the simulator. The self-directed learning group received lecture and orientation plus together worked through scenario and received a debriefing at end. The instructor-modeled group received lecture and orientation as	*Knowledge Assessment Test* (KAT) given at pre-test, post-test 1 (after lecture), and post-test 2 (after simulation experience one week after post-test 1). *Self-Efficacy Tool* (SET) given at same time as KAT.	• No significant difference on the KAT between groups. • The results of the SET showed significant differences at all three times. • Significant difference as to when to start Albuterol on TET. • Significant differences in 8 or 10 parts of BAT. • Needs to be redone on larger sample size.

Table 2-1   Characteristics of Existing Nursing Research Studies Using High-Fidelity Patient Simulators (n = 26) (continued)

				Technical Evaluation Tool (TET) / Behavioral Assessment Tool (BAT)	
			control group plus observed three faculty conduct scenario and then could ask questions of faculty.		
Nehring, W. M. (2008). U.S. boards of nursing and the use of high-fidelity patient simulators in nursing education. *Journal of Professional Nursing, 24,* 109–117.	"To ascertain the use of high-fidelity patient simulators for clinical time in current regulations" (p. 109).	Conducted in U.S. Each board of nursing in the 50 states, District of Columbia, and Puerto Rico	Survey Representatives from the boards of nursing completed and returned a mailed survey in 2006.	Completed survey	• 5 states and Puerto Rico have made regulation changes; only Florida indicated a percentage of time. • 16 states gave approval for simulation substitution. • 17 states may consider making changes.
Nehring, W. M., & Lashley, F. R. (2004a).Current use and opinions regarding human patient simulators in nursing education: An international survey. *Nursing Education Perspectives, 25,* 244–248.	"To examine the use of high-fidelity patient simulators in nursing education, specifically addressing courses and percentage of use, training of faculty and staff, how the simulator is used	Conducted internationally. 34 nursing programs (33 in U.S. 1 in Japan) and 6 simulation centers around the world who	Survey Participants completed and returned a mailed survey.	Completed survey. Results were divided by Community College, University, and Simulation Center.	• Simulation was used predominantly ≤ 5% of the curriculum in all types of programs. • Was used most often to teach physical assessment and medical-surgical content in community colleges and universities, and basic nursing skills in simulation centers.

Table 2-1 Characteristics of Existing Nursing Research Studies Using High-Fidelity Patient Simulators ($n = 26$) (continued)

Study	Purpose	Participants	Design and Interventions	Outcome Measures	Outcomes
Nursing Education					
	for evaluating specific competencies, other uses for this technology, and student opinions" (p. 44).	use Medical Education Technologies, Inc. (METI) simulators.			• Specific curricular content is delineated. • 25% or less of faculty were involved. • 58.1% of faculty were receptive to technology. • Student opinions were positive. • Competency evaluation was most often done in the university setting.
Radhakrishnan, K., Roche, J. P., & Cunningham, H. (2007). Measuring clinical practice parameters with human patient simulation: A pilot study. *International Journal of Nursing Education Scholarship*, 4, article 8.	"To identify the nursing clinical practice parameters influenced by high-fidelity patient simulation" (p. 1).	Conducted in U.S. 12 senior second-degree baccalaureate nursing students	Post-test only Students were divided equally into control and experimental group. Experimental group participated in two simulation practice sessions each lasting 1 hour. At the end of the course, all students	Clinical Simulation Evaluation Tool developed and completed by faculty.	• Students in the experimental group scored significantly higher in safety (45 vs 34, $X^2 = 10.81$, p = .001) and basic assessment skills (43 vs 33, $X^2 = 6.76$, p = .009).

Table 2-1 Characteristics of Existing Nursing Research Studies Using High-Fidelity Patient Simulators (n = 26) (continued)

Citation	Purpose	Sample/Setting	Design/Methods	Instruments	Findings
			participated in simulation exercise and faculty completed evaluation tool.		
Rystedt, H., & Lindstrom, B. (2001). Introducing simulation technologies in nurse education: A nursing practice perspective. *Nurse Education in Practice, 1,* 134–141.	"To explore how simulation technologies may contribute to learning in advanced education programs for nurses" (p. 135).	Conducted in Sweden. 15 nurses who were practicing in (a) critical and/or emergency care, and (b) anesthesia, as well as students studying in these areas (both are one-year programs)	Qualitative Participants participated in group interviews. Three groups were composed of practicing nurses and the other two of students. The interviews took place one month after receiving introduction on simulation technologies from low to high fidelity. Participants were asked to discuss what skills were difficult to learn, difficult to master, and which skills could be improved with use of simulation.	Group interviews (n = 5)	"Six critical aspects of nursing practice: • Judging the patient's health status. • Monitoring care interventions. • Prioritizing and carrying out interventions efficiently. • Communicating with patients and their relatives. • Cooperating with other members of the staff. • Managing complexity" (p. 136).
Scherer, Y. K., Bruce, S. A., & Runkawatt, V. (2007). A comparison of clinical simulation and case study presentation on nurse practitioner students' knowledge and confidence in managing a	"To compare the efficacy of control simulation mannequin assisted learning and case study presentation	Conducted in U.S. 23 NP students	Pre-test, post-test design "Participants were divided into control and experimental groups. Each received instruction on atrial arrhythmias and then a pre-test on knowledge and	Pre-tests and post-tests Confidence scale Evaluations by students	• No significant differences between tests for either group on knowledge. • Control group was more confident at post-test (p = 0.040).

43

Table 2-1 Characteristics of Existing Nursing Research Studies Using High-Fidelity Patient Simulators (n = 26) (continued)

Study	Purpose	Participants	Design and Interventions	Outcome Measures	Outcomes
Nursing Education					
cardiac event. *International Journal of Nursing Education Scholarship, 4*, article 22.	on knowledge and confidence of nurse practitioner (NP) students in managing a cardiac event" (p. 1).		confidence, and took the same test again as a post-test and completed an evaluation of the experience. The experimental group participated in a simulation scenario and the control group participated in a case study" (p. 1).		• Both groups rated the experience as positive.
Schoening, A. M., Sittner, B. J., & Todd, M. J. (2006). Simulated clinical experience: Nursing students' perceptions and the educators' role. *Nurse Educator, 31*, 253–258.	"To examine students' experience as a method of instruction, emphasizing the importance of the educators' role in promoting positive student	Conducted in U.S. 60 junior baccalaureate nursing students during their high-risk obstetrical experience	Pilot evaluation study Participants participated in a high-fidelity patient simulation orientation, two weeks of scenario practice,	10-item evaluation tool	• Students felt that they were able to practice appropriate skills and had hands-on learning and practice. • Students felt they experienced increased confidence in a safe environment. • Students felt that their critical thinking skills were improved, the environment was

outcomes" (p. 253).		followed by a debriefing session.			real, and that they had practice in their clinical decision-making skills. • Students found value and satisfaction in the experience and felt they could transfer the skills to the practice setting. • Students enjoyed the communication and teamwork experience.
Wong, T. K. S., & Chung, J. W. Y. (2002). Diagnostic reasoning processes using patient simulation in different learning environments. *Journal of Clinical Nursing, 11,* 65–72.	"To explore the diagnostic reasoning process among nursing students with different learning environments" (p. 65).	Conducted in China 20 nursing students: 10 from a university and 10 from a nursing program	Case-study design Participants completed the *Bigg's Study Process Questionnaire* and listed the differential diagnoses for three scenarios (peptic ulcer, hypoglycemia, and shortness of breath).	*Bigg's Study Process Questionnaire* (evaluates styles of studying) Results of problem behavior graphs drawn to show clinical reasoning to determined differential diagnoses.	• No significant differences between two groups on study approaches. • University students used both horizontal and vertical reasoning patterns, whereas the nursing program group showed only horizontal reasoning.

Table 2-1 Characteristics of Existing Nursing Research Studies Using High-Fidelity Patient Simulators ($n = 26$) (continued)

Study	Purpose	Participants	Design and Interventions	Outcome Measures	Outcomes
Team Management					
				Analyses were done/between two groups	
Davis, D. P., Buono, C., Ford, J., Paulson, L., Koenig, W., & Carrison, D. (2007). The effectiveness of a novel, algorithm-based difficult airway curriculum for air medical crews using human patient simulators. *Prehospital Emergency Care, 11*, 72–79.	"To evaluate the effectiveness of a simulator-based difficult airway curriculum in a large, aeromedical company" (p. 72).	Conducted in U.S. 120 flight nurses and paramedics	Pre-test, post-test design The pre-test consisted of the results of the final test from previous airway management curriculum that did not include simulation. The post-test was the final results after implementation of the new curriculum that does include simulation.	Results of the two final tests before and after implementation of simulation into the difficult airway curriculum Confidence rating	• Improvement was obtained on first attempt and overall endotracheal intubation success. • Incidence of hypoxic arrests also decreased. • Participants felt greater confidence with simulation as part of curriculum.
Gilligan, P., Bhatarcharjee, C., Knight, G., Smith, M., Hegarty, D., Shenton, A., et. al. (2005). To lead or not to lead?	"To investigate whether emergency nurses with previous advanced life	Conducted in UK 57 participants: 20 ALS	Post-test only Each participant first had their pulse and blood pressure taken.	Pre-intervention pulse and blood pressure of participants	• Nurses had the highest mean score (73.7%) followed by ALS trained

Table 2-1 Characteristics of Existing Nursing Research Studies Using High-Fidelity Patient Simulators (n = 26) (continued)

Prospective controlled study of emergency nurses' provision of advanced life support team leadership. *Emergency Medicine Journal, 22*, 628–632.	support (ALS) training provided good team leadership in a simulated cardiac arrest situation" (p. 628).	[similar to advanced cardiac life support (ACLS) in U.S.] trained nurses, 19 ALS trained emergency doctors, and 18 emergency doctors without ALS training.	They then had to lead the team which was composed of the investigators in a mock cardiac arrest situation. Their performance was scored.	"Performance score based on scenario understanding, team orientation to tasks, preparation, rhythm recognition, sequencing of interventions, appropriateness of interventions, and performance of defibrillation" (p. 629).	doctors (72.3%) and non-ALS trained doctors (69.5%). • Nurses found the experience to be less stressful than the non-ALS trained doctors did.
Jankouskas, T., Bush, M. C., Murray, B, Rudy, S., Henry, J., Dyer, A. M. et al. (2007). Crisis resource management: Evaluating outcomes of a multidisciplinary team. *Simulation in Healthcare, 2*, 96–101	"To evaluate improvement in the nontechnical skills of a multidisciplinary team of pediatric residents, anesthesiology residents, and pediatric nurses following participation in the crisis resource management	Conducted in U.S. "40 participants divided into seven multidisciplinary groups composed of three pediatric nurses, two pediatric residents, and one anesthesia resident" (p. 97).	Test-retest method Each group attended a 3-hour CRM program that included an orientation to the simulation laboratory and simulator; performance on a pediatric scenario, measurement of the collaboration and satisfaction with the scenario, a presentation of key concepts of CRM with	*Satisfaction about Care Decisions* instrument — measures perceived collaboration and perceived satisfaction. *Anesthetists' Nontechnical Skills System* (ANTS) — measures task management, teamworking, situation awareness, and	• There was significant differences in collaboration (1.42, $p < .0001$) and satisfaction (1.27, $p < .0001$) from the first to second scenario timeframe. • Teamwork was the only significant factor on the ANTS (0.8, $p = 0.03$).

Table 2-1   Characteristics of Existing Nursing Research Studies Using High-Fidelity Patient Simulators (*n* = 26) *(continued)*

Study	Purpose	Participants	Design and Interventions	Outcome Measures	Outcomes
Team Management					
	(CRM) educational program" (p. 96).		debriefing of initial scenario, performance on a second pediatric scenario, and final measurement of collaboration and satisfaction and ANTS rating.	decision-making" (p. 97–98).	
Morgan, P. J., Pittini, R., Regehr, G., Marrs, C., & Haley, M. F. (2007). Evaluating teamwork in a simulated obstetric environment. *Anesthesiology, 106,* 907–915.	"To determine whether the *Human Factors Rating Scale* (HFRS) and a *Global Rating Scale* (GRS) could be used to reliably assess obstetric team performance" (p. 907).	Conducted in Canada 34 participants: 16 nurses, 6 obstetricians, 6 anesthesiologists, and 6 residents. Also, included 9 external raters.	Correlational study to determine reliability of two tools Groups of health professionals were mixed to perform obstetrical scenarios using high-fidelity patient simulator.	*"Human Factors Rating Scale* is a behaviorally based performance evaluation scale. *Global Rating Scale of Performance* is a performance-based evaluation of overall team performance on the scenario" (p. 908).	• "Some scenarios were more difficult to assess performance. • The HFRS was not found to be useful for the assessment of obstetric teams. • The GRS did show promise as a summative evaluation tool" (p. 907).

Ten articles addressed the use of high-fidelity patient simulation as complementary to more traditional methods of instruction (Bremner, Aduddell, Bennett, & VanGeest, 2006; Childs & Sepples, 2006; DeCarlo, Collingridge, Grant, & Ventre, 2008; Henrichs, Rule, Grady, & Ellis, 2002; Jeffries & Rizzolo, 2006; King, Moseley, Hindenlang, & Kuritz, 2008; Lasater, 2007b; Nehring & Lashley, 2004a; Rystedt & Lindstrom, 2001; Schoening, Sittner, & Todd, 2006). The researchers examined the value of high-fidelity patient simulation, student or staff and/or faculty satisfaction with this technology, and student or staff attitudes. All of the research took place in the United States, except for one study in Sweden (Rystedt & Lindstrom, 2001). Five of the studies involved pre-licensure nursing students (Bremner et al., 2006; Childs & Sepples, 2006; Jeffries & Rizzolo, 2006; Lasater, 2007b; Schoening et al., 2006), two studies involved graduate students (Henrichs et al., 2002; Rystedt & Lindstrom, 2001), two studies involved practicing nurses (DeCarlo et al., 2008; Rystedt & Lindstrom, 2001), one study involved nursing faculty (King et al., 2008), and one study involved nursing programs (Nehring & Lashley, 2004a). The number of participants in these studies ranged from 12 to 523, with a median of 44.5. Surveys were used in seven of the studies (Bremner et al., 2006; Childs & Sepples, 2006; DeCarlo et al., 2008; Jeffries & Rizzolo, 2006; King et al., 2008; Nehring & Lashley, 2004a; Schoening et al., 2006), focus groups in three studies (Henrichs et al., 2002; Lasater, 2007b; Rystedt & Lindstrom, 2001), and pre- and post-tests in one study that also used surveys (Jeffries & Rizzolo, 2006). The nurse researchers found that the participants using high-fidelity patient simulation generally were satisfied and felt that they contributed to learning.

Competence in the performance of skills was assessed in eight studies (Alinier, Hunt, & Gordon, 2004; Alinier, Hunt, Gordon, & Harwood, 2006; Feingold, Calaluce, & Kallen, 2004; Hoffmann, O'Donnell, & Kim, 2007; Kuiper et al., 2008; Radhakrishnan, Roche, & Cunningham, 2007; Scherer, Bruce, & Runkawatt, 2007; Wong & Chung, 2002). Five of the studies took place in the United States (Feingold et al., 2004; Hoffmann et al., 2007; Kuiper et al., 2008; Radhakrishnan et al., 2007; Scherer et al., 2007), two in the United Kingdom (Alinier et al., 2004; Alinier et al., 2006), and one in China (Wong & Chung, 2002). Pre-licensure nursing students were the subjects in seven of the studies, with graduate nursing students participating in one study (Scherer et al., 2007) and faculty participating in one of the studies involving pre-licensure nursing students (Feingold et al., 2004). The number of participants in these studies ranged from 12 to 99, with a median of 36.5. Quasi-experimental studies involving pre- and post-tests predominated (Alinier et al., 2004; Alinier et al., 2006; Hoffmann et al., 2007; Kuiper et al., 2008; Scherer et al., 2007), with two studies employing surveys (Feingold et al., 2004; Radhakrishnan et al., 2007), and one study employing case studies (Wong & Chung, 2002). In general, performance on skills was improved. Alinier, Hung, Gordon, and Harwood (2006) found that there was no significant improvement in student confidence after practice with a high-fidelity patient simulator. Kuiper, Heinrich, Matthais, Graham, and Bell-Kotwall (2008) found no significant difference in student clinical reasoning abilities after clinical experience in a healthcare setting as compared to after a high-fidelity patient simulation experience, and Wong and Chung (2002) found no significant difference in diagnostic reasoning in nursing students using high-fidelity patient simulation as compared to students using a case study. In addition, Scherer, Bruce, and Runkawatt (2007) found no significant differences in knowledge level between nursing students who participated in high-fidelity patient simulation experiences as compared to students who participated in a case study.

Two nursing research studies examined the use of high-fidelity patient simulation as a substitute for clinical time in a healthcare setting (Bearnson & Wiker, 2005; Nehring, 2008). Bearnson and Wiker (2005) examined the possibility of substituting one clinical day in the junior year with experience with high-fidelity patient simulators in a nursing program in the United States. The nursing students filled out a survey at the completion of this experience, which revealed that students felt they had increased their knowledge and skills and were more confident about their ability to administer medications. Nehring (2008) surveyed the boards of nursing in all 50 states in the United States, the District of Columbia, and Puerto Rico to ascertain whether regulations in that state or territory allowed for substitution of clinical time with the use of high-fidelity patient simulation, and if not, whether future consideration would be made on this issue. Such regulation changes had been made in five states and Puerto Rico. Approval by the state board of nursing for substitution with high-fidelity patient simulation was given in 16 states, and future regulatory changes were being discussed in 17 states.

Lasater (2007a) examined clinical judgment in pre-licensure nursing students in the United States. Through her experiences observing and interviewing the students who took part in high-fidelity patient simulation experiences, she developed a clinical judgment rubric that can be used by nursing schools for the evaluation of this construct.

Finally, LeFlore and colleagues (2007) examined whether nurse practitioner students in a U.S. nursing program learned more from an instructor-driven high-fidelity patient simulation experience as compared to a student-driven high-fidelity patient simulation experience. This study involved three groups of students: traditional lecture, instructor-driven simulation experience, and student-driven simulation experience. Because the total sample consisted of 16 students, the authors recommended replication of the study with a larger sample size to ensure valid outcomes.

Team Management Nursing Research Studies

Four nursing research studies examined team management in the practice setting (Davis, Buono, Ford, Paulson, Koenig, & Carrison, 2007; Gilligan et al., 2005; Jankouskas et al., 2007; Morgan, Pittini, Regehr, Marrs, & Haley, 2007). Two studies were conducted in the United States (Davis et al., 2007; Jankouskas et al., 2007), one study in the United Kingdom (Gilligan et al., 2005), and one study in Canada (Morgan et al., 2007). All studies involved nurses and at least one other discipline. These disciplines included paramedics (Davis et al., 2007); emergency department physicians (Gilligan et al., 2005); pediatric residents and pediatric anesthesia residents (Jankouskas et al., 2007); and obstetricians, anesthesiologists, residents, and external raters (Morgan et al., 2007). The number of participants ranged from 34 to 120, with a median of 48.5. Two of the studies involved pre- and post-tests (Davis et al., 2007; Jankouskas et al., 2007), one study involved a post-test only design (Gilligan et al., 2005), and one study had a correlational design (Morgan et al., 2007). In general, team performance improved with experience with high-fidelity patient simulators, as well as confidence to some degree. Morgan and colleagues (2007) found one of the scenarios that they used to be more difficult to evaluate.

RECOMMENDATIONS FOR FUTURE NURSING RESEARCH

As nursing faculty from across the country learn more about the advantages of using simulation, including high-fidelity patient simulation, in their curricula, the rationale for initial and continued expenditure of scarce funds to support a simulation program is needed for post-secondary college and university administrators. In all of the health professions, the key question is: How can research prove the efficacy of high-fidelity patient simulation in education programs? A review of the current nursing research on this topic is at best inconclusive with regard to efficacy. Like their counterparts in the medical research literature (see Issenberg et al., 2005), current nursing researchers have found that the use of high-fidelity patient simulation in nursing education is valuable, provides positive experiences, and may improve knowledge, skill performance, and confidence. Unfortunately, the current data are based on small sample sizes and have not had the benefit of a power analysis; use variable samples consisting of pre-licensure, graduate, and practicing nurses; measure a variety of constructs; and were gathered with a number of instruments, including some that have not been subjected to validity or reliability testing. Similar study characteristics can be seen in a comparison of all nursing research involving all forms of simulation (see Chapter 1).

Where must nursing research on the use of high-fidelity patient simulation go from this point? Nursing research in this area should focus on three areas: educational efficacy, competency testing, and practice improvement. Ideally, a meeting should be convened among the current nurse researchers in this area so that they might collectively construct a plan for nursing research in high-fidelity patient simulation that covers these three areas.

Under the topic of educational efficacy, nursing research should be designed not only to examine whether the use of high-fidelity patient simulation has validity in assisting nursing students to increase their knowledge base, competently perform skills, and increase confidence in their practice as future nurses, but also to examine what makes an expert nurse educator. Benner's theory, in addition to other learning theories can be used for this area of research. Medical educators have discussed the different forms of validity in reference to high-fidelity patient simulation, including content, face, concurrent, construct, and predictive (Patel & Gould, 2006; Reznek, 2004). These authors believe that predictive validity will be the most difficult to demonstrate given the problems in comparing performance in a standardized situation and in a highly variable clinical environment. Multisite studies are needed to ensure such validation. In addition, further testing, as exemplified by the work of Jeffries and Rogers (2007), will add to this evolving area of nursing research.

As discussed in Chapter 1, nursing as a field has long debated how best to measure competency in nursing. The use of high-fidelity patient simulation would be beneficial for both an objective process and a summative evaluation of competency for nursing students across either the pre-licensure or graduate curriculum. Assessment and evaluation of performance can also take place on an individual or team level. Evaluation of the theory of mastery learning, in which students are graded on mastery of knowledge and skills at a predetermined level, could influence changes in nursing curricula in future years and would influence the amount of time nursing students take to complete a program based on individual learning levels (McGaghie, Miller, Sajid, & Telder, 1978). This idea has been proposed and implemented for nursing practice (del Bueno, Weeks, & Brown-Stewart, 1987). Could we see a competency-based curriculum for nursing in the future? If so, the use of high-fidelity patient simulation would play a major role in its evolution. Scenarios could be designed that reflect evidence-based practice, cover the critical behaviors and conditions that nursing students should know, and meet the educational goals or program objectives of the program.

Practice improvement can be influenced by educational efficacy and competency, but this area encompasses the total practice of a nurse individually and as a member of a healthcare team. Multisite, intradisciplinary, and interdisciplinary studies are needed to fully capture results in this area of research.

Additional studies on team management will further develop this area of research, as well as testing of the Nehring and Lashley (2004a) model.

In addition, we need to understand how to develop and maintain a successful simulation program in a nursing program. This book provides many examples of how simulation programs have been developed and what goes into the development of a scenario. This knowledge should be synthesized to create a workable process that can be adopted by nursing programs around the world. In turn, we should continue to share our experiences in the literature, at conferences, and in conversations.

CONCLUSION

This chapter has summarized the emerging nursing literature on the use of theoretical frameworks and research using high-fidelity patient simulation. The outcomes of this work by nurses around the world are promising. As the need for and popularity of high-fidelity patient simulation in nursing education and practice settings continues to grow in response to calls for better quality and safety in education and practice, more nurses will publish their work on theoretical development and/or research. We must continue to provide forums for nurses to communicate their experiences and findings. In turn, more funding must be made available for intradisciplinary and interdisciplinary research involving individuals and teams. It is hoped that the body of literature in these areas will grow exponentially and relate significant findings that will influence changes in how we educate nursing students and practice in the real world.

References

Alinier, G., Hunt, W. G., & Gordon, R. (2004). Determining the value of simulation in nurse education: Study design and initial results. *Nurse Education in Practice*, *4*, 200–207.

Alinier, G., Hunt, B., Gordon, R., & Harwood, C. (2006). Effectiveness of intermediate-fidelity simulation training technology in undergraduate nursing education. *Journal of Advanced Nursing*, *54*, 359–369.

Bearnson, C. S., & Wiker, K. M. (2005). Human patient simulators: A new face in baccalaureate nursing education at Brigham Young University. *Journal of Nursing Education*, *44*, 421–425.

Benner, P. (1984). *From novice to expert*. Menlo Park, CA: Addison-Wesley.

Bradley, P., & Postlethwaite, K. (2003). Simulation in clinical learning. *Medical Education*, *37*(suppl 1), 1–5.

Bremner, M. N., Aduddell, K., Bennett, D. N., & VanGeest, J. B. (2006). The use of human patient simulators: Best practices with novice nursing students. *Nurse Educator*, *31*, 170–174.

Childs, J. C., & Sepples, S. (2006). Clinical teaching by simulation: Lessons learned from a complex patient care scenario. *Nursing Education Perspectives*, *27*, 154–158.

Davis, D. P., Buono, C., Ford, J., Paulson, L., Koenig, W., & Carrison, D. (2007). The effectiveness of a novel, algorithm-based difficult airway curriculum for air medical crews using human patient simulators. *Prehospital Emergency Care, 11,* 72–79.

DeCarlo, D., Collingridge, D. S., Grant, C., & Ventre, K. M. (2008). Factors influencing nurses' attitudes toward simulation-based education. *Simulation in Healthcare, 3,* 90–96.

Decker, S. (2007). Integrating guided reflection into simulated learning experiences. In P. R. Jeffries (Ed.), *Simulation in nursing education: From conceptualization to evaluation* (pp. 73–85). New York: National League for Nursing.

del Bueno, D. J., Weeks, L., & Brown-Stewart, P. (1987). Clinical assessment centers: A cost-effective alternative for competency development. *Nursing Economics, 5*(1), 21–26.

Feingold, C. E., Calaluce, M., & Kallen, M. A. (2004). Computerized patient model and simulated clinical experiences: Evaluation with baccalaureate nursing students. *Journal of Nursing Education, 43,* 156–163.

Ferguson, S., Beeman, L., Eichorn, M., Jaramillo, Y., & Wright, M. (2004). High-fidelity simulation across clinical settings and educational levels. In G. E. Loyd, C. L. Lake, & R. B. Greenberg (Eds.), *Practical health care simulations* (pp. 184–203). Philadelphia: Elsevier.

Gaba, D. M., Fish, K. J., & Howard, S. K. (1994). *Crisis management in anesthesiology.* New York: Churchill Livingston.

Gilligan, P., Bhatarcharjee, C., Knight, G., et al. (2005). To lead or not to lead? Prospective controlled study of emergency nurses' provision of advanced life support team leadership. *Emergency Medicine Journal, 22,* 628–632.

Henrichs, B., Rule, A., Grady, M., & Ellis, W. (2002). Nurse anesthesia students' perceptions of the anesthesia patient simulator: A qualitative study. *AANA Journal, 70,* 219–225.

Hoffmann, R. L., O'Donnell, J. M., & Kim, Y. (2007). The effects of human patient simulators on basic knowledge in critical care nursing with undergraduate senior baccalaureate nursing students. *Simulation in Healthcare, 2,* 110–114.

Issenberg, S. B., McGaghie, W. C., Petrusa, E. R., Gordon, D. L., & Scalese, R. J. (2005). Features and uses of high-fidelity medical simulations that lead to effective learning: A BEME systematic review. *Medical Teacher, 27,* 10–28.

Jankouskas, T., Bush, M. C., Murray, B., et al. (2007). Crisis resource management: Evaluating outcomes of a multidisciplinary team. *Simulation in Healthcare, 2,* 96–103.

Jeffries, P. R., & Rizzolo, M. A. (2006). *Designing and implementing models for the innovative use of simulation to teach nursing care of ill adults and children: A national, multi-site, multi-method study.* New York: National League for Nursing.

Jeffries, P. R., & Rogers, K. J. (2007). Theoretical framework for simulation design. In P. R. Jeffries (Ed.), *Simulation in nursing education: From conceptualization to evaluation* (pp. 20–33). New York: National League for Nursing.

King, C. J., Moseley, S., Hindenlang, B., & Kuritz, P. (2008). Limited use of the human patient simulator by nurse faculty: An intervention program designed to increase use. *International Journal of Nursing Education Scholarship, 5*(1), Article 12.

Kolb, D. A. (1984). *Experiential learning.* Englewood Cliffs, NJ: Prentice-Hall.

Kuiper, R., Heinrich, C., Mattias, A., Graham, M. J., & Bell-Kotwall, L. (2008). Debriefing with the OPT model of clinical reasoning during high fidelity patient simulation. *International Journal of Nursing Education Scholarship, 5*(1), Article 17.

Larew, C., Lessans, S., Spunt, D., Foster, D., & Covington, B. G. (2006). Innovations in clinical simulation: Application of Benner's theory in an interactive patient care simulation. *Nursing Education Perspectives, 27,* 16–21.

Lasater, K. (2007a). Clinical judgment development: Using simulation to create an assessment rubric. *Journal of Nursing Education, 46,* 496–503.

Lasater, K. (2007b). High-fidelity simulation and the development of clinical judgment: Students' experiences. *Journal of Nursing Education, 46,* 269–280.

Leddy, S. (2008). Curriculum development. In B. A. Moyer & R. A. Wittmann-Price (Eds.), *Nursing education: Foundations for practice excellence* (pp. 66–86). Philadelphia: F. A. Davis.

LeFlore, J. L., Anderson, M., Michael, J., Engle, W. D., & Anderson, J. (2007). Comparison of self-directed learning versus instructor-modeled learning during a simulated clinical experience. *Simulation in Healthcare, 2,* 170–177.

Long, R. E. (2005). Using simulation to teach resuscitation: An important patient safety tool. *Critical Care Nursing Clinics of North America, 17,* 1–8.

McGaghie, W. C., Miller, G. E., Sajid, A., & Telder, T. V. (1978). *Competency-based curriculum development in medical education: Public health paper no. 68.* Geneva, Switzerland: World Health Organization.

Morgan, P. J., Pittini, R., Regehr, G., Marrs, C., & Haley, M. F. (2007). Evaluating teamwork in a simulated obstetric environment. *Anesthesiology, 106,* 907–915.

Nehring, W. M. (2008). U. S. boards of nursing and the use of high-fidelity patient simulators in nursing education. *Journal of Professional Nursing, 24,* 109–117.

Nehring, W. M., & Lashley, F. R. (2004a). Current use and opinions regarding human patient simulators in nursing education: An international survey. *Nursing Education Perspectives, 25,* 244–248.

Nehring, W. M., & Lashley, F. R. (2004b). Using the Human Patient Simulator™ in nursing education. *Annual Review of Nursing Education, 2,* 163–181.

Nehring, W. M., Lashley, F. R., & Ellis, W. E. (2002). Critical incident nursing management using human patient simulators. *Nursing Education Perspectives, 23,* 128–132.

Patel, A. A., & Gould, D. A. (2006). Simulators in interventional radiology training and evaluation: A paradigm shift is on the horizon. *Journal of Vascular Interventional Radiology, 17,* S163–S173.

Pesut, D. J., & Herman, J. (1999). *Clinical reasoning: The art and science of critical and creative thinking.* Albany, NY: Delmar.

Radhakrishnan, K., Roche, J. P., & Cunningham, H. (2007). Measuring clinical practice parameters with human patient simulation: A pilot study. *International Journal of Nursing Education Scholarship, 4,* Article 8.

Reznek, M. A. (2004). Current status of simulation in education and research. In G. E. Loyd, C. L. Lake, & R. B. Greenberg (Eds.), *Practical health care simulations* (pp. 27–47). Philadelphia: Elsevier.

Rystedt, H., & Lindstrom, B. (2001). Introducing simulation technologies in nurse education: A nursing practice perspective. *Nurse Education in Practice, 1,* 134–141.

Scherer, Y. K., Bruce, S. A., & Runkawatt, V. (2007). A comparison of clinical simulation and case study presentation on nurse practitioner students' knowledge and confidence in managing a cardiac event. *International Journal of Nursing Education Scholarship, 4,* Article 22.

Schoening, A. M., Sittner, B. J., & Todd, M. J. (2006). Simulated clinical experience: Nursing students' perceptions and the educator's role. *Nurse Educator, 31,* 253–258.

Schon, D. A. (1983). *The reflective practitioner: How professionals think in action.* New York: Basic Books.

Tanner, C. A. (2006). Thinking like a nurse: A research-based model of clinical judgment in nursing. *Journal of Nursing Education, 45,* 204–211.

Waldner, M. H., & Olson, J. K. (2007). Taking the patient to the classroom: Applying theoretical frameworks to simulation in nursing education. *International Journal of Nursing Education Scholarship, 4*(1), Article 18.

Wong, T. K. S., & Chung, J. W. Y. (2002). Diagnostic reasoning processes using patient simulation in different learning environments. *Journal of Clinical Nursing, 11,* 65–72.

Unit 2

Setting Up a Simulation Program

Developing and Implementing a Simulation Program: Baccalaureate Nursing Education

Patricia Ravert

Brigham Young University (BYU) is a private university (owned by the Church of Jesus Christ of Latter-day Saints), established in 1875. The main campus is located in Provo, Utah, 45 miles south of Salt Lake City at the base of the Wasatch Mountains and serves approximately 33,000 students. The College of Nursing (CON) was founded in 1952. The CON offers two programs, the undergraduate Bachelor of Science and the Master of Science; the latter program prepares family nurse practitioners. The CON programs are approved by the Utah State Board of Nursing and are accredited by the National League for Nursing Accrediting Commission and the Commission on Collegiate Nursing Education.

The theme for the CON is "Learning the Healer's Art," and its defined mission is to develop professional nurses who promote health, care for the suffering, engage in the scholarship of the discipline, invite the Spirit into health and healing, and lead with faith and integrity. The baccalaureate program prepares students with the knowledge, competencies, values, and leadership abilities to enter into professional nursing practice. The CON builds on a broad liberal foundation of arts, sciences, and humanities. All but 3 of the 15 nursing courses incorporate didactic, clinical, and laboratory components, which all figure into the grade for the course. Three courses—Pharmacology in Nursing, Ethics in Nursing, and Scholarly Inquiry in Nursing—do not have a clinical or laboratory component.

Throughout the course of the CON's existence, there have been areas designated to support the development of psychomotor skills. In the 1970s, a single room was furnished with hospital beds and basic care models so students could practice basic skills. In the 1990s, a Nursing Learning Center (NLC) was created to facilitate student learning in a variety of settings such as critical care, pediatric health, and maternal health. The current 6000-square-foot NLC was completed in 1998 and serves as the hub of student activity in the CON, as suggested by Hodson-Carlton and Worrell-Carlisle (2005). The NLC includes several rooms for a variety of student uses (see Figure 3-1). The initial area of the NLC is an open student study area with computer stations, two group student study rooms, and a satellite nursing library and circulation desk. The remaining areas include a four-bay exam area and four nursing skill laboratories designed for advanced, basic, pediatric, and maternal health nursing skills teaching and learning. The NLC is open approximately 70 hours each week and is staffed by student workers, a full-time supervisor, and a faculty coordinator. Other faculty members and approximately six part-time registered nurses hired as teaching assistants work with students in the NLC each week.

Figure 3-1   Nursing Learning Center

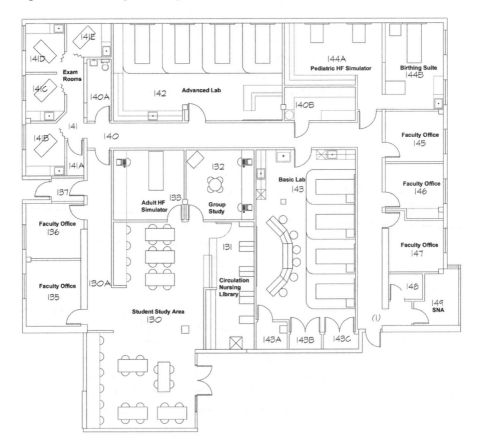

The CON has used clinical simulation for many years, as part of its efforts to replicate the clinical environment. When the NLC was completed in 1998, the computer programs, manikins, equipment, and medical supplies were state-of-the-art. The laboratory hours are a required part of the curriculum and are figured into the clinical and laboratory requirements for 7 of the 15 courses. A faculty member, Professor Sandra Mangum, was the NLC coordinator for more than 20 years and led the CON through the construction of the NLC in the 1990s. She was instrumental in the development of the laboratory experiences for BYU nursing students. Professor Mangum planned a retirement for mid-2001, and I took the NLC coordinator position beginning in January 2001 to allow for time for orientation to the position.

At the end of 2000, Dean Elaine Marshall creatively used instructional technology/computer funds to order a high-fidelity patient simulator, the Human Patient Simulator (HPS) from Medical Education Technology Incorporated (METI). At that time, the simulators were constructed as ordered and BYU's high-fidelity patient simulator was scheduled for a mid-2001 delivery. During my orientation to the NLC, Professor Mangum informed me of the purchase and stated I would have to figure out how to use the high-fidelity patient simulator and integrate it into the curriculum. I was not familiar with high-fidelity patient simulators, so I investigated the matter further and found that the University of Utah, Department of Anesthesia, had an HPS. I made a visit to the University of Utah and then attended the Human Patient Simulator Network (HPSN) 2001 presentation sponsored by METI in February. Thus BYU's journey of high-fidelity simulation began in 2001.

THE BYU EXPERIENCE: PLANNING AND INTEGRATION

To prepare for the high-fidelity patient simulator, one of the two group student study rooms was remodeled to function as a high-fidelity adult simulation room. A door was added to facilitate access to supplies and medical gases. The medical gases and compressed air were piped in from another storage room, and cabinets and shelving were added. Later a headwall unit was added.

The HPS was delivered and set up in spring 2001. Initially the technicians taught me how to operate the high-fidelity patient simulator. I practiced throughout the summer and learned much, but knew there was much more to learn if the CON staff and students were to effectively use the high-fidelity patient simulator. An educator from METI came to the CON in September 2001, and 10 faculty members attended the 2-day education course. Faculty members were selected from each of the basic courses. During the school year, none of these faculty members used the high-fidelity patient simulator. During the next year, I worked on a plan to use the high-fidelity patient simulator with students in the basic medical–surgical course.

Basic medical–surgical nursing scenarios had not been developed for the HPS. As a consequence, I spent many hours programming two or three scenarios. I also networked with other nurse educators; obtained programming for scenarios that would teach and facilitate learning of ideas; and shared the ones I developed. As a result of this work, I came to realize that I needed more help: I could not set up programming, run the high-fidelity patient simulator computer, and facilitate all scenarios for a class of 48–64 students.

To obtain funding for assistance in the integration of simulation, I applied for a Mentored Environment Grant and research funds from BYU. I planned a research project (doctoral project) using the high-fidelity patient simulator. Part of the grant and research funds were used to hire undergraduate students as research assistants. The research assistants were taught to run the high-fidelity patient simulator computer, act as the patient voice, act as the health-care provider's voice, set up and take down the simulation environment, and perform typical research activities of data collection and entry.

During fall 2002, we practiced running scenarios with volunteers. We decided to use five patient scenarios: a male medical–surgical patient admitted following a motor vehicle accident, a female experiencing a postpartum hemorrhage, an antepartum female experiencing pregnancy-induced hypertension, a male experiencing chest pain, and a male experiencing disseminated intravascular coagulation. These scenarios were chosen because programming and supporting documents were available, rather than because the scenarios correlated with course objectives. After the initial implementation, scenarios were selected through survey of course and program objectives.

In 2003, the five scenarios became available for students in the medical–surgical course. Some were part of the study (Ravert, in press) regarding critical thinking; others were not. Once the study was completed, I met with the medical–surgical course coordinator to determine which scenarios would better fit the course objectives. It was determined that all students should have experience with a core group of patient diagnoses/experiences: assessment of the medical–surgical patient, diabetic ketoacidosis, cerebral vascular accident, congestive heart failure, chest pain in a medical–surgical patient, and gastrointestinal bleeding. The computer programming and supporting documents were developed or found for these scenarios. The medical–surgical scenarios were facilitated by a registered nurse hired as a teaching assistant with support from the student workers (former research assistants). The students involved in the study enjoyed doing the simulations and especially liked the maternal health scenarios (postpartum hemorrhage and pregnancy-induced hypertension), even though they had not taken the obstetrical course and the content was not part of the medical–surgical curriculum. During the next semester, the scenarios were changed to better fit with the medical–surgical course objectives.

During the next school year, I met with the course coordinator for the Care of the Child-bearing Family course to facilitate high-fidelity simulation experiences with maternal health. A plan was developed to orient the faculty for this course on how to facilitate the simulation sessions and how to use student workers to assist in setting up for the sessions and running the computer. The first semester we planned to have all students experience the postpartum hemorrhage scenario. Later the pregnancy-induced hypertension scenario was added to the schedule. The schedule for the course lab was revised to allow for the simulation sessions without decreasing clinical hours.

During the 2004–2005 school year, scenarios were added for students in the advanced medical–surgical course (which covered intensive and critical care concepts and experiences). These scenarios focus on "code" situations, including a respiratory arrest from exacerbation of congestive heart failure, a classic myocardial infarction, a respiratory arrest from sedation medication, and an arrest of an alcoholic patient with gastrointestinal bleeding. The students find these scenarios helpful in utilizing the concepts they have learned in the didactic, lab, and clinical components of their courses. These experiences are sometimes observed in the clinical component, but most students have an opportunity to participate only through simulation.

METI began selling the Program for Nursing Curriculum Integration (PNCI) in 2005. The PNCI includes 90 simulated clinical experiences for the company's adult, pediatric, and baby high-fidelity patient simulators. The majority are geared toward the adult high-fidelity patient simulator. The package includes the programming, supporting documents, and consulting to assist in integrating plans. BYU purchased the PNCI as soon as it became available. The PNCI is worth the investment: Learning to develop and program scenarios is extremely time-consuming, and the PNCI saves much in time and effort, thereby allowing faculty to easily use a variety of scenarios with little start-up time. After purchasing the PNCI, BYU has converted most of the simulations to those developed by METI.

In 2006, a high-fidelity pediatric simulator, PediaSIM from METI, was purchased through donor funds. At the CON, the pediatric content is taught in the Care of the Child-rearing Family course, which students take during the same semester as the Care of the Child-bearing Family course. The pediatric clinical experiences vary according to assignment. There is a large pediatric facility in Salt Lake City, but not all students are able to have clinical experiences in the facility; the remaining students have pediatric clinical experiences in local hospitals, which sometimes do not have patients with much variation in their patient populations. The simulation integration plan included using clinical time for simulation. Each clinical group is scheduled to come to the NLC and participate in two pediatric simulations, which replace a clinical day in the curriculum. The faculty members (full-time and part-time adjunct) have been trained to facilitate the simulation sessions. Some faculty members enjoy facilitating more than others, and occasionally negotiation of coursework occurs so that some faculty members act as facilitators for other clinical groups.

By 2007, the adult HPS system that BYU obtained in 2001 had begun to have a variety of problems during use, most notably with the respiratory system. A decision was made to replace the HPS with a METI Emergency Care Simulator (ECS). The ECS system meets all the needs of a baccalaureate program. The new system was put into service prior to the fall 2007 semester.

During the latter part of 2005 and 2006, Colleen Tingey, the NLC supervisor, learned to use a Noelle birthing simulator (Gaumard Scientific) that BYU had purchased several years before but had not utilized. Several birthing simulations were done with students. Some sessions could not be completed due to technical problems with the simulator. After consulting with the manufacturer, Colleen and the course coordinator traveled to Florida for further training from the Gaumard Scientific personnel. During this training, they were introduced to the updated tetherless Noelle childbirthing system. In late 2007, BYU purchased the new system along with the Newborn Hal. An educator from Gaumard came to BYU and conducted a two-day training session on the new system. BYU also had two personnel from the campus instrument shop go to Florida for technical training; they can now perform most of the adjustments and repairs without having to send the system to Florida. The BYU technicians have been extremely helpful to the CON. When we have experienced problems, they have been able to immediately respond and get the system up and running usually within 15–20 minutes.

During the winter 2008 semester, the postpartum hemorrhage and pregnancy-induced hypertension simulations were done on the Noelle simulator. The faculty members had found it difficult to get everything ready (equipment, supplies, and patient documentation forms) for the simulation experience and to run the computer, making changes to the patient as needed, as well as facilitate the sessions. To assist the faculty, one of the experienced student workers completed her senior project by programming the computers for birthing, postpartum hemorrhage, and pregnancy-induced hypertension simulations; developing the supporting documentation; setting up procedures; and filling boxes of supplies and items to set the scene. The student worker also assisted in several scenarios to help faculty to use the items she had developed.

In 2008, the BYU baccalaureate students participated in 15 high-fidelity simulation experiences throughout the curriculum. The masters of nursing students did not use the high-fidelity patient simulators. There has been some interest from a new faculty member, so the future may include integration of the graduate students into the simulation program.

At the outset of implementation of the high-fidelity patient simulation system, a decision was made to use the simulation sessions as part of a teaching/learning strategy rather than as part of an evaluation process. Students are required to attend, and preparation is highly encouraged. Most students prepare by completing 5–10 questions on the type of patient or disease entity, and they have reported that they have a better experience when they have prepared. Throughout the implementation, students have been surveyed regarding their perception and satisfaction of the simulation experience. Focus groups have been conducted with the students during most semesters, and several key themes have been identified. The data from written surveys are evaluated through SPSS, with the software-analysis results and focus-group themes being shared with faculty members, student workers, and teaching assistants. Overall, the students report they enjoy and value the simulation experiences and suggest more experiences be included. The results of the evaluations have been used to improve the sessions across the curriculum.

SUGGESTIONS FOR SUCCESSFUL IMPLEMENTATION

Simulation Specialist

If a program is contemplating integrating high-fidelity simulation experiences into the curriculum, it is recommended that a simulation specialist or champion be appointed. The simulation specialist needs to have designated time to facilitate the integration. Initial helpful tasks are to visit other programs that use high-fidelity simulation experiences and to watch others actually running sessions with students. The simulation specialist also ought to attend conferences and workshops where much networking occurs.

Simulation Integration Team

The simulation specialist will need others to assist in the integration work. Many programs develop a team or task force to deal with this issue. Members may include an administrative representative, faculty members who have expressed an interest in simulation, a faculty member from each major clinical course, and technical/computer support personnel. The team tasks may include performing a curriculum review, determining scheduling of simulation activities, setting student expectations, and determining a simulation integration timeline and plan.

Curriculum Review

The simulation specialist will lead the team in reviewing the curriculum to determine which concepts or objectives could or should be taught through simulation. An important part of the curriculum is "to assist students in obtaining the body of knowledge, attitudes, and skills necessary to practice as a registered nurse" (Jeffries & Norton, 2005). The curriculum is developed by faculty members and should be reviewed if simulation will be used. At BYU, care of the patient experiencing postpartum hemorrhage is taught only through high-fidelity simulation. Other concepts are taught partially through didactic content, with the patient care and management elements being taught through simulation.

Another decision is to determine which types of patients and situations to simulate. Some programs choose to simulate high-risk and low-frequency situations so that students will have an opportunity to experience these situations in a safe, simulated environment.

Scheduling Time for Simulation

The team must also discuss and determine where the time for simulation will come from within the program. Programs vary in this regard: Some use didactic time for simulation, others devote clinical or lab hours to the simulation activities. This decision may also vary from course to course. Once the decision is made about how the time for simulation will be allocated, the team should discuss how groups will be scheduled.

Scheduling of student groups can be accomplished in a variety of ways and may also vary from course to course. Some programs have all students in a clinical group come together. The students then participate in two or more different patient scenarios, with some of the students observing while the remainder do the actual patient care. The observing students may be involved by completing observation sheets, acting as resources for the group, or looking up information on the Internet or in books (such as information about drugs). Partway through the scenario, the students giving care may be instructed to give reports to the observing students, who then take over the care. Throughout the session, all students are involved, either through providing direct care, making observations, or acting as resources in all the scenarios. At BYU, the pediatric course schedules the clinical groups to come to the NLC rather than to clinical sites, and students participate in two different pediatric scenarios (an asthma patient and a diabetic patient).

Another scheduling option is to provide opportunities at various times and allow students to sign up for the simulation in groups of four to six. The groups then participate in the assigned scenario at the selected time. At BYU, the basic medical–surgical students participate in five scenarios across the semester. At the beginning of the semester, students sign up with three other students to come at a specific time every other week for simulation activities. To accommodate the 64 students in the course, it requires two full days of simulation on our one adult high-fidelity patient simulator. The time for simulation is part of the scheduled lab hours for the course.

A third scheduling option is to determine specific dates and times that will accommodate the nursing students' schedules and then to either assign each student to a date and time or allow students to sign up on their own. The childbearing course at BYU uses this type of scheduling. If this option is selected, it is recommended that the dates and times be determined early in the semester so students may add the high-fidelity patient simulation experiences to their busy schedules.

A fourth scheduling option is to have the simulation experience be part of a lab day where several different lab stations are established. The students then rotate through the stations, one of which is a simulation activity. At BYU, this model is used with a group of students who are front-loading several essential skills at the beginning of the semester, with the simulation experience consisting of review and practice of assessment skills.

Other scheduling options can be developed that fit the unique needs of a particular course within a program. Whichever schedule or schedules are used, students should be informed early so they can plan for the simulation experience.

Student Expectations

Another task the simulation integration team may choose to discuss is expectations for students regarding attendance, preparation work, and student dress (Spunt & Covington, 2008). Many programs use the simulation experiences as a teaching/learning strategy and expect students to come prepared for the particular patient case. Some assign reading, questions to answer, or packets of information to read and complete. Other programs require students to develop care maps or care plans, as in a regular clinical experience. At BYU, students are given basic written information on the patient situation prior to the simulation activity, usually one to two weeks before their session. The information also contains 5–10 questions which students answer, either individually or as a group, to prepare for the high-fidelity patient simulation experience. The preparation work is not collected but serves to assist the students in getting ready for the experience.

The team should also discuss the expectations of attendance. In particular, it should determine whether the simulation experiences will be required or optional and whether grades or points for attendance will be given. At BYU, students are required to attend the simulation experiences and are given a small number of points for attendance, which are then incorporated into their overall course grade.

Expectations for student dress during simulation activities vary from program to program. It has been observed that students act in a more "professional" role when they are dressed as a "nurse." Some programs require students to follow clinical uniform guidelines whenever they work in the skill lab. Other programs require students to wear uniforms only when they participate in high-fidelity simulation experiences. For many years, BYU students wore street clothes in the NLC for their lab experiences. In 2007, after watching several videos of groups of students (some in uniforms and some in street clothes), I brought up the issue of wearing uniforms in the NLC during faculty assembly. The faculty members were mixed on their opinions and recommended the issue be addressed by the Student Nurses' Association. The students understood the rationale but didn't want to have the requirement for another day for a "clean and crisp" uniform; instead, they suggested the college purchase lab coats that students would put on as they came into the high-fidelity simulation room. The college obtained inexpensive lab coats and required students to wear them. Now students automatically pick up the lab coats and actually choose to wear them in other labs as well. The first-semester students wear uniforms for any lab pass-off/competency evaluation.

Integration Timeline

An integration timeline and plan for implementation of the simulation also need to be developed. Some programs decide to implement one high-fidelity patient simulation experience in each course during the initial semester or year. Other programs start with those courses in which the faculty are willing to learn to facilitate high-fidelity patient simulation sessions. These faculty members may choose to integrate one or more different simulations within the course. After successful integration in the first course, another course is selected to begin high-fidelity patient simulation use. Still other programs choose to simulate patient conditions that they believe all students should have experience with, such as postpartum hemorrhage, chest pain in medical–surgical patients, and "code" situations.

Simulation Support Staff

Besides designating a simulation specialist, it is necessary to determine who will provide the needed services for simulation experiences, such as scheduling of simulation equipment and rooms/areas, operating the computer (i.e., "running the computer"), facilitating and debriefing sessions, and providing technology support.

Scheduling of Equipment and Simulation Areas

Some colleges or programs have centralized scheduling programming, so that the simulation areas and equipment are simply added to the existing programming. Others do the programming through a designated person in the laboratory area. The scheduling may be done electronically or in paper format. The advantage to an electronic schedule is faculty members can see whether the resource is available without having to track down an actual person and make inquiries. Policies regarding scheduling, such as priority in scheduling, may need to be developed as the use of simulation equipment and areas increases.

Computer Operators

Running the computer is often an intimidating task for many faculty members. If faculty members are expected to operate the computer, they must have adequate training and practice to feel comfortable. Jones and Hegge (2007) suggest the simulation specialist organize high-fidelity patient simulation demonstrations initially and then provide training and practice for faculty to become familiar with the equipment and programming. Other colleges or programs hire a nonfaculty staff member to "run the computer." This person may have a medical or a computer/technology background that enables him or her to assist in simulation activities.

BYU uses nursing students to run the computer and assist in setting up and cleaning up for simulation experiences. Students apply to act as a student simulation worker after they have completed several medical–surgical simulations. Usually we have two to three students employed, each of whom works 5–10 hours per week. The student simulation workers assist with nearly all the simulation activities in the college, which relieves the faculty from having to both run the computer and facilitate the session. This strategy has supported the faculty and greatly decreased their anxiety.

Facilitators/Debriefing

In most colleges and programs, the faculty members do the facilitating and debriefing of the simulation activities. Some programs have faculty members who are assigned to the simulation laboratory as part of their workload. These faculty members facilitate and debrief sessions for the majority of the simulation activities. In most programs, faculty members do the facilitating/debriefing for their own course, sometimes with each person doing his or her own clinical section. In other programs, one faculty member is assigned to do the facilitating/debriefing for all students in the same course.

Another option is to hire nonfaculty registered nurses to assist in the simulation activities. In their study, Foster, Sheriff, and Cheney (2008) reported that using nonfaculty registered nurses in simulation activities (as facilitators and in debriefing) resulted in nearly all of the students experiencing high self-confidence, satisfaction, and acquisition of knowledge with this learning methodology. The students also reported that the nonfaculty registered nurses were highly effective in the simulation activities.

BYU uses full-time faculty, part-time adjunct faculty, and nonfaculty registered nurses for facilitating and debriefing. The nonfaculty registered nurses have clinical experience, and students frequently state they enjoy the sharing of current and "real-life" patient experiences as related to the scenario.

Technology Support

Successful colleges and programs using high-fidelity patient simulators have adequate technology support. This support can be provided in a variety of ways. Some programs hire a technician to assist with the simulation activities. The technician may run the computer, program the computer for specific scenarios, and/or troubleshoot and fix problems with the equipment. Some technicians without medical background may struggle with programming, however, and need supervision and direction from the nursing faculty. Many programs rely on the information technology personnel from the college or school to assist with technology issues. Keeping the information technology personnel up-to-date and informed is a key to success.

The manufacturers of the simulation equipment provide support (some in person, others through phone consultation) and often training for those involved in support. Most manufacturers also offer warranties for the simulators. Although these warranties are costly, most programs view them as a needed insurance policy to ensure the ongoing functioning of the equipment.

Faculty/Staff Education

One of the most important keys to success with a high-fidelity patient simulator is education for faculty and staff. Given that high-fidelity simulation as a teaching/learning pedagogy is new to many nursing faculty, education and training are necessary to teach successful ways to use this technology. The education plan should be based on the expected role of the faculty and staff. If faculty members are expected to run the computer as well as facilitate and debrief simulation activities, then the plan would be different than that for those faculty members who will only facilitate sessions and debrief students.

If the expectation is that personnel will perform scenario development and editing as well as programming, the education will need to include instruction and practice in these tasks. The technology support personnel need a different education plan as well.

Many colleges and programs begin the education plan with an overview of high-fidelity simulation for all faculty and staff. The plan then includes sections based on the expectations for particular groups of personnel. Those expected to run or operate the computers need training in basic operation of simulator/computer/gases, basic troubleshooting, and assisting in role-play (such as healthcare providers). Those expected to facilitate sessions and debrief students need education in the principles of facilitating and purpose of debriefing. They also need to practice facilitating and debriefing, initially with other faculty members, then with a group of students while being supported by a faculty member with experience in high-fidelity simulation pedagogy. Those expected to develop scenarios will need education and training from the manufacturer of the specific simulation equipment. Depending on the extent of programming (i.e., programming of original scenarios versus editing existing scenarios), the training will need to be customized for the staff members who will undertake this role. Many colleges and programs purchase preprogrammed scenarios (such the METI PNCI) or obtain programming through the sharing of original scenarios through simulator user groups (program to program).

Jones and Hegge (2007) found that faculty members thought repeated education and training was preferable to in-depth initial training. The pedagogy has many aspects that must be learned; by providing ongoing updates and training, faculty members may better be able to integrate the concepts into their courses.

Costs

High-fidelity patient simulators are fairly expensive initially when compared to static manikins and task trainers. Most nursing colleges or programs use models that cost approximately $60,000. The initial purchase may be funded through donors or college/program funds.

During the purchase process, most manufacturers suggest purchase of a warranty as well. Keeping warranties in place will ensure that parts, repair, and maintenance of the unit will be covered. The warranty fee varies according to the manufacturer and the type of warranty. A basic warranty may include replacement parts and assistance with replacing parts, whereas an extended or supreme warranty may include having a technician visit the site to perform routine maintenance. Some colleges/programs decide not to purchase a warranty and instead hire manufacturer technicians on an as-needed or hourly/daily charge basis.

The cost of the gases and compressed air required to run the high-fidelity patient simulator is often discussed in simulation literature. With the HPS, BYU did have construction costs to pipe the gases into the simulation area from a room across the hall (air is piped through the ceiling and walls). The HPS uses compressed air, carbon dioxide, oxygen, and nitrogen—it has a normal gas exchange. BYU utilizes gases provided by an on-campus source that is piped to all labs on campus. When BYU was running the HPS one to two days per week, the cost was $20–30 per month, which also included oxygen used in all other labs. With an ECS system, which uses only compressed air, no costs for gases are associated with the high-fidelity patient simulator.

As new scenarios are started with the high-fidelity patient simulator, new batches of disposable supplies will be needed. This increase in supplies is related to an increase in labs and the desire to have the simulation imitate the clinical site as closely as possible, rather than solely because a high-fidelity patient simulator is used. BYU does not require students to purchase laboratory packs; instead, the entire cost for lab experiences is part of its operating budget. With the use of a Microsoft Office Access database created for the NLC, in the past year we have determined how much is spent per student per semester for disposable medical supplies; this amount ranges from $10 to $104 depending on the semester. The highest cost is associated with the fundamental course, which teaches basic nursing skills and for which BYU provides actual medical supplies for each student. Very few supplies are reused during this course.

Depending on which equipment is already available, high-fidelity patient simulation activities may lead a program to purchase additional or new equipment, such as a crash cart, defibrillator, or additional intravenous pumps. At BYU, most of the equipment was already available. We did purchase a replacement defibrillator and an additional crash cart, rather than moving equipment from one lab to another, because this equipment is frequently used in both areas.

One of the goals of high-fidelity simulation activities is to mimic the actual clinical situation and patients involved. To set the scene in an attempt to "suspend disbelief," many programs obtain clothing, wigs, and items to make the scene more realistic. Initially, I gathered used clothing from family and friends. I also purchased jewelry and clothing, including shoes, eyeglasses, purses, and other items, from a used-clothing store. In addition, I purchased several wigs from a wig shop to simulate women and men of different ages. Halloween season provides a treasure trove of opportunities to find additional items such as tattoo sleeves, fake blood, and inexpensive artificial wounds.

BYU EVOLUTION AND FUTURE PLANS

After the CON obtained a METI HPS in 2001, BYU personnel took about a year to learn how to use the high-fidelity patient simulator, with one faculty member initially practicing on the unit and then adding other faculty to the training over time. We then invited students to volunteer to participate in simulation sessions. When BYU officially implemented scenarios into coursework, five scenarios were integrated in the basic medical–surgical course. Over the next five years, ten more simulation experiences were implemented in the remainder of the undergraduate clinical courses using adult, pediatric, and birthing simulators.

Our future plans include an expanded NLC with additional space for an additional adult simulator and an infant simulator. The college today is raising funds for this purpose, with a goal of obtaining $4 million to expand and remodel the NLC. The new area will include dedicated space for the additional simulators as well as the pediatric simulator and a control center. The control center will include the METI product METI LiVE, which facilitates the simulation of multiple patients from one control panel. The simulation may involve individual patients on one unit or may simulate the process of patient care (from emergency department, to operating room, then to patient care unit). The new simulation area will also include debriefing rooms so students can move out of the simulation room to participate in the debriefing session while the simulation room is prepared for the next group of students. Currently, the debriefing takes place in the simulation room because another area is not available.

Brigham Young University's College of Nursing is committed to excellence in nursing education, and one of our strategies is to have a state-of-art Nursing Learning Center to serve our students. High-fidelity patient simulation is an important aspect of these efforts. As we are able to expand the simulation areas, students will be able to have more high-fidelity patient simulation experiences. Until we are able to expand, the faculty and staff will continue strive to use our current resources in an effective manner to best accommodate students.

References

Foster, J. G., Sheriff, S., & Cheney, S. (2008). Using nonfaculty registered nurses to facilitate high-fidelity human patient simulation activities. *Nurse Educator, 33*(3), 137–141.

Hodson-Carlton, K. E., & Worrell-Carlisle, P. J. (2005). The learning resource center. In D. M. Billings & J. A. Halstead (Eds.), *Teaching in nursing: A guide for faculty* (pp. 187–212). St Louis, MO: Elsevier Saunders.

Jeffries, P. R., & Norton, B. (2005). Selecting learning experiences to achieve curriculum outcomes. In D. M. Billings & J. A. Halstead (Eds.), *Teaching in nursing: A guide for faculty* (pp. 187–212). St Louis, MO: Elsevier Saunders.

Jones, A. L., & Hegge, M. (2007). Faculty comfort levels with simulation. *Clinical Simulation in Nursing Education: Journal of International Association for Simulation and Clinical Learning, 3*(1). Retrieved July 5, 2008, from: http://www.inacsl.org

Ravert, P. (in press). Patient simulator sessions and critical thinking. *Journal of Nursing Education.*

Spunt, D., & Covington, B. G. (2008) Utilizing clinical simulation. In B. K. Penn (Ed.), *Mastering the teaching role: A guide for nurse educators* (pp. 233–251). Philadelphia: F. A. Davis.

CHAPTER 4

Developing and Implementing a Simulator Program: Associate Degree Nursing Education

Karen Mayes

The process of adding high-fidelity patient simulation to the curriculum of our Associate Degree Nursing Program at St. Louis Community College began in the summer of 1999. The campus leaders of our college had the vision that simulation would be of great value in teaching and learning. Potential funding for establishing simulation was sought through Regional Technical Education Council (RTEC) funds. Bids were received and Medical Education Technologies, Inc. (METI), became our successful bidder. The final decision to purchase three METI simulators was made in March 2000 and delivery of our first set of high-fidelity adult Human Patient Simulator (HPS) "triplets" occurred in August 2000.

ENVIRONMENTAL AND SPACE CONCERNS

Delivery of the simulator triplets at St. Louis Community College, located in St. Louis, Missouri, was making history in an already history-laden institution. St. Louis Community College was approved by voters in 1962. It is the largest community college district in Missouri and one of the largest in the United States. It is also a member of the League for Innovation in the Community College and is accredited by the Higher Learning Commission of the North Central Association of Colleges and Schools.

St. Louis Community College has four campuses: Florissant Valley, Forest Park, Meramec, and Wildwood. It also has four education centers: William J. Harrison Northside Education Center, South County Education and University Center, Joseph P. Cosand Community College Center and Downtown Education Center, and the Center for Business, Industry, and Labor.

St. Louis Community College services an area of 718 square miles. Maintaining its policy of open admissions, the college had a spring 2008 enrollment of 23,425 credit students. Enrollment in continuing education brings the total number of students to approximately 65,000 per semester. The college offers 11 college-transfer options and more than 90 career programs.

Environmental and space concerns are common with the delivery of any triplets, and the delivery of our triplets—that is, our simulators—to an already well-established institution was no different. Each simulator was to be housed on a different geographical campus of the college. Building facilities on each campus were approximately 40 years old.

The simulator housed on the Florissant Valley Campus was placed in the already very full nursing laboratory. Study carousels that had become obsolete were removed to provide a dedicated space for the simulator. The very noisy air compressor that is necessary to run the simulator was located in the lab faculty member's office that was adjacent to the simulator's location. Stan, the simulator at the Florissant Valley Campus, was up and running. (See Figure 4-1.)

The simulator housed on the Forest Park Campus was placed in a room formerly used as a conference room. Although we were very fortunate to

---

Figure 4-1   Florissant Valley Campus Simulation Lab

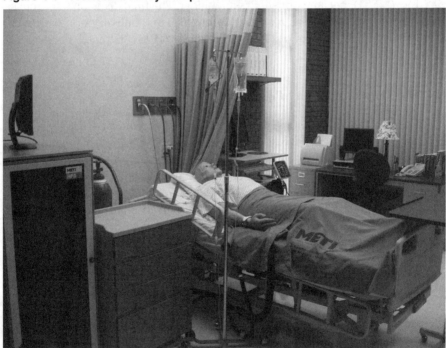

Source: Courtesy of the Work, Education, and Lifelong Learning Simulation Center.

Figure 4-2 Forest Park Campus Simulation Lab Being Constructed

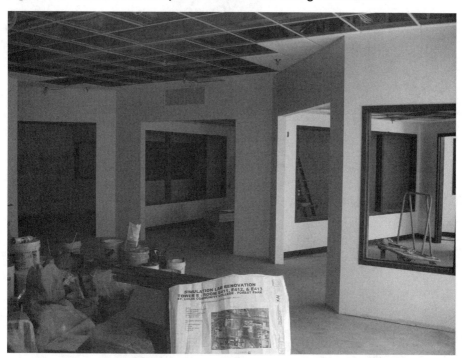

Source: Courtesy of the Work, Education, and Lifelong Learning Simulation Center.

obtain that space, we sorely missed the availability of a conference room. The room size was adequate for instruction but the tile walls and the air compressor resulted in a very noisy environment. Regardless of the drawbacks, Stan, the simulator at the Forest Park Campus, was now operational. (See Figure 4-2.)

The simulator housed on the Meramec Campus was placed in our extremely crowded nursing laboratory. In addition to the space limitations, the noise issue was a problem, as it was on both of the other campuses. In spite of these issues, Sydney, the simulator at the Meramec Campus, was also implemented in the curriculum. (See Figure 4-3.)

PROGRESS WITH ENVIRONMENTAL AND SPACE CONCERNS

As previously mentioned, limited space and excessive noise were initially issues of concern on all three campuses designated as sites for the high-fidelity

Figure 4-3   Merrimac Campus Simulation Lab

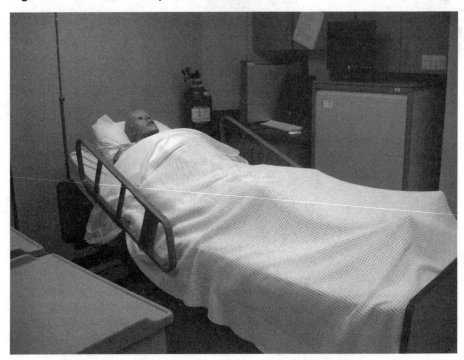

Source: Courtesy of the Work, Education, and Lifelong Learning Simulation Center.

patient simulators. Since the installations of the simulators in 2000, extensive physical changes have occurred that allow for a greatly improved environment. The Florissant Valley Campus nursing laboratory moved into a renovated room during the summer of 2004 that has a dedicated area for the simulator. This area can easily be separated from the rest of the lab by accordion wall partitions that allow for great versatility. The air compressor is located in a soundproof closet, which resolved the space and noise problems associated with this unit.

The Forest Park Campus underwent a renovation that included development of a dedicated 1700-square-foot simulation laboratory that consists of a simulated three-bed hospital unit along with an adjacent classroom that seats 24. The three-bed unit is fully visible from the adjacent classroom via cameras and monitors. The noisy air compressor is located in a soundproof closet, again remedying both the space and noise problems. The project was completed in August of 2008.

The Meramec Campus underwent a renovation of its nursing laboratory during the summer of 2007. Approximately 1200 square feet of space was added during this renovation, which allowed a room to be dedicated to the simulator. The noisy air compressor was placed in a closet, so both the space and noise problems have been greatly improved.

Although the existing setup is not a perfect situation, the environmental and space concerns have been greatly improved through extensive renovations on each of the three campuses. St. Louis Community College's leadership has always been very supportive of the simulation project, both in locating initial space to house the simulators and in supporting the renovations to improve on the make-do initial environments. The most immediate challenge now is faculty education and the effective use of the simulators.

FACULTY EDUCATION AND SIMULATOR USE

The next challenge became how to educate faculty to use the simulators in their teaching once the decision was made where to house the simulators. This has been a very slow process, as the integration of simulation into the curriculum is very time-consuming. Prior to the arrival of the simulators, faculty observed simulation labs at other institutions to begin assimilating how to utilize them at St. Louis Community College. Our initial multidisciplinary training occurred immediately after the first installation in August 2000 and included faculty from the areas of nursing, respiratory therapy, radiologic technology, emergency medical services, dental hygiene, physical education, and biology. Faculty from the nursing and respiratory therapy programs emerged as the users of the simulators following the multidisciplinary training and remain so today. Interest is beginning to increase from other disciplines, however, which is a very encouraging development.

The simulators were not used to full capacity for several years for multiple reasons. As mentioned, lack of space and excessive noise were initially problematic. Additionally, college faculty faced the challenges of personnel changes, structural changes, a national accreditation report to prepare, and a lack of time for our already extremely busy faculty to devote to becoming comfortable with the simulator and developing scenarios. For the few nursing program faculty members who did write their own scenarios, it was a tremendous time-consuming effort to learn the skills needed for scenario development using the former DOS-based system. One advantage to writing their own scenarios, however, is that these personnel more intimately understood the workings of the scenario as opposed to using a scenario written by someone else.

When St. Louis Community College leaders noted the underutilization of the simulators, additional on-site training was scheduled in March 2003. This education was very valuable in that it provided more detail for faculty on how to use the simulator. The next step in formal training occurred when faculty attended two more days of training in August 2004. Because of the large number of faculty participating in the training, it was more cost-effective to bring the METI education staff to St. Louis Community College than to send so many personnel to the METI location in Florida. The one exception to this practice occurred when the eight faculty leaders using the high-fidelity patient simulators went to the METI location for the focused Level 1 and Level 2 training in January 2006.

Each session of additional training provided ever more opportunities for faculty to expand usage of the simulator, but we were still not where we felt we needed to be. Approximately three faculty members on each campus were regular users, and college leaders wanted to increase that number. Our goals were to have more faculty involved and to more fully incorporate the high-fidelity patient simulation experiences into the curriculum. Additional opportunities to gain expertise in using the simulator were afforded via attendance at many workshops that offered sessions on simulation, being members of a simulator users' listserv, hosting the Mid-America Regional Simulation Workshop in October 2006, and forming a local Simulation Implementation Group at St. Louis Community College.

Faculty attendance at the annual Human Patient Simulator Network (HPSN) conference hosted by METI has provided an extremely helpful opportunity for further education. This conference is aimed at simulator users of all levels, from the rawest novice users to the most expert users. Approximately 22 of our 33 full-time nursing faculty have attended this conference at least once, as have 3 respiratory therapy faculty.

PLANNING FOR A SECOND SET OF TRIPLETS

The lifespan of our simulator technology, as with many other types of technology, appeared to be approximately five years. When that point was reached, the operating system was becoming outdated. Repair was becoming more challenging because some replacement parts were difficult to acquire due to their relatively old age. The warranty became obsolete as our triplets matured with longevity. The need to replace the high-fidelity patient simulators soon became obvious, so we approached the task replacing them through our capital process.

St. Louis Community College has a capital process that begins each fall when initial requests are made for selected items. This process entails setting priorities at the department, division, campus, and district levels. It also involves campus budget hearings and a district capital committee. Final approval of recommendations for capital expenditures rests with the board of trustees and occurs each June. As part of the capital process, capital requests can be channeled toward many accounts. The request for replacement of the three simulators was channeled to RTEC funding, as it was with the purchase of the original simulators.

The second set of high-fidelity adult HPS triplets were delivered in September 2005. It was sad to see the original set of triplets being returned as trade-ins; however, that emotion could not stand in the way of progress. Of course, with the delivery of the new high-fidelity patient simulators came the need to learn how to operate them. It also seemed to be the right time to purchase the Program for Nursing Curriculum Integration (PNCI), a decision that followed in October 2005. This program is extremely valuable to faculty because it eliminates the very time-consuming task of writing original scenarios.

Two consultation visits by METI education staff were included along with the PNCI purchase. The first consultation visit occurred in March 2006, with 30 nursing faculty members participating in the training session. A report from the METI educational consultant followed, which outlined the barriers to integration of simulation at St. Louis Community College, made recommendations for handling those barriers, and presented a fairly detailed plan for integration of simulation into each nursing course using the PNCI's Simulated Clinical Experiences (SCEs).

The second consultation visit occurred in January 2008, again with 30 nursing faculty members attending. This visit began with faculty from each campus sharing information on how high-fidelity patient simulation was implemented in their respective courses. This session proved to be a very valuable learning experience. The consultation visit also included a review of simulation concepts such as use of varying roles, increasing realism, managing death of the simulator, debriefing concepts, role of the facilitator, and evaluation. Various examples of different models that have been used for scheduling students with the simulators were shared, and simulation research was discussed. Finally, recommendations were made regarding how to achieve further integration of simulation into the curriculum.

Integrating the simulators into our curriculum varies somewhat by campus and has progressively increased each year. We currently use high-fidelity patient simulation in all four semesters of our four-semester Associate Degree Nursing Program. Often the students are videotaped to assist them in their debriefing and evaluation, which allows them to self-identify strengths and areas in need of improvement.

The first semester nursing course, Fundamentals of Nursing, uses the simulators to evaluate assessment skills, injections, and medication administration. We specifically use the Postoperative Assessment of the Gastrectomy Patient SCE, focusing on respiratory and abdominal assessment. This simulation replaces clinical time, with students participating in groups of six or seven members. One campus uses a physical assessment scenario developed by the faculty. The Skills Validation SCE is also used in first semester.

The second semester nursing course, Nursing of Adults and Children I, uses the Anaphylactic Reaction SCE, the Postpartum Hemorrhage SCE, and the Pulmonary Embolism SCE. The Skills Validation SCE has also been used at the beginning of the semester as a review of students' fundamental skills. Another faculty-designed scenario concentrates on preoperative/postoperative nursing care with a focus on communication and teamwork.

The third semester nursing course, Nursing of Adults and Children II, uses the Acute Renal Failure SCE, the Chronic Diabetic SCE, the Diabetic Ketoacidosis SCE, and/or the GI Bleed SCE. The Chronic Diabetic SCE is especially valuable because it provides an opportunity to role-play the responsibilities of ancillary personnel.

The fourth semester nursing course, Nursing of Adults and Children III, utilizes the Acute Exacerbation of COPD SCE and the Myocardial Infarction SCE. The three-bed simulation lab being developed at the Forest Park Campus will provide an invaluable opportunity to simulate delegation and prioritization skills with multiple patients by our fourth-semester students.

During the process of implementing the PNCI, faculty interest in the use of this technology has varied widely. Many faculty members are very enthusiastic users and believe time is probably the only factor preventing them from even greater use of the simulators. The ease of use provided by the PNCI, along with the growing number of faculty who are using the simulator and are able to provide support to one another, have provided an enriching environment for increased usage of the simulator. A much smaller number of faculty members are not nearly as enthusiastic about using the simulators and feel totally comfortable with an approach to teaching that does not include simulation.

INITIAL COSTS

Now that the simulators are located in an adequate space and a quiet environment, and the faculty members have had multiple educational opportunities related to implementing the simulators, a discussion of cost is in order. Again, using the analogy of the triplets, there must be unexpected initial costs associated with their arrival, just as we found unexpected initial costs associated with our simulators.

The initial cost of the simulators in 2000 was approximately $125,000 per simulator, which included a cost reduction for purchasing three units at one time. This amount included the full body mannequin, the computer and monitor, computer rack, software, system manuals, technical support, trauma package, ACLS package, hand-held remote PC, genitourinary subsystem, drug recognition subsystem, two-year extended warranty with software upgrades during this time period, technical support, copies of system manuals, and faculty training.

In addition to these initial costs, many other items were necessary to prepare our simulators for actual use. An air compressor was necessary to run the simulators. Each compressor cost approximately $2000. Medical-grade gases (oxygen, carbon dioxide, and nitrogen) needed to be purchased along with regulators. This entailed monthly tank rentals and the purchase of tank stands for ease in transporting the tanks. The ongoing cost of the tanks of gas is approximately $25–30 each, depending on the type of gas and the size of the tank. The length of time a tank lasts varies greatly on usage of the simulator. Tank rental is another ongoing cost and, at our location, amounts to approximately $6 per tank per month. The tanks needed to be safely secured to the walls with wall brackets, which required a one-time maintenance cost. The tank stands cost approximately $75 each. The tank regulators required a one-time cost of $130 per tank per campus.

Other costly supplies were purchased including hospital beds with mattresses, side rails, and IV rods, for an approximate total of $1500 per campus. Defibrillators and pulse oximeters were purchased at a cost of $6000 per campus. A computer table, two chairs, and a surge protector cost another $2000 per campus. Two medical storage cabinets were purchased for each campus at $1000 per campus.

Many other day-to-day medical supplies were needed to run the simulators, including oxygen masks, endotracheal tubes, blood pressure cuffs and sphygmomanometers, stethoscopes, intubation stylets, nasal cannulas, various types of laryngoscope blades and handles, manual resuscitator bags, bags of saline, bags of sterile water, boxes of syringes, Foley tray urine collection bags, chest tubes, portable IV poles, tools, and a tool box. Collectively, these items cost approximately $3000 per campus.

The PNCI required an outlay of $28,000 for the initial campus plus $2000 per additional campus for the site license; it was a one-time expense, not counting future releases of newer and expanded versions. The cost of the new replacement simulators in 2005 was $100,000 per campus, including trade-in. The enhanced warranty is $12,500 per year per campus and allows for technical support and annual on-site maintenance. We currently fund this annual warranty fee through a student technology fee.

ONGOING COSTS

Our second set of triplets is here, and their nurseries are stocked as described earlier. The main ongoing costs are the gases, the annual enhanced warranties, professional development support of faculty, and replacement of medical supplies as the others wear out. The enhanced warranties are the greatest ongoing expense but are worth the money because of the complexity of the simulator technology.

MAINTENANCE

Over the lifespan of our simulators, we have had relatively few maintenance concerns. Some of this good fortune is because of the annual maintenance that occurs with the warranty. The adage "An ounce of prevention is worth a pound of cure" seems very appropriate when talking about high-fidelity patient simulation. The telephone technical support provided by METI has been incredibly helpful, from the simple troubleshooting that quickly remedies a concern to the more complex troubleshooting of describing how to remove the head of the simulator for transport back to METI when one of the simulators quit blinking. Each campus has kept a log of the simulator's medical history with the maintenance concerns.

STUDENT INVOLVEMENT

Most of our faculty members are avid believers in simulation—but how do the students perceive this technology as part of their learning? The comments on the student evaluations tell the story and confirm that most of them are avid believers as well. Their comments are overwhelmingly positive:

- "This was great practice. Wish we had more time with it."
- "Loved it!!!"
- "This was better than clinical because you can try different interventions with the patient to see what happens without really harming them."
- "This provided a great learning experience because it made us put everything together we have learned."
- "It was nice to really see how [the high-fidelity patient simulator] responded to drugs, and how he responded to dosage calculations that were WRONG! Those decimal places really make a difference and that was good to see!"
- "Wish we had it more often."

- "It was good to have to critically think with the simulator. I learned a lot and can carry that over to my patient care in the hospitals."
- "Good place to practice my therapeutic communication."
- "Very interesting how real life it is."

One of our campuses hosted fourth-semester nursing students from a rural school located several hours away that does not have simulators. The students and faculty felt they greatly benefited from the experience and were hopeful that their own school could someday purchase simulators to benefit their future students.

EVOLUTION AND FUTURE PLANS

We have evolved over the past several years from being users of the traditional static mannequins to users of high-fidelity simulators with simulated clinical experiences. What lies in our future? Our main goal is to secure a full-time position for either a technical professional or a faculty member dedicated to direct simulation use. We firmly believe this step would greatly assist our faculty in more fully utilizing the simulators. Another goal is to increase use of the simulators by other disciplines. We have many allied health programs that could benefit, in addition to the many offerings in the Allied Health Continuing Education Department that could benefit from this technology. Another goal is to develop a six-bed simulation unit that would allow students to simulate delegation and prioritization of patient care for multiple patients. We are well on our way with the renovation of the simulation area at the Forest Park Campus, which includes a three-bed simulation lab. Our final goal is to increase communication among our campus simulator users to further assist in increasing our implementation of the simulation system. Great activities are happening on each campus, and we sometimes fail to share them with our colleagues.

CHAPTER 5

Graduate Nurse Anesthesia

Margaret Faut-Callahan, Keith Marino, and Judith Wiley

INTRODUCTION

Patient simulators have become more common in the education of health-care students and practitioners over the past two decades (Good, 2003). The use of simulators for medical education dates back to the early 1960s, with the creation of Resusci-Annie for training in cardiopulmonary resuscitation and mouth-to-mouth resuscitation (Cooper & Taqueti, 2004). In the mid-1960s, Sim One was created by Drs. Judson Denson and Stephen Abrahamson at the University of Southern California. Sim One was the first lifelike, computer-controlled mannequin. This simulator was used for training anesthesia residents to perform induction of general anesthesia, laryngoscopy, and endotracheal intubation without compromising patient safety. Unfortunately, Sim One was not acceptable for commercial production at the time because computer technology was too expensive for mass production and anesthesia training of that era was based on the apprenticeship model (Cooper & Taqueti, 2004).

In the late 1980s, Dr. David Gaba and colleagues at Stanford University created the first human mannequin simulator for anesthesia training. Real-time anesthesia simulation evolved over the past 20 years to include mannequins with lifelike cardiovascular, respiratory, pharmacokinetic, and pharmacodynamic responses replicating many disease processes (Cooper & Taqueti, 2004).

The real-time characteristics of human patient simulation have allowed for better training of anesthesia personnel, including nurse anesthetists, at various levels of experience in role determination, proper communication skills, standards of care, and effective crisis management. Further, these skill sets advance patient safety initiatives that have become a high priority for the nurse anesthesia community.

The development of these advanced simulators has clearly facilitated the training of anesthesia providers in role determination and communication skills. Role determination is an important concept in proper crisis management and establishes who is in charge of the situation. The leader of the team is responsible for evaluating the current environment, allocating proper resources, and communicating the roles and tasks for other ancillary personnel in the operating room. Effective communication begins with addressing each team member by name, being precise about the task to be done, and having the receiver close the communication loop by repeating the orders back to the leader. Without proper role determination and communication, a calm situation can turn into chaos, with everybody "doing their own thing" and not focusing at the proper tasks at hand (Gallagher & Isenberg, 2007).

Simulation promotes proper training in the standards of care for anesthesia practice and "provides the opportunity to observe and evaluate the technical performance of anesthesia personnel" (Zausig et al., 2007, p. 673). According to Schwid et al. (1999), the use of computer training improves retention of medical guidelines better than standard textbook review. In the Rush University Simulation Laboratory, the student registered nurse anesthetists (SRNAs) are introduced to the proper standards of care prior to beginning clinical practice in the operating rooms; that experience is the focus of this chapter.

ENHANCING PATIENT SAFETY

Gaba and DeAnda (1988) were early pioneers in the development of a simulated environment that would promote patient safety through research and education. Crisis resource management (CRM) was first described by Gaba, Fish, and Howard (1994). CRM, which was based on the aviation industry "cockpit resource management" approach, is a model of the processes used by anesthetists to make decisions based on the information presented to them. Given that major airline pilots are required to be proficient at handling crises in the air, anesthetists can certainly learn from this model. Anesthesia providers, who typically have varying degrees of experience, often miss key bits of information that would assist in making a better clinical decision. Even if the critical incident is recognized, the anesthesia provider might not organize the team in an effective manner to treat the patient problem. These issues were documented by Kremer, Faut-Callahan, and Hicks (2002), who noted that nurse anesthetists in crisis situations might hold on to "biases" based on previous clinical situations and miss important clinical information. The ability to educate nurse anesthetists in a simulated environment, and to demonstrate that information might be present but overlooked, is a powerful teaching tool.

Gaba and his team (Stanford University School of Medicine, VA Simulation Center, 2008a) noted that "sound medical and technical knowledge is not enough. Anesthesiologists need to know how to manage a variety of resources effectively, bringing them together in concert as necessary to deal with the situation" (p. 1). Specifically, training focused on the following areas is essential for the management of perioperative crises (Stanford University School of Medicine, VA Simulation Center, 2008b):

- Use of all available information and cross-checking of redundant data
- Anticipation and planning
- Communication
- Leadership and assertiveness
- Use of all available resources
- Anesthetist utilizing a cognitive aid during anesthesia crisis resource management (ACRM) training
- Distribution of workload and mobilization of help
- Reevaluation of situations

Building on the principles of CRM, Cox (2008) developed the *Aspects of Anesthesia Care Team Crew Resource Management Training Program* to enhance perioperative care and address key concepts related to effective patient care and safety. Cox (2008) proposed that:

> The purpose of the Anesthesia Care Team Crew Resource Management Training Program is to optimize the safety and effectiveness of the Anesthesia Care Team service delivery model. The program accomplishes its mission through human resource team performance training, and development and dissemination of clinical methods and tools, to achieve optimal utilization of the professional knowledge and skill sets inherent to the multidisciplinary providers who participate in the Anesthesia Care Team service delivery model. (p. 3)

Using clinical simulation for the purpose of enhancing team performance and communication is an essential component of patient safety initiatives (Awad et al., 2005; Grogan et al., 2004; Pizzi, Goldfarb, & Nash, 2001).

Gordon, Wilkerson, Shaffer, and Armstrong (2001) demonstrated both student and faculty satisfaction with a simulated learning environment that would allow "practice without risk" (p. 469). Nishisaki, Keren, and Nadkarni (2007) noted that "simulation training is an essential educational strategy for health care systems to improve patient safety" (p. 233). Evidence is mounting that simulation training enhances team communication and procedural skills in simulated environments. More work must be done to ensure that these results can be replicated in the clinical environment.

O'Donnell, Fletcher, Dixon, and Palmer (1998) were early adopters of CRM and adapted CRM so that it could be integrated into nurse anesthesia education. Recognizing the improbability that all students would see critical incidents and crises in their clinical studies, O'Donnell and colleagues (1998) developed a curriculum plan that allowed every student to play a role in the care of critically ill patients undergoing an anesthetic crisis. Students and faculty embraced this addition to the curriculum, and today this program is a leader in the field.

Turcato (2005) reported that 48% of nurse anesthesia programs used CRM in the curriculum. The amount of CRM in curricula varied, but 30% of respondents in Turcato's study reported that it was used throughout the curriculum. Twenty-seven percent of programs said they used CRM in a limited way, such as a course module.

Jankouskas et al. (2007) utilized a CRM framework in evaluating interdisciplinary teams. The authors noted that previous studies often evaluated a single discipline, yet rarely do crises occur that fail to include members from various disciplines. The participants completed the *Perceived Collaboration and Satisfaction about Care Decisions* (CSACD) instrument (Baggs, 1994), which rates answers to six questions on a seven-point, Likert-type scale. Additionally, the *Anesthetists Nontechnical Skills System* (ANTS; Fletcher, Flin, McGeorge, Glavin, Maran, & Patey, 2003), an observational scale, was used to assess this aspect of care. Whereas the CSACD demonstrated statistically significant improvement between pre- and post-training outcomes, the ANTS showed a significant difference in teamwork.

CRM is a strategy to engage the learner in rare clinical experiences with the goal of enhancing clinical decision making, communication, and teamwork. Patient safety initiatives are built on these principles, and evidence exists to suggest that CRM improves practitioner response to crises. The Consolidated Risk Insurance Company (CRICO), the medical malpractice carrier of the Harvard University medical community, has initiated an incentive program for anesthesiologists who participate in a CRM program (McCarthy & Cooper, 2007). The program has been successful, with CRICO reporting that the training is so effective that the differential premium has been increased to 19%. CRICO also reports that some hospitals are now requiring CRM for credentialing purposes.

NURSE ANESTHESIA PROGRAM USE OF SIMULATED LEARNING

Turcato (2005) surveyed nurse anesthesia programs to determine the use of clinical simulation in educational programs. Ninety-six percent of programs reported the use of some form of clinical simulation within the curriculum, including use of manikins for intubation, radial artery cannulation, central line placement, spinal models, SimMan, METI Man, and standardized patients. The most commonly used models were manikins for intubation (98%), central-line models (81%), and spinal models (93%). Fifty-one percent of respondents re-

Table 5-1   Barriers to the Use of Clinical Simulation in Nurse Anesthesia Programs*

1. **Time**
   – Not enough time for faculty to develop and implement scenarios
2. **Cost**
   – Equipment and faculty development
3. **Distance from program**
   – Need to travel to another institution so students can access simulation
4. **Scheduling**
   – Competition with other learners
5. **Technician support lacking**
6. **Lab space lacking**
7. **Faculty**
   – Not enough FTEs to "run" simulations
8. **Faculty development**
   – Not properly trained to use simulation technology
9. **Administration not supportive**

*Areas identified in order of frequency.
Source: Turcato, 2005.

ported the use of SimMan; 44% used METI Man. Turcato also identified nine major barriers to the use of simulation; these obstacles are listed in Table 5-1.

Cannon (2008) reported that nurse anesthesia programs that use clinical simulation typically receive positive feedback on this technology from students. She also noted that strong face validity exists in the use of simulation and suggested that various methods of simulation be used in combination to promote full integration of simulation into existing courses.

VALID OUTCOME MEASURES/EVALUATION PLANS

Establishing valid outcome measures to assure the attainment of clinical competencies is often a challenge. Jankouskas et al. (2007), however, demonstrated that effective evaluation of multidisciplinary teams in a crisis situation is possible. Nurse anesthesia programs use a variety of approaches to evaluate student performance in simulated learning experiences. Some use simulation to ensure that students achieve mastery of content. Others use simulation to actually determine student competency in specific clinical situations. Typically, competency is measured by a simple checklist method that confirms students have completed all appropriate interventions and by an observational assessment that evaluates whether the students verbalized thought processes and ability to explain actions during the simulation.

Progress is being made in the area of expected performance behaviors and the relationship to specific time frames, although more work in this area is needed. Research is being done to determine expectations of novice, intermediate, and experienced nurse anesthetists as it relates to the establishment of expected response times in simulations (Bevans, 2008).

CLINICAL SIMULATION CONSORTIA

Turcato (2007) formed a workgroup to establish a simulation consortium within the New England Assembly of Nurse Anesthesia Faculty. Its creation involved a lengthy process of needs assessment, resource identification, curriculum development, and faculty education.

To confront the extraordinary costs of high-fidelity simulation, collaboration among nurse anesthesia programs is essential. Mechanisms to share resources for faculty training, scenario development, and simulation-based teaching can be negotiated among programs with geographic or institutional similarities. For example, a faculty member of one program might attend a formal simulation-based training program, and subsequently offer an informal debriefing to a consortium of educators based on the content of the course. Additionally, nurse anesthesia programs without access to high-fidelity simulation can share resources with those that already have adequate infrastructure and curriculum by arranging fee-for-service contracts and sending students to engage in specific learning activities, such as ACRM. These arrangements can be mutually beneficial, as students from one institution are afforded meaningful learning experiences, while the simulation center of the other institution can use external fees to offset the often-high maintenance costs associated with high-fidelity simulation. This additional revenue source can be essential to a simulation center's survival, given that equipment often needs to be updated or replaced after five years of use. The cost of maintenance could translate into tens of thousands of dollars, given the fact that the initial costs associated with outfitting high-fidelity simulation laboratories amount to approximately $1.5 million.

Other mechanisms for intradisciplinary promotion of advanced simulation may involve the recruitment of clinical preceptors from affiliated clinical sites to serve as simulation instructors. Nurse anesthesia faculty can provide or subsidize the training of affiliated anesthetists to staff the simulation scenarios, thereby solidifying the link between the simulation curriculum and the clinical arena, and addressing the staffing issues in an already overburdened program. Links may also be extended between anesthesia programs by the formation of simulation task forces or committees, whose functional imperative is collaboration and sharing of resources to promote simulation among the member programs. The pooling of energies for faculty development, scenario development, and special topics instruction can be further enhanced by obtaining external funding via center grants to support collaborative teaching enterprises.

Interdisciplinary collaboration may function similarly to reduce costs and pool resources for integration of stimulation across multiple disciplines. "Strength in numbers," for example, keeps simulation on the radar screen of administrators and decision makers. The University of New England's College of Health Professions in Portland, Maine, developed a simulation user group, consisting of simulation advocates from the six disciplines that make up the college: nursing, nurse anesthesia, dental hygiene, physician assistants, occupational therapy, physical therapy, and social work. This group meets monthly to share ideas and expertise. Areas of collaboration include the development of interdisciplinary research projects and case scenarios. These scenarios can then be shared with all students of the college during the quarterly Grand Rounds, as a means of promoting simulation-based learning and collaborative practice among disciplines.

The simulation user group at the University of New England also offers the staff of the simulation center (Clinical Simulation Program) an opportunity to update faculty members on policies, equipment, software, and Web resources. Taped learning cases can be presented at meetings and give faculty participants an opportunity to discuss the nuts-and-bolts of advanced simulation teaching and learning. The mutual support facilitated by user groups helps members maintain their enthusiasm for simulation and fosters interest among other faculty who may be less motivated to embrace this technology. Members also cross disciplines to participate as "actors" in one another's clinical scenarios and as facilitators in the debriefing process. Cross-staffing offsets the time and costs associated with simulation-based instruction throughout the institution.

The creation of collaborative alliances with fellow nurse anesthesia educators and colleagues from other disciplines may help surmount the current barriers to universal use of advanced simulation-based instruction in our programs. Overcoming the time and financial constraints associated with simulation-based teaching is essential, so that more student nurse anesthetists can be exposed to this valuable teaching tool and the unique and important learning experiences it offers.

ROLE OF ACCREDITATION AGENCIES RELATED TO SIMULATED ACTIVITIES

The Council on Accreditation of Nurse Anesthesia Educational Programs (COA, 2007) allows for the use of simulated experiences to count as clinical experience in two areas: fiber-optic intubation and central line placement. Although the National Council of State Boards of Nursing (NCSBN) has recently funded several studies to look at the ability to substitute simulated clinical experiences for traditional clinical experiences, data from these studies are not yet available. The COA itself has not undertaken research in this area.

SIMULATION IN CONTINUING EDUCATION AND CREDENTIALING

The National Board on Certification and Recertification of Nurse Anesthetists (NBCRNA) currently requires nurse anesthetists to certify that they have completed a rigorous program of study accredited by the COA. Initial certification requires the individual to have graduated from a COA-accredited program and to successfully complete the national certification examination administered by the NBCRNA Council on Certification. CRNAs must recertify every two years; currently, 40 continuing education units (CEUs) are required for recertification.

Today, some continuing education programs use various forms of clinical simulation within the context of the course offering. Devices such as task trainers and low- and high-fidelity simulators, for example, may be incorporated into the programs. To date, the NBCRNA has not required a standardized approach to certification or recertification utilizing human patient simulators. Nevertheless, the organization plans to consider the potential applications of the simulator as it moves forward in credentialing. For example, simulation may prove useful for educating nurse anesthetists in the NBCRNA's refresher programs (Plaus, 2008).

The American Society of Anesthesiologists (ASA) formed a group to investigate the use of human patient simulation in continuing medical education and credentialing (see ASA, 2006a). A survey of graduating residents suggested that 76% found simulation-based instruction valuable; 70% said they would seek simulation experiences for CME upon completion of the residency (ASA, 2006c). The positive response by residents reflected the fact that 76% had experiences with simulated learning in their programs.

When the American Society of Anesthesiologists (ASA) surveyed practicing anesthesiologists, it found that physicians would most likely choose the following simulation-based CME training: difficult airway management (13%); cardiovascular/hemodynamic events (12%); diverse selection of infrequent, life-threatening events (12%); events related to equipment failure/malfunction (9%); and pulmonary events (7%) (ASA, 2006b). When asked if simulation-based CME should be standardized, 49% thought the "entire course content, including the individual cases and learning objectives" should be the same, and another 22% believed that the individual cases and learning objectives should be the same (ASA, 2006b, p. 3).

The ASA has developed a mechanism and criteria for endorsement of simulation laboratories (ASA, 2006a). Intrinsic to the use of this type of assessment is the establishment of valid and reliable measures as well as the

Table 5-2　ASA Simulation Program Endorsement Criteria

ASA endorsement will be granted to programs that demonstrate:

1. ASA member value
2. Policies and procedures commensurate with high quality educational offerings
3. An infrastructure that is consistent with the proposed/described services
4. Equipment and space that supports the educational objectives
5. An evaluation process for the course, the instructors and the program
6. Policies and procedures to provide ASA members with a confidential and secure environment
7. Sound education process for course development and evaluation
8. The ability to provide CME

Source: American Society of Anesthesiologists, 2006a.

credentialing of appropriate centers to conduct such assessments. ASA-endorsed programs must meet eight criteria, which are outlined in Table 5-2. Although no specific standards are available, the development of these criteria is a first step in assuring the educational credibility of simulation laboratories.

The feasibility of initiating a mandatory, competency evaluation using human patient simulation requires finding solutions for many of the barriers identified by Turcato (2007). Establishing a *voluntary* process for CRNAs to recertify using this technology is simply a more realistic first step.

SIMULATION IN A NURSE ANESTHESIA CURRICULUM

Simulation learning environments should be designed to mesh with the expected learning activities that will occur in the simulation laboratory. When developing a plan for simulation, the overall philosophy of the laboratory must be considered. The Rush University Simulation Laboratory (RUSL), for example, promotes the vision of "Patient Safety Without Patient Risk" (see Figure 5-1). The RUSL faculty believe that the simulator is a teaching environment. Thus, although assessment of competency certainly occurs, the overall goal is to provide the student with opportunities for mastery of skills and critical thinking. Because of this overarching belief, debriefing is an integral part of the RUSL program. Students actively support and critique one another during clinical simulations, and a positive learning environment is maintained.

The RUSL simulation area consists of a conference/debriefing room, airway management room, invasive procedure room, and a realistic clinical environment that can be set up to mimic an operating room, an intensive care room, or a general patient room. The conference/debriefing room is equipped with audiovisual equipment for presenting lectures, watching training videos, and observing activities in the simulated operating room. The airway management room consists of multiple intubating models with realistic airway anatomy. These models provide SRNAs with an opportunity to perform and validate competency in direct laryngoscopy, fiber-optic intubation, one-lung ventilation (double-lumen and bronchial-blocker endotracheal tubes), intubating and original laryngeal mask airway and airway exchange catheters, and other advanced airway management techniques. In the invasive procedure room, SRNAs are able to practice and validate competency in IV catheter, arterial line, central line, epidural, and spinal anesthesia placement and management (see Figure 5-2).

The simulated operating room is equipped with a Medical Education Technologies, Inc. (METI) Patient Simulator (Sarasota, Florida), Drager Medical Apollo anesthesia machine (Lubeck, Germany), General Electric Marquette monitors (United Kingdom), end-tidal carbon dioxide monitoring, and anesthesia cart with all the available drugs for anesthesia and advanced cardiac life support (ACLS) practice. The METI patient simulator enables us to simulate rare situations not commonly observed in the operating room. The simulator can simulate patients of either gender, of different ages, who are healthy or critically ill. The students are able to perform fiber-optic intubation and transtracheal jet ventilations on difficult airway scenarios, and run advanced cardiac life support scenarios and complex patient management scenarios. Invasive monitoring and other techniques, such as circothyrotomy, are discussed during the scenario and practiced on other low-fidelity devices.

Preclinical Education

Clinical simulation is an integral part of nurse anesthesia education, beginning in the first clinical course. The goals of clinical simulation during the preclinical phase of nurse anesthesia education are to improve patient safety and to enhance student learning.

The RUSL faculty believes that learning psychomotor skills such as intravenous catheter placement and direct laryngoscopy on skill trainers and a human patient simulator improves patient safety. For example, patients do not receive multiple IV sticks or the complications of laryngoscopy (e.g., dental injury, arterial oxygen desaturation). When trainees learn the step-by-step process of induction of anesthesia on the simulator, the process can be repeated again and again until they are completely familiar with the sequence. The students can then give a return demonstration of these skills in the simulation lab.

Learning psychomotor skills in the simulation lab also allows the faculty to manipulate time—for example, stopping time to allow for discussion and speeding it up to get to another critical moment in the anesthetic process. This approach can deepen a student's knowledge and allows the faculty to understand a student's thought processes. Videotaping a simulation session and discussing it afterward can serve a similar purpose. Practicing psychomotor skills until they are familiar, breaking down a clinical procedure into multiple steps, and discussing student performance allows a first-year anesthesia student to become familiar with a new environment, enhances learning (Gordon et al., 2001), and improves patient safety.

During the first clinical course, the SRNAs are taught and practice the proper standards of care in anesthesia machine setup and checkout, anesthesia cart setup, direct laryngoscopy, standard intravenous and inhalational induction, rapid sequence induction, and extubation techniques on the METI patient simulator. When practicing standard IV inductions, RUSL instructors begin with a case discussion, including formulating an anesthetic plan with backup plans, choice and dosing of anesthetic agents, and potential complications (how to prevent them and how to manage them) (see Table 5-3). Scenarios focus on expected tasks and sequencing.

In the second and third clinical courses, the first-year SRNAs use the METI patient simulator to learn the management of advanced principles of anesthesia. These advanced concepts include management of hypoxemia,

---

Table 5-3   Standard Induction of General Anesthesia

Expected tasks and sequence
Standard and patient specific monitors in place*
Effective pre-oxygenation *
Patient specific narcotic dosing (if appropriate)*
Patient specific defasciculation/priming NMB (optional)*
Patient specific induction agent dosing*
Eye/Consciousness check*
Checks baseline neuromuscular function
Establishes mask ventilation
Patient specific NMB dosing
Protects eyes
Confirms absence of neuromuscular function
Blade off the teeth
Effective ETT depth
Effective balloon inflation
Confirm ETT placement (BBSE & ET CO_2)
ETT taped

*Maintains verbal communication with patient, explaining actions and reassuring

hypercarbia, hypotension, hypertension, dysrhythmias, myocardial ischemia, malignant hyperthermia, bronchospasm, laryngospasm, air and fat embolisms, blood transfusion reaction, and anaphylaxis under anesthesia. Scenarios focus on tasks, sequencing, planning, and decision making (see Table 5-4). Also, first- and second-year students use the invasive procedure room for formal training

---

Table 5-4   Standard Scenario for a Novice Learner

26 y/o male presents to the OR for a L2-L4 lumbar laminectomy. He has c/o RLE numbness and tingling. The patient denies past medical history. He had a tonsillectomy as a child with no anesthetic complication. He is 5'7", 176 lbs. Airway assessment reveals Mallanpati II. Normal heart and lung sounds, and grossly intact neuro exam (other than RLE numbness/tingling).

Faculty teaching points

Preoperative evaluation and preparation

Objectives:

1. Identify ASA status.
2. Discuss preoperative medication.
3. Discuss anesthetic plan based on preoperative assessment and diagnostic tests.
4. Discuss how to prepare for induction of anesthesia.

What is the ASA status?
What is your preoperative instruction for this patient?
Discuss with patient risk and benefits of general anesthesia, especially possibilities of blood transfusion. Establish IV.
What medications should be considered preoperatively?
What lab exams should be ordered?
What type of anesthesia is required for this surgery?

Induction:
Objectives

1. Discuss how to approach induction of anesthesia.
2. Discuss the induction medications.
3. Discuss induction agents and doses for general anesthesia
4. Perform mask ventilation and intubation.

After several minutes of managing the patient's airway, the patient's HR increases to 123 and BP decreases to 76/30. What is your intervention?

in advanced airway techniques (e.g., fiber-optic intubation, double-lumen tubes for one-lung ventilation), as well as arterial/central line placement and management. Once first-year SRNAs have demonstrated a high level of competence in these areas of simulated practice, they are allowed to perform these procedures in the operating room environment, under the direct supervision of a CRNA and an anesthesiologist.

Enhanced Didactic Coursework

In addition to the technical skills learned and reinforced in the RUSL, faculty members use simulation technology to teach principles of advanced pharmacology, complex patient management, communication, and teamwork. For example, managing an intraoperative hypotensive crisis is more easily demonstrated in the simulation laboratory. The process involved in weighing the complex pharmacologic actions of various interventions is also clearly shown in the laboratory. Should students choose a drug that has a concomitant effect of bradycardia in an already bradycardic patient, the drug effect is dramatically demonstrated. Lessons such as these make pharmacology come alive.

Advanced Clinical Scenarios

SRNAs are in an intensive clinical residency for the final 15 months of the program, in which they rotate through various clinical sites and attend class on a weekly basis. In the first four months, the second-year SRNAs participate in simulation laboratory by reviewing and validating their previous learned skills in handling crises, advanced airway techniques, and invasive monitoring management. Advantages of the simulation laboratory environment in the second year of training include advanced exploration of uncommon but serious intraoperative complications, and opportunities for SRNAs to practice their differential diagnoses and administer appropriate treatment modalities with no risk of death or injury to a patient (Devitt, Kurrek, Cohen, & Cleave-Hogg, 2001).

Crisis Resource Management

CRM is a training concept integrated into the second-year curriculum. Gaba, Fish, and Howard (1994) first wrote about the complexity of clinical decision making in the specialty of anesthesia. They liken anesthesia to a series of potential crises: "anesthesiology, by its nature, involves crises" (Gaba et al., 1994, p. 5). The basis for CRM is that the "anesthetist, while under stress and time pressure, optimally implements standard techniques of diagnosis and treatment to the patient." Fundamental to this complex decision making are the issues of stress and time.

Replication and manipulation of these variables are obviously possible with human patient simulation. It is important for all students to have experience with those infrequent, yet potentially serious intraoperative crises. Such things as true anaphylaxis, cardiac arrest, and malignant hyperthermia are rarely seen in the OR. However, if they occur, rapid response is necessary to protect that patient. In the final phase of the program, all students go through key scenarios to assure that their response is accurate, appropriate, and timely. Decision making, treatment, and team communication are evaluated throughout the scenario. Students must master the scenarios before the completion of the program.

Capstone Projects

Prior to graduation, the second-year SRNAs are required to participate in a capstone experience. The capstone project evaluates the student's ability to use case studies to analyze patient clinical problems, integrate theory and research, and develop a comprehensive plan of care with appropriate interventions. Students are required to write a scholarly paper on a complicated disease state, demonstrating syntheses of physiology, pathophysiology, pharmacology, and anesthesia principles. After writing the paper, the students are placed in groups of two and give a PowerPoint presentation on the anesthetic implications of the complicated disease states to the anesthesia faculty and a group of their peers. Finally, the students complete scenarios based on their co-morbidities for a hypothetical patient on the METI patient simulator.

The second-year SRNAs are given specific patient scenarios based on the co-morbidities they have studied while their peers in the conference room evaluate their performance. These scenarios include detailed histories in which the students have to seek additional patient information through physical assessment and laboratory data. This approach requires them to conduct a thorough preoperative interview. The students then develop an anesthetic plan of care and implement their plan throughout the simulated perioperative period.

Students work in the team approach model and manage the induction, maintenance, and emergence of the simulated scenario patient. They are evaluated on their ability to implement the anesthetic plan based on the standards of care, co-morbidities of the patient, and responses to clinical problems that may arise during the simulated scenario. The sessions are videotaped for review and debriefing with clinical faculty and students. During the debriefing period, the anesthetic clinical decisions are discussed, in an open forum, to facilitate brainstorming on clinical actions that others may have taken if the given situation presented itself. Table 5-5 illustrates an example of a multisystem capstone scenario.

Table 5-5   Complex Scenario for a Capstone Experience

Scenario: Long Bone Fractures and Pulmonary and Fat Emboli

Pt is a 55 y/o male who was riding in the Toys for Tots motorcycle parade and was hit by a vehicle traveling at a high rate of speed. Pt presents to the OR boarded and c-collar in place, agitated and confused. You ask the trauma team for report and all they state is he has major pelvic and bilateral subtrochanteric femur fractures with multiple rib fractures. Limited information was available from a friend who was present at the time of the accident.

History
Patient Medical History: Unknown
Patient Social History: Unknown
Allergies: Penicillin
Social History: Smokes 1 pack per day $\times$ 30 years, Alcohol use = none, Drugs: marijuana.
Medications: 10 mg of MSO_4 in ER

Physical Exam:
T = 100.4, RR = 37 with splinting, B/P 85/30, P = 140, SpO_2 = 90% on 2 L nasal cannula
Neuro: Pt agitated and confused, R pupil is 5 mm–3 mm sluggish and L pupil is 3–2 mm brisk. He does not follow commands, moving all extremities (MAE), but not purposefully. 5 cm $\times$ 3 cm expanding hematoma posterior skull noted

Respiratory: Pt is tachypenic, using accessory muscle to breathe with chest x-ray (CXR) showing elevated diaphragms, R 2–10th rib fractures, + HEMOTHORAX R noted, no cardiomegaly.

MPC unable to determine d/t pt agitation.

Cardiovascular: Weak thready pulse noted, with skin pale, cool, and diaphoretic.

LABS: $14.8 > \dfrac{5.0}{18} < 130$

$\dfrac{139}{5.0} | \dfrac{105}{25} | \dfrac{18}{1.0} < 200$ PT = 13.9 , PTT = 37.5, INR=1.12

ABG: 7.01/56/90/-15/90% Ionized Ca .85
+ DPL noted in ER

EKG: NSR with conduction delay, consider digitalis effect.

Planned Procedure. Exploratory laparotomy and IM nailing of femurs by the orthopedic surgeons.

Table 5-5   Complex Scenario for a Capstone Experience *(continued)*

EXPECTED STUDENT OUTCOMES

- Support cardiopulmonary function and prevent extension and recurrence of the embolus.
- IV heparin works promptly to prevent extension of venous thrombus or recurrence of additional embolization to the lungs and improves outcome.
- TpA may be considered, but is undesirable in the postoperative patient.
- Hypotension from low CO may require treatment with isuprel, dopamine, or dobutamine.
- 90% of pulmonary emboli originate from thrombi in the legs; surgical treatment may include placement of a Greenfield filter in the IVC.
- 5% of patients have migration of the filter—this is a serious hazard.
- Pulmonary artery embolectomy using CPB is reserved for patients with massive PE who are unresponsive to medical therapy.
- Avoid hypoxemia and N_2O; may increase PVR
- The cardiopulmonary status of these patients is perilous before surgery, significant hemodynamic improvement occurs postoperatively.

FACULTY TEACHING POINTS

Long Bone and Pelvic Fractures
- Some lung dysfunction occurs in all patients after long bone fractures.
- Fat embolism occurs in 10–15% of patients with clinical signs of:
    - Hypoxia
    - Tachycardia
    - Mental status changes
    - Petechia
    - Fat globules in the urine and lung infiltrates (ARDS)
- Diagnosis of FES is suggested by petchiae on the chest, upper extremities, axilla, and conjunctiva.
- EKG in fat embolism may show ischemic appearing ST-segment changes and right heart strain.
- During GETA, S/S of fat embolism includes declining $ETCo_2$ and arterial oxygen saturation. If PA catheter present, may see increased PAP.
- Treatment of FES: prophylactic and supportive
    - Prophylactic being stabilization of the fracture.
    - Supportive: O_2 therapy and CPAP. Heparin treatment or alcohol have lacked clinical significance.
- Early operative repair cause decreased incidence of ARDS, reduced pulmonary shunting, decreased incidence of wound infections, less fat embolism.

Table 5-5   Complex Scenario for a Capstone Experience *(continued)*

Pelvic Fractures
- Pelvic ring and acetabular injuries are among the most serious involving the musculoskeletal system.
- Associated injuries include fractured skull, spine, face, or ribs (67% incidence); lower extremity fractures (54%); and liver or spleen injury (19%).
- Pt in auto vs pedestrian and motorcycle accident account for 75–90% of pelvic injuries.
- Injury patterns include severe hemorrhage, soft-tissue injury, colorectal disruption, GU injuries.
- Fractures of the posterior ring have the greatest incidence of vascular injury, major transfusion > 10 U PRBC and death.
- In hemodynamically unstable patients, occult intraabdominal or intrathoracic bleeding should be considered.
- MAST devices may help stabilize fractures in prehospital and emergency room settings and remains the only continued indication for application of MAST devices.
- Arterial embolizations techniques may be life-saving for stopping hemorrhage especially from branches of the hypogastric vessels.
- Repair of associated injuries—bowel and urinary tract lesions—may be necessary.

Pulmonary and Fat Emboli
- Clinical manifestations of PE are nonspecific and the clinical diagnosis is often difficult on clinical ground alone. The most consistent manifestation is an acute onset of dyspnea reflecting increased alveolar dead space and decreased pulmonary compliance.
- Breathing is usually rapid and shallow and wheezing may be heard upon auscultation of the lungs.
- Hypotension, tachycardia, and increased CVP are consistent with the diagnosis of life-threatening PE with cor pulmonale.
- Pulmonary infarction occurs (hours–days after initial event) cough, hemoptysis, and pleuritic pain is often present.
- ABG: decreased PaO_2 and $PaCO_2$ and increased A-a gradient for O_2.
- PE during anesthesia is often nonspecific and transient.
- Arterial hypoxemia, hypotension, tachycardia, and bronchospasm Increased A-aDCO_2.
- TEE may demonstrate dilation of the R atrium, R ventricle, and PA may aid in diagnosis of a PE.

The University of Pittsburgh Nurse Anesthesia program has utilized simulated learning for over a decade. Its curriculum is mapped from basic skills through advanced, critical thinking simulations (see Table 5-6). A curricular map allows for easy tracking of skill development and knowledge acquisition across the curriculum. Progression is easily assessed with such a model.

SUMMARY

The use of simulated learning in nurse anesthesia education has been prevalent for the past three decades. As early adopters of low- and moderate-fidelity simulators, nurse anesthesia educators have used task trainers and computer-based simulation programs since their initial development. Over the years, the introduction and use of high-fidelity patient simulators has revolutionized clinical education of nurse anesthesia students and has enhanced continuing education of CRNAs.

High-fidelity patient simulators have taken some of the risk out of clinical education and have enhanced patient safety. Although they work in a very safe specialty, nurse anesthetists perform complex, technical patient care. Prior to the use of low- and high-fidelity simulators, educational activities took place in the operating rooms. Under close supervision, nurse anesthesia students, like anesthesiology residents, were trained while providing direct patient care.

Today, more than 50% of nurse anesthesia students receive clinical education that is enhanced with patient simulation (Tucato, 2005). At this time, simulated activities are not required by the COA, although the COA does allow programs to use simulation for fiber-optic intubation and central line placement. Nurse anesthesia programs, therefore, incorporate simulation into their individual curriculum plans in institution-specific ways. Many nurse anesthesia programs use clinical simulation as part of preclinical activities and orientation, as an adjunct to didactic coursework, for case scenarios, and as a component of crisis management and capstone projects.

Despite students' and faculty members' positive responses to clinical simulation, there remain many barriers that must be overcome before this technology will be more widely used (Turcato, 2005). These barriers and challenges to nurse anesthesia programs include the high cost of simulation devices, the expense of technical expertise and faculty with skills needed to optimally implement a simulation-based curriculum, the need for curriculum development skills, and the need for evaluation mechanisms. Novel strategies have been investigated that encourage the sharing of expertise and resources to surmount these obstacles.

Early research suggests that the use of clinical simulation is not only well received by learners, but also enhances patient safety through improved

Table 5-6   University of Pittsburgh, Nurse Anesthesia Program Simulation Curriculum Map

Simulation events are integrated throughout the 52 didactic/60 clinical credit curriculum. The program started in 1994–1995 and has grown dramatically over time. Students experience the full spectrum of simulation context and fidelity. The average student receives 87 direct contact hours in simulation. Students may also choose to register for independent study in simulation with exposure to programming, curricular development, and assessment elements. Two simulation facilities are used; the School of Nursing Center for Instruction and Clinical Learning (CICL) and the Winter Institute for Simulation, Education, and Research (WISER). A total of 27 full body simulators are available across 14 simulation training areas. A wide array of part task trainers are also available and are integrated throughout the curriculum.

Part or Full Task Workshops	Course Name	Primary Objective— Students will:	Simulator(s) Used	Hours/ Student	Prep/ Turnover	Students/ Session	Faculty: Student Ratio	Evaluation Data: Knowledge, Attitude, Skill (KAS)	Formative and/or Summative Evaluation (F/S)	Debrief	Assessment Tool
Basic Principles of Airway Management	Basic Principles of Anesthesia	Develop standardized approach to airway management using a variety of approaches	Laerdal Intubation Training Heads— Adult and Pediatric	4	3	20	1:5	K, S	S	No	Checklist
IV Insertion Workshop	Basic Principles of Anesthesia	Develop standardized IV insertion skills	NASCO IV line insertion trainer and Laerdal VirIV	3	2	10	1:5	K, S	F	No	Checklist

Table 5-6   University of Pittsburgh, Nurse Anesthesia Program Simulation Curriculum Map *(continued)*

Part or Full Task Workshops	Course Name	Primary Objective— Students will:	Simulator (s) Used	Hours/ Student	Prep/ Turnover	Students/ Session	Faculty: Student Ratio	Evaluation Data: Knowledge, Attitude, Skill (KAS)	Formative and/or Summative Evaluation (F/S)	Debrief	Assessment Tool
Arterial Line Insertion Workshop	Basic Principles of Anesthesia	Develop standardized arterial line insertion skills	NASCO arterial line insertion trainer	3	2	10	1:5	K, S	F	No	Checklist
Patient Positioning Lab	Basic Principles of Anesthesia	Develop skill in safe patient positioning and use of OR table	Simulated Patient (SP)	3	2	7	1:3.5	K, S	F	No	n/a
Mock Induction Workshop	Basic Principles of Anesthesia	Develop skills in the process of written care plan development and IV induction	Laerdal SimMan	8	3	7	1:3.5	K,A,S	S	Yes	Checklist, Quiz
Mock Induction— Think on Your Feet	Basic Principles of Anesthesia	Develop skills in rapidly developing and implementing an anesthesia management plan	Laerdal SimMan	6	3	7	1:3.5	K, S	F	Yes	n/a

Table 5-6   University of Pittsburgh, Nurse Anesthesia Program Simulation Curriculum Map *(continued)*

Gas Machine Checkout and Trouble-shooting	Chemistry and Physics in Anesthesia	Develop skills in anesthesia machine check-out and troubleshooting for three different manufacturers	n/a	4	2	4	1:4	K, S	F	No	Checklist, Quiz
Problem-Based Simulation Adult	Applied Physiology and Pathophysiology	Develop management skills integrated with course content (autonomic dysreflexia, bronchospasm, hemorrhage, elevated ICP, myocardial depression)	Laerdal SimMan	8	2	12	1:6	K,A,S	F/S	Yes	Checklist, Survey, Quiz
Cardiopulmonary Exam	Physical Diagnosis Clinical	Develop skill in cardiac auscultatation, palpation, and diagnosis of cardiopulmonary findings	Harvey Cardiopulmonary Simulator	2	0.5	12	1:12	K, S	F	No	n/a
Problem-Based Simulation Pediatrics	Advanced Principles 1	Develop skill in pediatric set-up, induction, problem identification, and management	Laerdal SimBaby Laerdal SimMan Laerdal Megacode Kid	8	2	12	1:3	K, A, S	F/S	Yes	Checklist, Survey, Quiz

Table 5-6   University of Pittsburgh, Nurse Anesthesia Program Simulation Curriculum Map (continued)

Part or Full Task Workshops	Course Name	Primary Objective— Students will:	Simulator(s) Used	Hours/ Student	Prep/ Turnover	Students/ Session	Faculty: Student Ratio	Evaluation Data: Knowledge, Attitude, Skill (KAS)	Formative and/or Summative Evaluation (F/S)	Debrief	Assessment Tool
Regional Anesthesia Workshop	Advanced Principles 1	Develop skill in administration of regional anesthetic techniques including spinal, epidural, airway, and peripheral blocks	Simulated Patient (SP)-model NASCO Spinal and Epidural Simulator, Cadaver	6	2	20	1:4	K, S	F/S	No	Checklist, Quiz
Double Lumen Endobronchial Tube Placement	Advanced Principles 2	Develop skill in endobronchial tube placement with fiber-optic confirmation	Laerdal AirMan	2	1	5	1:5	K, S	F/S	No	Quiz
Jet Ventilation Workshop	Advanced Principles 2	Develop familiarity with high frequency jet ventilation skills including airway exchange catheters, insufflation catheters, various adaptors, and troubleshooting strategies	Laerdal SimMan	2	1	5	1:5	K, S	F/S	No	Quiz

Table 5-6 University of Pittsburgh, Nurse Anesthesia Program Simulation Curriculum Map (continued)

Central Venous Catheter Insertion	Advanced Principles 2	Develop skill in placement of central venous catheters including internal jugular and subclavian	Laerdal CVC Trainer	2	1	20	1:10	S	F	No	n/a
Trauma Rounds	Advanced Principles 3	Develop skills in assessment, triage, and management of diverse trauma patients	Laerdal SimBaby Laerdal SimMan Laerdal Megacode Kid Gaumard Birthing Simulator	4	2	25	1:6	K, S	F/S	No	Quiz/Audience Response System Evaluation
Difficult Airway Management	Advanced Principles 3	Develop skills in assessment, triage, and management of the difficult airway according to the ASA difficult airway algorithm	Laerdal SimMan	8	1	8	1:2	K, A, S	S	Yes	Survey, Quiz, Performance Exam
Anesthesia Crisis Leadership Training (SRNA + Resident)	Advanced Principles 3	Develop skills in assessment, triage, and management of anesthesia crisis events in combination with anesthesia residents	Laerdal SimMan	4	1	8	1:2	K, A, S	F	Yes	Survey, Quiz, Checklist

Table 5-6 University of Pittsburgh, Nurse Anesthesia Program Simulation Curriculum Map (continued)

Part or Full Task Workshops	Course Name	Primary Objective—Students will:	Simulator(s) Used	Hours/ Student	Prep/ Turnover	Students/ Session	Faculty: Student Ratio	Evaluation Data: Knowledge, Attitude, Skill (KAS)	Formative and/or Summative Evaluation (F/S)	Debrief	Assessment Tool
Anesthesia Crisis Resource Management (SRNA only)	CRNA Role Seminar	Develop skills in assessment, triage, and management of anesthesia crisis events focusing on crew resource management skills	Laerdal SimMan	8	1	10	1:5	K, A, S	F	Yes	Survey, Quiz, Checklist
Fiber-optic Bronchoscopy Workshop	Pediatric Clinical Rotation	Develop beginning Skill in fiber-optic bronchoscopy	Laerdal Airman	2	1	6	1:3	S	F	No	n/a

Source: Simulation curriculum map courtesy of John O'Donnell, CRNA, DrPh(c), from the Winter Institute for Simulation, Education, and Research (WISER) at the University of Pittsburgh.

communication, rapid clinical skill development, critical thinking demonstration, and crisis management (Bevans, 2008; Gordon et al., 2001; O'Donnell et al., 1998; Turcato, Robertson, & Covert, 2008). Use of clinical simulation in nurse anesthesia programs has provided a foundation for its use in other nursing and advanced practice nursing specialties. Creative strategies must be employed to add these activities to nursing educational programs.

Rystedt and Lindwall (2004) challenged educators to evaluate simulated learning in new ways. They suggest that educators should not only look at ways to apply simulation to their teaching for student benefit, but also focus on how learning activities are interactively developed. Rystedt and Lindwall (2004) further suggest that context, collaboration, technology, and learning be used to frame the learning experience. Similarly, Glavin (2007) has summarized key recommendations that must be considered when employing simulated learning experiences (see Table 5-7).

Looking to the future, Gaba (2007) has suggested that the healthcare industry prioritize "systematic training and assessment of healthcare personnel. . . . Simulation training will be applied not only to individuals, but more importantly also for crews, teams, work units, and organizations" (p. 133). According to this author, clinical simulation will be important for creating a culture of safety and competency-based practice.

Nurse anesthetists, in collaboration with other nurse faculty, must develop new models of nursing education, evaluation, and competency-based practice. So much of what has been done in the field of simulation is easily translated to nurse anesthesia practice. The barriers that have been described must be broken down, and innovative educational and practice models must be developed. Enhancing patient safety and provider accountability must be guiding tenets.

Table 5-7 Recommendations for the Use of Clinical Simulation

- Medical simulation should be thoughtfully used and supported as a complement to current teaching methods for medical students, resident trainees, and faculty.
- The integrated use of various modes of simulation should be a priority in simulation efforts.
- Medical simulation research should pursue performance-based and patient-centered outcomes, using robust quantitative and qualitative measures.
- Advocates of medical simulation should give a high priority to multicenter collaboration as a means to stimulate the use of simulation technology and to study efficacy.

Source: Glavin, 2008, p. 83.

References

American Society of Anesthesiologists (ASA), Workgroup on Simulation Education. (2006a). ASA approval of anesthesiology simulation programs. Retrieved September 25, 2008, from http://www.asahq.org/SIM/membersurvey.htm

American Society of Anesthesiologists (ASA). (2006b). American Society of Anesthesiologists follow-up survey on course development. Retrieved September 25, 2008, from http://www.surveyconsole.com/console/ShowResults?id=221049&mode=data

American Society of Anesthesiologists (ASA). (2006c). ASA senior resident poll on simulator CME. Retrieved September 25, 2008, from http://www.asahq.org/SIM/ResidentSurveyGraphic Results.htm

Awad, S., Fagan, S., Bellows, C., et al. (2005). Bridging the communication gap in the operating room with medical team training. *American Journal of Surgery, 190*(5), 770–774.

Baggs, J. G. (1994). Development of an instrument to measure collaboration and satisfaction about care decisions. *Journal of Advanced Nursing, 20*, 176–182.

Bevans, T. (2008). *Use of simulation for clinical competency assessment.* Unpublished paper. Chicago: Rush University.

Cannon, M. R. (2008). *Practical aspects of developing a simulator course.* Paper presented at the American Association of Nurse Anesthetists, Assembly of School Faculty. Newport Beach, CA. February 21–23, 2008.

Cooper, J. B., & Taqueti, V. R. (2004). A brief history of the development of mannequin simulators for clinical education and training. *Quality and Safety in Health Care, 13*, i11–i17.

Council on Accreditation of Nurse Anesthesia Educational Programs. (2007). *Standards for accreditation of nurse anesthesia educational programs.* Park Ridge, IL: Author.

Cox, G. (2008). *Development and implementation of a crew resource management-based training program designed to improve the attitudes and enhance the effectiveness and safety of the anesthesia care team.* Unpublished paper. Chicago: Rush University.

Devitt, J. H., Kurrek, M. M., Cohen, M. M., & Cleave-Hogg, D. C. (2001). The validity of performance assessments using simulation. *Anesthesiology, 95*(1), 36–42.

Fletcher, G., Flin, R., McGeorge, P., Glavin, R., Maran, N., & Patey, R. (2003). Anaesthetists' non-technical skills (ANTS): Evaluation of a behavioural marker system. *British Journal of Anaesthesia, 90*, 580–588.

Gaba, D. (2007). The future vision of simulation in healthcare. *Simulation in Healthcare, 2*, 126–135.

Gaba, D., & DeAnda, A. (1988). A comprehensive anesthesia simulation environment: Recreating the operating room for research and training. *Anesthesiology, 69*, 387–394.

Gaba, D., Fish, K., & Howard, S. (1994). *Crisis management in anesthesiology.* Philadelphia: Livingstone-Churchill.

Gallagher, C. J., & Issenberg, S. B. (2007). *Simulation in anesthesia.* Philadelphia: Saunders Elsevier.

Glavin, R. (2007). Simulation: An agenda for the 21st century. *Simulation in Healthcare, 2*, 83–85.

Good, M. L. (2003). Patient simulation for training basic and advanced clinical skills. *Medical Education, 37* (Suppl. 1), 14–21.

Gordon, J., Wilkerson, W., Shaffer, D., & Armstrong, E. (2001). "Practicing" medicine without risk: Students' and educators' responses to high-fidelity patient simulation. *Academic Medicine, 76*, 469–472.

Grogan, E., Stiles, R., France, D., et al. (2004). The impact of aviation-based teamwork training on the attitudes of health-care professionals. *Journal of the American College of Surgeons, 199,* 843–848.

Jankouskas, T., Bush, M., Murray, B., et al. (2007). Crisis resource management: Evaluating outcomes of a multidisciplinary team. *Simulation in Healthcare, 2,* 96–101.

Kremer, M., Faut-Callahan, M., & Hicks, F. (2002). A study of clinical decision making by Certified Registered Nurse Anesthetists. *American Association of Nurse Anesthetists Journal, 70,* 391–398.

McCarthy, J., & Cooper, J. (2007). Malpractice insurance carrier provides premium incentive for simulation-based training and believe it has made a difference. Retrieved February 22, 2008, from http://www.apsf.org/resource_center/newletter/2007/spring/17_malpractice.htm

Nishisaki, A., Keren, R., & Nadkarni, V. (2007). Does simulation improve patient safety? Self-efficacy, operational performance and patient safety. *Anesthesiology Clinics, 25,* 225–236.

O'Donnell, J., Fletcher, J., Dixon, B., & Palmer, L. (1998). Planning and implementing an anesthesia crisis resource management course for student nurse anesthetists. *CRNA: The Clinical Forum for Nurse Anesthetists, 9,* 50–58.

Pizzi, L., Goldfarb, N. I., & Nash, D. B. (2001). Crew resource management and its applications in medicine. In Agency for Healthcare Research and Quality, U.S. Department of Health and Human Services (Ed.), *Making health care safer: A critical analysis of patient safety practices.* Rockville, MD: Agency for Healthcare Research and Quality. Retrieved January 18, 2009, from: http://www.ahrq.gov/clinic/ptsafety/chap44.htm

Plaus, K. (2008). Personal communication (February 22, 2008).

Rystedt, H., & Lindwall, O. (2004). The interactive construction of learning foci in simulation-based learning environments: A case study of an anaesthesia course. *Psychology Journal, 2,* 168–188.

Schwid, H. A., Rooke, G. A., Ross, B. K., & Sivarajan, M. (1999). Use of a computerized advanced cardiac life support simulator improves retention of advanced cardiac life support guidelines better than a textbook review. *Critical Care Medicine, 27,* 821–824

Stanford University School of Medicine, VA Simulation Center. (2008a). Anesthesia crisis Resource management. Retrieved February 22, 2008, from http://med.stanford.edu/VAsimulator/acrm

Stanford University School of Medicine, VA Simulation Center. (2008b). Crisis resource management training in emergency medicine. Retrieved February 22, 2008, from http://med.stanford.edu/VAsimulator/center1.html

Turcato, N. (2005). *Nurse anesthesia program director survey on the use of clinical simulation.* Unpublished paper. Chicago: Rush University.

Turcato, N. (2007). *Developing simulation experiences to support the education of nurse anesthetists in the New England area.* Unpublished paper. Chicago: Rush University.

Turcato, N., Roberston, C., & Covert, K. (2008). Simulation-based education: What's in it for nurse anesthesia educators? *Journal of the American Association of Nurse Anesthetists, 76,* 257–262.

Zausig, Y. A., Bayer, Y., Hacke, N., et al. (2007). Simulation as an additional tool for investigating the performance of standard operating procedures in anaesthesia. *British Journal of Anaesthesia, 99,* 673–678.

CHAPTER 6

Statewide Nursing Simulation Program

Jana F. Berryman

INTRODUCTION

With the national focus on patient safety, nurse retention issues, and the looming nursing shortage, nursing programs and practice agencies need to work together to develop solutions. It has been estimated that there is currently an 11% shortage of nurses in Colorado, which is twice the national average; this shortage is projected to triple to 30% by 2020 (Colorado Center for Nursing Excellence, 2005). The lack of qualified, available faculty has made it increasingly difficult to accommodate greater numbers of students as workload and role expectations demand have swelled (American Association of Colleges of Nursing [AACN], 2004). Creating a statewide model for collaboration has proven to be a powerful strategy to bring practice and education together to embrace innovations that increase nurse educator knowledge, improve student nurse competence, and enhance patient outcomes in this time of shortage (Berryman & Roan, 2006).

The State of Colorado recognized the need to collaborate on these important issues and brought together many unique partners for this statewide project. In June 2004, the Colorado Center for Nursing Excellence, in partnership with the Colorado Department of Labor and Employment (CDLE) and the Colorado State Workforce Development Council, convened multiple healthcare forums (see Table 6-1) around the state; their task was to formulate a solution designed to support the development and utilization of technology to train workers for the high-demand nursing industry. That collaboration brought unique partners to the table, such the public and private sectors, Colorado's schools of nursing, hospitals, Area Health Education Centers, the Public Broadcast System, and other healthcare partners (i.e., School of Medicine and Paramedic programs). From that work, the CDLE submitted a proposal to the U.S. Department of Labor and Employment

(USDoLE) to provide funding for this statewide initiative with the overall goals of (1) enhancing the state's workforce development infrastructure for health-care education pre- and post-licensure and (2) for faculty development, utilizing innovative technologies and state-of-the-art practices to expand and strengthen the workforce.

After a two-year proposal process, the USDoLE funded the first phase of the statewide simulation center. The Colorado Center for Nursing Excellence contracted with CDLE for development and operations of the future statewide simulation center. Besides the funding received from the USDoLE, additional organizations assisted with the design and provided grant matching funds (see Table 6-2). A key element of the proposal during Year 1 was to design and model a 5000-square-foot simulation center, equip the center with high-

---

Table 6-1   Participant Institutions

Adams State College
Banner Health
Centura Health Systems
Colorado Community College System
Colorado Permanente Medical Group
Columbine Health System
Craig Hospital
Denver Health Medical Center
Emily Griffith Opportunity School
Exempla Healthcare
HealthONE
Kaiser Permanente
Memorial Hospital
Mesa State College
Metropolitan State College of Denver
Platt College
Poudre Valley Hospital
Regis University–Loretto Heights, Department of Nursing
University of Colorado Hospital
University of Colorado at Denver Health Sciences Center
University of Colorado, Colorado Springs, Beth El College of Nursing and Health Sciences
University of Northern Colorado
T.H. Pickens Technical Center
San Luis Valley Regional Medical Center
St. Mary's Hospital

Table 6-2   Organizations Who Assisted with Proposal Design and Matched Funding

Colorado Department of Labor and Employment
Colorado Center for Nursing Excellence
University of Colorado Hospital
University of Colorado Health Sciences Simulation Center
Touch of Life
State Workforce Development Council
Colorado Department of Education
Rocky Mountain Public Broadcasting System
Colorado Area Health Education Centers

fidelity patient simulators, VH Dissector virtual anatomy, medical supplies, and debriefing space, along with the development of learning scenarios to implement the collaborative faculty learning environment.

Today, Colorado's statewide simulation center is a resource for faculty training in both practice and schools of nursing, training for pre-licensure nursing students in a multidisciplinary environment, and both on-site and off-site simulation training events for experienced nurses.

BACKGROUND: STATEWIDE NURSING SIMULATION PROGRAM

The scarcity of resources has increased the demand for collaboration, particularly as it relates to the nursing shortage and healthcare worker clinical competency enhancement. The State of Colorado identified this unmet need in 2002 and established a nonprofit organization, the Colorado Center for Nursing Excellence, to fulfill that need. Since its establishment, the Colorado Center for Nursing Excellence has been recognized as a statewide resource for collaborative and strategic work among nursing stakeholders. It is the only organization in Colorado exclusively dedicated to ensuring that the state has adequate numbers of highly qualified nurses. To this end, it has brought together educational institutions, hospitals, government agencies, and foundations to investigate the sources of the nursing shortfall and has assisted in the development of strategies to address and secure funding to implement solutions to this ongoing problem.

The Colorado Center for Nursing Excellence, in partnership with the CDLE and State Workforce Development Council, convened a stakeholder group that consisted of chief nursing officers, deans of schools of nursing, and other healthcare leaders throughout Colorado to investigate next steps to developing a collaborative simulation center. The Colorado Center for Nursing Excellence provided technical expertise for the establishment of objectives for a statewide simulation center as well as investigated staffing requirements, equipment needs, space planning, and course offerings for the new facility.

The stakeholders recognized that an increasing number of schools and practice settings were acquiring high-fidelity patient simulators and other innovative technology to assist with the competency/skill development of students and practicing nurses. Unfortunately, few nurse educators and faculty were equipped with the technical knowledge or had enough time to fully utilize these technologies. Those barriers left much of the equipment underutilized. To make full and effective use of these innovative simulated technologies, collaboration was identified as a vital component in ensuring the success of the proposed simulation center.

Phase I of the statewide simulation center focused on making innovative technologies available to nursing faculty statewide. Development of best practices, standardization of scenario development, creation of a simulation scenario library, and provision of technical support and assistance were all incorporated into the model.

STAFFING

Staff composition of the statewide simulation center during Phase I of the work consisted of daily operation staff (see Table 6-3) along with an additional Partner Oversight Committee. The simulation center was staffed with 5.25 full-time equivalents (FTEs), which allowed for adequate project oversight, contract management, space design/construction, curriculum development, and implementation of project work. As this type of collaboration was unique, a key role of staff personnel was the ability to invent and create new solutions as the project unfolded.

The Partner Oversight Committee included project partner organizations such as CDLE, Workforce Development Council, Rocky Mountain Public Broadcast System, Area Health Education Centers, and Touch of Life Technologies (see Table 6-2). This Committee met on an ongoing basis during the development and implementation of the simulation center. Its main purpose was to direct grant functions and contractors.

The Project Director was charged with overall oversight of the simulation center. Critical components of the Project Director's role included facilitating discussions with key stakeholders regarding equipment needs, overseeing building design/construction, and working on the development of services.

Table 6-3   Colorado Center for Nursing Excellence Operation Staff Roles

Project Director (1.0 FTE) — responsible for overall daily operations, project oversight, and partnership building.

Simulation Technical Coordinator (1.0 FTE) — computer and high-fidelity mannequin operation and troubleshooting oversight.

Administrative Assistant (1.0 FTE) — administration support to project director, organization of course materials, data tracking, and reporting.

Curriculum Coordinator/Grant Writer (0.75 FTE) — conductor for curriculum development and design, coordinator of content experts, and scenario training development. Conducts environment scan, coordinates, and writes for grant opportunities.

Simulation Clinical Coordinator (1.0 FTE, implemented after 6 months) — clinical expertise for simulation training, provides coaching and mentoring for facilitators and leads workshops.

*0.25 FTE was provided by the Center's CEO/President who oversaw the Project Director, contract with CDLE and participated on variety of committees.
**0.25 FTE was provided by the Center's Director of Operations who managed operations budget, payroll and human resource responsibilities.

The success of the collaborative model was evident in the Project Director's ability to gain buy-in and input from stakeholders for each of the work areas. For example, an environmental scan was conducted with end-users of high-fidelity patient simulation partners, and the results of that survey then assisted with the strategic decision to equip the simulation center with all high-fidelity patient simulators and to provide resources for technical support of the equipment.

As Phase I of the project was intended to itself be a resource for technical development end-users, a Simulation Technical Coordinator role was formulated. The background desired for this role was a healthcare paraprofessional with computer operational expertise. Ultimately, this combination of skills proved difficult to find in a single recruit. Eventually, efforts focused on recruiting the computer operational expertise; education was then provided in the staff member's initial orientation for basic healthcare knowledge, such as an online medical terminology course and certified nursing assistant experience.

During the first 6 months of the project, the Simulation Technical Coordinator and Project Director worked closely together to gain understanding of and insight into equipment needs, purchasing decisions, and space design/

construction requirements. Once the simulation center was functioning, the Simulation Technical Coordinator role transitioned to even more in-depth knowledge of operations of the equipment, including high-fidelity patient simulators, audiovisual devices, and the other equipment that was integrated into the simulation center.

Another transition point occurred within six months of operations, when a Simulation Clinical Coordinator was added to the staff. The background required for this staff member was a registered nurse (RN) with both clinical and educational backgrounds. As scenarios were being developed and faculty were being trained, an RN was critical to the work with the partners for development of simulation scenarios, facilitation of simulation training events, and provision of coaching to faculty to enhance their skill sets.

The organizations and programs served by the simulation center vary in level of nursing content. The unique skill set of the Simulation Clinical Coordinator and the Simulation Technical Coordinator, plus the fact that they work closely together, has allowed for the facilitation of individual program needs. For example, the Simulation Clinical Educator works with the nursing program educators (content experts) to write scenarios that are then programmed by the Simulation Technical Coordinator.

From the inception of the project, the simulation center was staffed with an expert in curriculum design and development process. This role was crucial for the collaborative model. Owing to the limited number of staff, the development of the curriculum was dependent on outside content experts; this role allowed for coordination of these content experts and provided standardization and consistency across all elements of the curriculum.

As the project evolved and templates were established, a portion of time was then dedicated for searching and writing project grants for the simulation center. One successful grant gave the simulation center an opportunity to hire two additional staff for a patient safety initiative. The staffing for that project included a full-time Simulation Clinical Coordinator and a full-time Simulation Technical Coordinator/Administrative Assistant (60% technical, 40% administration).

Considerations When Hiring

Because this type of learning methodology was relatively new to the field of nursing, as was the very idea of a statewide collaborative model, flexibility was a critical component of all staff positions. During the project, a notable saying was that "The sidewalk was being paved along the way, not paved for us." This philosophy directed Phase I of the project and provided future direction.

Throughout the implementation, a best practice for the staff was holding regular debriefing sessions about the project work. The team developed a debriefing worksheet that each member would complete immediately following every event. These worksheets would then be reviewed at regularly scheduled staff meetings, where each staff member was able to discuss items that went well and make suggestions for improvement. Each team member's input was vital to the enhancement of the scenarios, faculty development courses, and outreach and training events.

EQUIPMENT

Training Equipment

As part of the collaborative model, staff members engaged in in-depth discussions with end-users of the high-fidelity patient simulators. These users were asked to give input on purchase decisions with the mannequin vendors. It was determined that the statewide simulation center would include high-fidelity patient simulation mannequins from a variety of vendors, such as Laerdal, METI, and Guamard.

A unique, innovative tool for the statewide simulation center was an anatomy teaching methodology called VH Dissector. VH Dissector is a cutting-edge, interactive computer program for learning anatomy and virtual dissection. Utilizing data from National Library of Medicine's Visible Human Project, it provides the ability to interact with correlated three-dimensional (3-D) and cross-sectional views of more than 2000 anatomical structures through identification, dissection, assembly, and rotation (see Figure 6-1). Through the collaborative efforts of the center staff and Touch of Life Technologies, VH Dissector has now been used with clinical scenarios using high-fidelity patient simulators. Specifically, it has been configured to work in conjunction with the mannequins. With this approach, the healthcare professional not only learns how to respond to a specific clinical situation, but also gains an understanding of the underlying concepts that contribute to the decision-making process.

Audiovisual Equipment

The simulation center is equipped with video cameras and microphones throughout the simulation training area. Each simulation training area has two cameras for recording and incorporating information into the debriefing session. Figure 6-2 provides a complete list of the audiovisual equipment.

Figure 6-1   A three-dimensional view from the VH Dissector program.

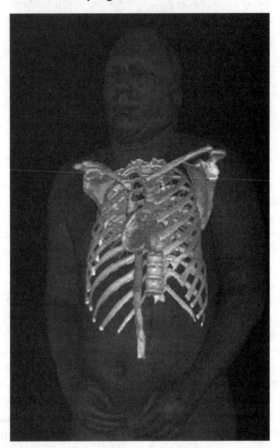

General Equipment

As part of the initial funding, not only was high technology equipment purchased, but part of the funds also assisted in the purchase of hospital beds, IV pumps, tables, chairs, and other equipment that was required for a simulation training space. Although consumable equipment has always been part of the operations budget, multiple partners have donated expired medications and unused equipment as well. The collaborative nature of the statewide simulation center has also allowed for borrowing and integrating high-cost equipment, such as ventilators and x-ray machines, into the simulation training events without breaking the bank.

Figure 6-2   WELLS Center Floor Plan and Equipment List

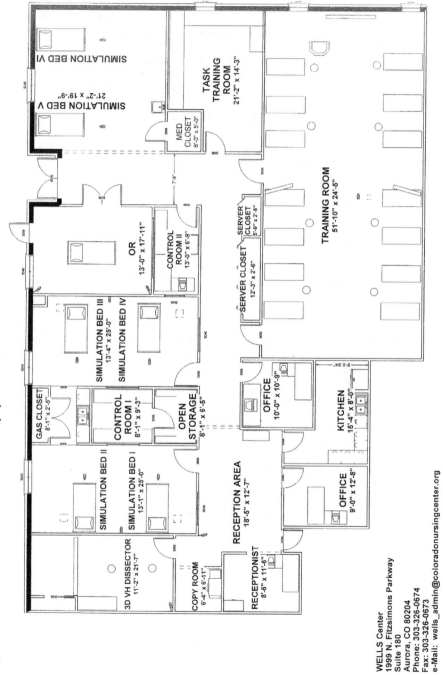

WELLS Center
1999 N. Fitzsimons Parkway
Suite 180
Aurora, CO 80204
Phone: 303-326-0674
Fax: 303-326-0673
e-Mail: wells_admin@coloradonursingcenter.org

Figure 6-2   WELLS Center Floor Plan and Equipment List *(continued)*

WELLS Center
Building Vital Statistics

Total square footage: 43827 (does not include perimeter walls; finish interior space to interior dry wall only)
Construction duration: April 1, 2006 through June 30, 2006; 2 months

High-fidelity patient simulator mannequins:
  Laerdal SimMan
  Laerdal SimBaby
  Noelle (birthing simulator)
  METI ECS
  METI HPS
  METI ECS BabySim
  METI ECS PediaSim

13 video cameras with video servers: $1\times$ reception area; $1\times$ debriefing room; $3\times$ simulation lab 1; $3\times$ simulation lab 2; $2\times$ operation room; $2\times$ nursing station; and $1\times$ training room.

28 omnidirectional ceiling microphones: $2\times$ reception area, $2\times$ debriefing room, $4\times$ simulation lab 1, $4\times$ simulation lab 2, $2\times$ operation room, $2\times$ nursing station, and $14\times$ training room.

WELLS Center is Ethernet and wireless ready.

Receptionist area:
1 50″ plasma display
1 Canon VC-C50i communication camera
1 AXIS 241 video servers

3D VH Dissector:
1 Custom Display 120″ diagonal vista black 130 rear screen system
2 Hitachi high-resolution 1400×1050 3500-lumen LCD projectors
2 Hitachi short throw lens 8
1 G5 Mac computer for VH Dissector
1 30″ Mac monitor display
1 Canon VC-C50i communication camera
1 AXIS 241 Video servers
2 Ceiling mount speakers
1×2 way in-wall LCD touch panel

Figure 6-2   WELLS Center Floor Plan and Equipment List *(continued)*

Control room l:
 3 7″ Preview LCD monitors
 1 12″ LCD touch panel
 1 Pro camera joystick controller
 2 G5 Mac computers (for VH Dissector)
 Options—Laerdal and METI operational systems

Simulation bed I and II:
 4 omnidirectional ceiling microphones
 3 Canon VC-C50i communication camera
 3 AXIS 241 Video servers
 1 30″ Mac monitor display (for VH Dissector)
 2 Power columns
 Space for compressors to assist with noise control

Simulation bed III and IV:
 4 omnidirectional ceiling microphones
 3 Canon VC-C50i communication camera
 3 AXIS 241 Video servers
 1 30″ Mac monitor display (for VH Dissector)
 2 Power columns
 Space for compressors to assist with noise control

Gas closet:
 3 Oxygen tanks (1 in use and 2 reserve); E cylinder
 3 Carbon dioxide (1 in use and 2 reserve); E cylinder
 3 Nitrogen (1 in use and 2 reserve); E cylinder
 3 Compressed air (1 setup for when needed and 2 reserve); E cylinder

Operation room (OR):
 2 omnidirectional ceiling microphones
 2 Canon VC-C50i communication camera
 2 AXIS 241 Video servers
 1 30″ Mac monitor display (for VH Dissector)

Control room II:
 2 7″ Preview LCD monitors
 1 12″ LCD touch panel
 1 G5 Mac computer (for VH Dissector)
 1 G5 Mac computer (for METI HPS)
 Options—Laerdal operational system

Figure 6-2   WELLS Center Floor Plan and Equipment List *(continued)*

Simulation bed V and VI:
>   2 omnidirectional ceiling microphones
>   2 Canon VC-C50i communication camera
>   2 AXIS 241 Video servers
>   2 Head wall units with oxygen and suction

Task training room
>   1 Laerdal Virtual IV
>   5 Haptic devices—arriving winter 2006
>   Training room
>   64 Seating
>   1 120″ Recessed electric screen
>   2 50″ Plasma displays
>   8 Ceiling mount speakers
>   14 Ceiling omnidirectional microphones
>   1 Lapel microphone
>   1 Hitachi high-resolution 1400 × 1050 3500-lumen LCD projector
>   1 DVD/VCR combo
>   1 Podium
>   2 LCD touch panels
>   34 Ethernet setup for VH Dissector

Server closet:
>   3 8 Mic mixer
>   1 Dialer
>   1 6 Input 4 output switcher
>   1 Crestron PRO-2 control system
>   1 Volume control equalizer
>   Rocky Mountain PBS datacast server
>   VH Dissector servers

Kitchen/moulage area:
>   1 Full size refrigerator
>   1 Utility sink
>   1 Dishwasher
>   Storage area

ENVIRONMENT AND SPACE CONSIDERATIONS

The 5000-square-foot space for the simulation center is located on the BioScience Campus (formerly Fitzsimons Army Hospital), which also houses the University of Colorado Hospital (UCH), the Children's Hospital, and the University of Colorado at Denver Health Sciences Center Schools of Nursing, Medicine, and Dental Medicine, as well as the Physical Therapy Program. A partnership between CDLE, the Colorado Workforce Center, and UCH provided funding for space build-out and the ongoing lease cost. As the statewide simulation program was planned to have multiple functions, the build-out was designed to incorporate flexibility for training. As Figure 6-2 demonstrates, the center has two offices, a reception area, a kitchen/moulage area, seven simulation training room areas, a 3-D projection room (also used as a small debriefing room for a maximum of 15 participants), and a large classroom that holds as many as 64 participants.

The following subsections describe the spaces that are included in the simulation center. Key characteristics have been noted regarding utilization, functionality, and flow.

Reception Area

The reception area is where the Administrative Assistant is stationed. This welcoming area is also large enough for small debriefing sessions, impromptu meetings, and as an overflow area for guests, thereby encouraging discussion and networking. This area has also been utilized as a walk-in triage station for simulation training.

3-D Projection Room

A space that allowed for backscreen projection was provided to enable VH Dissector to be seen in 3-D perspective. This technology allows participants to view the virtual anatomy in three dimensions with special glasses. As with all of the space in the simulation center, flexibility was key. This space is utilized for both 3-D anatomy training and simulation debriefing.

Classroom (Training Room)

As mentioned earlier, the classroom holds 64 people. The tables are on rollers, allowing the space to be rearranged efficiently for workshops, meetings, presentations, and simulation training. The classroom has two plasma displays and a projector/screen where participants can watch a simulation training event live; this technology is used for debriefing sessions. The room is also equipped with ceiling microphones and a built-in telephone conferencing system. The telephone conferencing system has been useful during meetings, presentations, and task forces that have allowed increased participation from all areas of Colorado.

Critical Care/Emergency Room Training Areas (Simulation Beds I, II, III, and IV)

This area hosts four beds, with a power column being provided for each bed. Monitors on each power column display vital signs for the high-fidelity patient simulators. There is also a 30-inch monitor between simulation beds I and II and simulation beds III and IV that displays lab readouts, x-ray, ultrasound, VH Dissector anatomy, and other adjunct needs.

Medical Surgical (M/S) Training Areas (Simulation Beds V and VI)

Two training areas have headwall units with compressed air to simulate oxygen and live suction. These areas have also been used as a multiple-bed trauma unit, for which additional beds and equipment were brought into the space, and as a labor and delivery room.

Operating Room (OR)

The operating room has been the last area to be targeted for equipment support, as work has recently begun with OR partners to develop a specialty course. As the METI Human Patient Simulator is nonmobile, its permanent location is in this space. Oxygen, carbon dioxide, nitrogen, and compressed air are permanently piped into this room from the gas closet, as shown in Figure 6-2. A best practice learned from another simulation center was to cut a trench in the floor to hide the mannequin's umbilical cord. As this area is not yet fully equipped with OR equipment, it has also been used as a trauma bay area.

Control Rooms

The simulation center has two control rooms. The larger of the two rooms is located between simulation beds I and II and simulation beds III and IV (see Figure 6-2). The Simulation Technical Coordinator, Simulation Clinical Coordinator, and clinical expert faculty occupy this space during the actual simulation event. The ability to record the training is also set up in both control rooms.

Kitchen/Moulage Area

The kitchen is equipped with a work sink, dishwasher, and refrigerator. It is primarily used for equipment cleaning and moulage setup.

Storage

Storage was a primary consideration, as simulation requires abundant storage space. The center has taken advantage of a storage shed and two large closets to provide this space.

Challenges

Space challenges have primarily centered on staff growth, which has led to the need for more office space and storage areas. The Simulation Technical Coordinator's office space was moved to the smaller control area, along with other staff members needing to share office and training space. As the simulation projects expand, this will be an ongoing challenge.

Collaborative Nursing Educational Programs

All curricula designed and developed at the simulation center are created collaboratively. The expertise of various partners is used either individually or in a group process to take advantage of the breadth and depth of their knowledge. For example, work carried out by the Colorado Simulation Development Group has focused on template standardization for scenario writing. Task forces have been important vehicles for this work (see Table 6-1).

To overcome some of the challenges inherent in any collaboration, it has been important for the simulation center to provide acknowledgment of and credit to the partners who contribute to the work. All scenarios and curricula developed by a simulation center task force or by an individual reflect that philosophy.

A lack of faculty time and a shortage of technical expertise were the greatest barriers to the integration of simulation into the nursing curriculum, both at the academic and practice levels. The recognition of this shortfall inspired the early development of educational workshops. The first of these workshops focused on assisting faculty to understand how best to use clinical experts to provide content for scenario development in areas where faculty were not specifically content experts. Templates that facilitated this process were executed in this workshop and disseminated to partners to achieve ease of simulation development as well as standardization.

To support the integration of simulation into nursing education at both the pre- and post-licensure levels, simulation development and facilitation workshops were developed. These workshops were designed to be interactive and flexible enough to focus on the specific needs of the individual participants. Typical topics include writing simulations utilizing high-fidelity patient simulators, providing a technical overview of the simulators, learning how to troubleshoot, developing a debriefing skill set, and facilitating a training event. These workshops are offered to faculty in both practice and education and are facilitated by the Simulation Clinical Coordinator and the Simulation Technical Coordinator.

Focused simulation training events have also been held at hospitals for competency training. In such an event, the Simulation Clinical Coordinator and the Simulation Technical Coordinator transport the high-fidelity patient simulators to the hospitals. Prior to the training event, staff work with the content experts to integrate specific hospital policies and procedures.

Recognizing that clinical site experiences are often lacking in variety for nursing students, the Simulation Center developed a multidisciplinary student-focused simulation training event. This training event involves both medical and nursing students in a pediatric clinical environment. The training methodology includes a high-fidelity patient simulator and integration of two actors—one serving as a healthcare technician for x-ray, lab, or other services, and the other acting as the mother of the child. This event has not only facilitated increased communication between family and team members, but has also served as a clinical make-up day for nursing students who missed clinical hours or who are short on pediatric clinical hours.

EVOLUTION AND FUTURE DIRECTION

In the past few years, there has been an increased focus on patient safety, especially as it involves team communication and training in health care. Part of the future work of the Colorado collaboration will be to expand beyond nursing to include instruction of other healthcare professionals. As mentioned previously, early work in that arena has been completed, although there remains the need for even more collaborative training.

Sustainability considerations have also been a concern of the team. As the simulation center evolves, a governing board will be established to move the simulation center from a project to a 501(c)3, nonprofit entity. The governing board will be a public and private entity, and its members will be representatives from across the state, ensuring that both metropolitan and rural needs are addressed by the board.

As future business plan development strategies unfold, critical nursing training areas, as identified by the Colorado Center for Nursing Excellence, will reside in specialty areas such as critical care, emergency nursing, labor and delivery, and perioperative training. Curricula will be developed to include high-fidelity patient simulators, VH Dissector, and other innovative methodologies. The courses will be developed through the work of task forces whose members represent both hospitals and schools of nursing, along with professional organizations.

A number of challenges have emerged and been overcome along the path establishing the statewide simulation center. The staff and partners of the center have viewed many of these challenges as opportunities to create a system change. Continued efforts will be directed toward seeking out funding opportunities to support operations, projects, and maintenance of equipment. The ongoing focus on patient safety has kept the work alive, and residents of Colorado should benefit from this model.

References

American Association of Colleges of Nursing (AACN). (2004). Nursing faculty shortage fact sheet. Retrieved May 23, 2005, from http://www.aacn.nche.edu/Media/Fact-Sheets/NursingFaculty Shortage.htm

Colorado Center for Nursing Excellence (2005). *The 2004 Colorado nursing faculty supply and demand study*. Denver, CO: Author.

Berryman, J., & Roan, L. (2006). Innovative collaborative strategies for nursing practice and education: Creating a simulation development group alliance. *Clinical Simulation in Nursing. 2*, e33-e40.

CHAPTER 7

Creating an Interdisciplinary Simulation Center

Robert L. Kerner, Jr.

INTRODUCTION

Almost a decade ago, the Institute of Medicine (IOM) published its findings pertaining to the state of health care in the United States. The failure of teams to work effectively together was identified as a factor contributing to medical errors (Kohn, Corrigan, & Donaldson, 2000). While an individual nurse, physician, or allied health professional may have received the highest-quality education, there is no guarantee that members of the various disciplines will function effectively as a team. Nurses, for example, often have relatively little sustained contact with physicians during the course of their undergraduate clinical education because the traditional models of nursing and medical education do not emphasize interdisciplinary teamwork. This phenomenon is often referred to as "training in silos," where each component of the patient care team behaves as if it is in its own universe. Not surprisingly, teams that train in silos often do not perform well together in times of crisis.

This chapter discusses the steps needed to build a successful interdisciplinary simulation center. These steps include identifying the need, identifying stakeholders, establishing goals, selecting faculty, developing faculty, developing the curriculum, and moving forward based on our experiences.

IDENTIFYING THE NEED

In response to the identified need to improve teamwork, the IOM has recommended "establish[ing] interdisciplinary team training programs, such as simulation, that incorporate proven methods of team management" (Kohn et al., 2000, p. 156). Many healthcare organizations have acted on this recommendation and established multidisciplinary simulation centers to "train in teams those who are expected to work in teams" (Kohn et al., 2000, p. 173). A recent survey of the Society for Simulation in Healthcare's Web site revealed 113 registered simulation centers that provide interdisciplinary training (Society for Simulation in Healthcare, 2008). Many more facilities are also in operation in the United States that have not registered with this site.

The IOM report calling for team training is but one reason to build an interdisciplinary simulation center. Coming in as a close second reason to build a center serving many disciplines is practicality. For a hospital or major healthcare system, it will very often be easier to secure funding and capital resources for an enterprise that will serve more than one discipline. In the current economic climate, it makes sense to build a center that will see consistent use by a number of professions and disciplines, rather than one that will be visited by only a limited number of users.

Assume, for the moment, that you are the CEO of Local Hospital and you have $1 million with which to construct a moderate-size simulation center with fully outfitted rooms, high-fidelity mannequins, and state-of-the-art audiovisual equipment. Will you build the center for the exclusive use of the nursing department? Don't the physicians and surgeons deserve a center of their own? Putting aside the IOM report for a moment, common business sense would suggest that the center should be shared by as many users as possible to maximize the return on investment. Creating an interdisciplinary center also means access to human resources, such as instructional faculty and subject matter experts, that might otherwise be lost.

IDENTIFYING STAKEHOLDERS

Having identified the need to have an interdisciplinary simulation center, it is now time to identify the key stakeholders who will support the endeavor. Stakeholders are the core professions and disciplines that will become the center's initial users. It goes without saying that the financial support of the organization will be needed, but it is also helpful to secure commitments to use the center before seeking financial backing. When selecting stakeholders, be on the lookout for individuals who pride themselves in being pioneers and risk takers. It is also helpful, although not absolutely necessary, if the initial stakeholders are technologically inclined. In keeping with the theme of this chapter, it is strongly recommended that the initial stakeholder group have representatives from a variety of professions and disciplines. There are countless options for selecting initial stakeholders but any institution can likely employ the following two options to get a center open and running: letting the stakeholder find the center and establishing a new program dependent on the center.

Let the Stakeholder Find the Center

The most common reactions to the announcement that an organization is planning a simulation center are "That's great—how do I get onboard?" and "Yeah, so what?" You definitely want the support of the people who want to get onboard; very often, they are looking for innovative solutions to clinical and educational problems. Sometimes the problem is finding a creative way to foster performance improvement; at other times, it is a corrective action that must be implemented with all deliberate speed. In either case, some potential stakeholders will probably need assistance executing their educational plan. If they have read the IOM report and kept abreast of current literature, chances are they will find their way to planning meetings. They may need a little coaxing but the audience is already there; all that has to be done is to provide the technology and guidance.

Take, for example, the situation of Dr. Jones, the well-respected chief of obstetrics at Anywhere Hospital. This past year his department has been sued four times for misadventures involving patients with shoulder dystocia. Dr. Jones is confident that his staff—doctors and nurses alike—is knowledgeable about how to handle obstetric emergencies; however, he has noticed that the delivery room often appears chaotic during emergencies. The state health department, meanwhile, has demanded a corrective action program targeted at team training in crisis situations. Dr. Jones has a history of finding innovative solutions to problems; therefore, when he hears that Anywhere Hospital is considering a simulation center, he volunteers to help establish the center in exchange for the opportunity to bring his staff to the center for team training.

Everyone benefits from this approach to identifying stakeholders. Dr. Jones can implement his team training educational plan using simulation, the department of health gets its corrective action, and the center gets its initial stakeholders (obstetricians and obstetrical nurses) and subject matter experts. Dr. Jones is the first one on board but word spreads fast and soon others are at your door looking for innovative solutions to their challenges.

Grow Your Own

If no initial stakeholders appear on their own, an individualized program can be created. This step is not as difficult as it sounds and can be as simple or complex as you want it to be. The basic premise is that once you have the center open and running, others will hear about the wonderful work you are doing and want to use the center, too.

The least complicated method of growing one's own program is to identify an existing course and modify it to incorporate simulation. For example, most institutions, whether they are hospitals or professional schools, conduct some degree of cardiac life support training, such as basic life support or advanced cardiac life support. These are excellent gateway courses: They teach essential skills, they are not too burdensome to organize and teach, the information is readily available, and, most importantly, they are multidisciplinary by design. The didactic content of the course is provided by the American Heart Association in the form of books and instructional CDs. The course is easily adapted to include simulation during the teaching and evaluation stations.

One word of caution here: Simulation must be a key, indispensable component of the program; otherwise, the people who are funding your center will be extremely skeptical of the capital investment. If the new program looks just like an existing program but with a $35,000 mannequin and some video cameras, you are unlikely to win the full support of the organization for the new venture. Be prepared to defend the proposal to create an interdisciplinary simulation center with research and data that support the position that simulation will improve the quality of the educational experience.

A more ambitious method to grow one's own program would be to create an original course with a curriculum grounded in experiential learning. Nurse residency programs are uniquely suited to this approach. At the Patient Safety Institute, for example, simulation is an essential and required component of a blended learning experience that includes didactic presentations and closely supervised clinical practice. Each group of nurse fellows (our term for new graduate nurses entering a critical care area) spends two days a week engaged in knowledge acquisition and two days a week in clinical practice. The didactic material consists of a very structured review of body systems and the care of patients with illnesses found in those systems. During the two clinical days, the fellows examine patients with the conditions covered in the didactic material; however, they are not expected to independently care for the patients during the initial phase of the fellowship. The fifth day is a culminating experience in the simulation center, during which the fellows care for patients independently or with minimal coaching from an instructor. The fellowship proceeds in this manner for eight weeks, covering all of the body systems, with a particular emphasis on teamwork and communication.

The fellowship was designed to meet a particular need for intensive care unit nurses. The designers of the program knew that an experiential learning component was necessary to prepare new graduate nurses for the rigors of the intensive care unit. They also had the foresight to recognize that by incorporating simulation into the fellowship program, they would be laying the groundwork for a thriving interdisciplinary center. They started with a small program whose size and quality they controlled, and then let word of mouth spread the good news about simulation. The fellowship program has been enormously successful for the fellows who participated and has generated great interest from other professions. An effort that started in an unused hospital room with a handful of people has grown into an 8000-square-foot facility with full-time and adjunct faculty hosting three distinct nurse fellowship programs, several physician user groups, and a paramedic program. You really can grow your own.

ESTABLISHING GOALS

Short- and long-term goals should be established as stakeholders are identified. These goals should be relevant to the educational needs and clinical challenges faced by the stakeholders. A formal needs assessment that gathers input from staff may facilitate the process. The organization's leadership, including the risk manager, may have specific goals as well. It is important not to get ahead of oneself when establishing goals. Stakeholders may want to have every staff member participate in simulation within the first year; however, this is an unrealistic expectation for most new simulation centers.

Establish goals that are achievable, particularly when just starting out. Having achievable goals is essential for maintaining faculty morale. No one wants to have a job where the bar is set so high that success is impossible. The same principle should inform curriculum development: Students will not want to participate at the center if the expectations are unrealistic. Realistic and achievable goals will keep everyone's confidence level high. Likewise, having achievable goals—and meeting them—will allow you to demonstrate a track record of success when it is time to expand the operation. To see how this process works, let's examine a long-term goal and consider how to achieve it through short-term actions.

Suppose our long-term goal is to establish an interdisciplinary simulation center, one that draws upon faculty and staff resources from every profession in the organization: nurses, physicians, surgeons, respiratory therapists, surgical technologists, and so on. We want these professionals to have an educational experience in the same context as they would work together in the hospital: as a team. It is unrealistic, however, to expect all of these groups to commit to simulation education without some prior experience or track record of success. This is where the short-term actions enter the picture.

A reasonable and attainable short-term goal might be to invite the surgeons to the center to work through a difficult case they encountered in the hospital. All of the surgeons do not need to be involved at first—just the influential ones who can appreciate the benefit of reviewing difficult cases to learn from mistakes. Those surgeons will return to the hospital and spread the word that the simulation center is not a scary place where people criticize past mistakes, but a safe haven in which to gain experience and identify opportunities for improvement. Similar small programs can be assembled for the other disciplines until a critical mass of users has been reached and a track record established.

Short-term goals can often be accomplished within a few months; in contrast, it may take a year or two to reach the long-term goal of interdisciplinary team education. In my experience, it is relatively easy to persuade members of individual specialties to participate in simulation. Our emergency department nurses and physicians, for example, appreciated the value of experiential learning almost immediately. The physicians were familiar with simulation because their department had a simulator. The nurses became acquainted with simulation through our center's nurse fellowship program. Although both groups are eager users and supporters of simulation education, true interdisciplinary education has eluded us, primarily due to scheduling issues. We have not met our long-term goal yet, but we will continue to pursue the short-term goal of running quality programs for the physicians and nurses until we reach the tipping point and are able to overcome the scheduling challenges. Rome wasn't built in a day.

It is very important to publicize successes, no matter how small. The organization no doubt spent a lot of money hiring faculty and purchasing equipment for the simulation center, and it will naturally look for evidence that the center is accomplishing what it was established to do. Take time to meet with benefactors, including the board of trustees, and update them on the progress of the center. If the organization has a newsletter, consider inviting the editor to the center to observe the good work being done. Likewise, consider sharing success stories with the local news media. It may be surprising that people within your organization will first learn about the simulation center by watching it on the local news broadcast. Publicizing successes, moreover, may open the door to new champions and benefactors. Perhaps most importantly, public recognition of their success makes the faculty and students feel good about going to work each day.

FACULTY SELECTION

Once you have established a basic business model including short- and long-term goals, it is time to begin the faculty selection process. It is very likely that faculty will be built incrementally, beginning with a core staff and adding subject matter experts as the program grows. Consider whether the long-term goal is to have a stand-alone faculty capable of teaching all of the courses that are being planned to offer or whether there will be a smaller, core faculty of simulation experts supported by an adjunct faculty of subject matter experts. For example, it may be impractical to have a full-time obstetrician on the faculty if obstetrical programs are taught only once or twice a month. In such a case, it may make more sense to affiliate with an obstetrician on a per diem basis.

The core faculty members should bring with them a wealth of clinical, educational, and leadership experience. Most of my colleagues at the Patient Safety Institute, for example, are experts in a particular clinical field and have served in various leadership capacities; consequently, they have a broad knowledge base to share with their students. Faculty members need to have excellent communication skills because they will be called upon to interact with the organization's leadership, other faculty members, and students. Perhaps most importantly, faculty should have some experience in evidence-based practice and curriculum development.

Depending on the scope of the operation, the core faculty must be subject matter experts in the areas most requested for training. If the simulation center offers courses targeted toward critical care providers, then at least some of your core faculty should have experience and credentials in that field. Specialty board certification in a particular subject adds even more credibility and demonstrates that the faculty member has achieved a certain level of expertise in that field. Additionally, specialty certification may be required if the simulation center plans to offer certain courses; for example, certification as an American Heart Association instructor is needed before one can administer an advanced cardiac life support course. By contrast, if the center will focus more on the behavioral and teamwork aspects of education, then it will be important to have experts in behavioral and human factors science.

Each new day in a simulation center brings with it new challenges and opportunities. Given this unpredictability, faculty members must have strong critical-thinking skills. Problem-solving skills are particularly important when dealing with the various technical aspects of simulation. There is no textbook on how to set up a simulation laboratory, hook up the wiring, and make the mannequin come to life for the students. There is no textbook to explain what to do when the mannequin stops breathing in the middle of a scenario. The solutions to these challenges will be arrived at through experience and trial and error. Faculty members ought to have a working knowledge of computer operating systems, basic computer interfaces, and the clinical equipment associated with patient care.

The core faculty should consist of visionaries. High-fidelity patient simulation is currently in its infancy. We are where we are today thanks to the efforts of a small group of visionaries who recognized the value of simulation in health care. Each center needs to have faculty capable of anticipating future needs and developing a curriculum that remains on the cutting edge of evidence-based education. It is very easy to fall into a "grindstone mentality" of thinking only about what is being done today while losing sight of long-term goals and hoped-for achievements. At my center, we hold biweekly meetings during which we discuss the future plans for the center.

If the center plans to engage in research, consider adding research experience to the list of qualifications required of the faculty. Keep in mind that not all physicians and nurses understand the finer points of conducting research. Where experience is lacking, there are often opportunities to send faculty members for additional education on research methodologies. For example, the annual Society for Simulation in Healthcare conference often includes workshops or special interest group sessions devoted to research.

As you assemble your list of essential skills and begin to interview candidates, give consideration to the titles you will give to your faculty members. "Simulation technician" seems to be a popular title; however, some professionals with advanced degrees may object to being referred to as a technician. Titles such as "educator," "faculty member," and "instructor" are less likely to cause controversy and also leave the door open for the faculty member to do more than operate the simulator. Consideration should also be given to the structure of the organization—in particular, whether it will be a relatively flat or multilayered hierarchy. Our center found that a relatively flat hierarchy works well. Although we have a director, who reports to our organization's chief learning officer, we all know that we are empowered to make decisions and conduct programs without the need for lengthy consultation with leadership. As a result, we do not get bogged down with minutia, as we might if we had a multilayered reporting system. Larger operations, of course, may require a more organizational structure. When you are just getting started, however, it is important to keep things simple.

FACULTY DEVELOPMENT

Initial faculty development will concentrate on acquiring the skills necessary to operate a simulation center. Simulation is a specialty skill and, as such, it is unlikely that many candidates who already possess the talents necessary to operate a simulation center will be found. Indeed, unless the candidate is coming from a position at another simulation center, there is almost no chance that the candidate will be familiar with the intricacies of operating a high-fidelity patient simulator. The same holds true for the audiovisual equipment in your center. The best way to learn to use the high-fidelity simulator is to have a manufacturer's representative conduct a class for your faculty. Most of the major manufacturers offer some form of training for organizations that buy their products. If you are opening a new simulation center and buying new equipment, the manufacturers should happily accommodate your request for a training session; if they don't, tell them you will buy their competitor's equipment!

It is vital to follow up the initial training encounter with continuing education. Approximately 50% of needed knowledge about operating the equipment will be learned during the initial encounter with the manufacturer's representative. Nevertheless, you should not expect to come away from the first session as an expert on the hardware and software—there is simply not enough time to learn all of the material at once. Attend workshops and conferences where faculty from other centers share their techniques and experiences on a regular basis. Networking with other users, along with practical experience with your equipment, is where the real learning takes place. While it is important to learn how the equipment operates, it is very easy to become distracted by the technical aspects of simulation.

When my center first opened, we were mesmerized by our simulator's graphical user interface and the various programming possibilities hidden behind it. We spent a great deal of time learning the fine art of scenario programming. Then we met someone at a national conference who told us that our time would be better spent designing realistic cases with a few simple objectives, rather than spending eight hours a day programming trends and handlers. We were fixated on the hardware and programming aspects of running a simulation center. Simulation, however, is about creating a realistic clinical environment. The graphical user interface and the mannequin are merely tools—they are not the reason we do simulation. It would have been easy to lose sight of this point were it not for the connections we made by attending conferences, such as those offered by the Society for Simulation in Healthcare and the Peter M. Winter Institute for Simulation Education and Research (WISER) at the University of Pittsburgh (Pennsylvania); the latter offers an annual symposium specific to nursing simulation.

The value of visiting other simulation centers cannot be understated. Almost all of what I know about simulation I learned by networking, visiting other centers, and asking questions. Some centers in the United States have been in operation for many years; these facilities have been on the cutting edge of simulation and have a proven track record of success. There is no need to reinvent the wheel. Visit other centers, and ask their staffs what they are doing and why they are doing it in that manner. The simulation community is for the most part an open source, meaning that centers share information and experiences openly with other members of the community. In fact, scenarios can be downloaded from a variety of Web sites for specific use in your center (e.g., see http://www.patientsimulation.co.uk/4680/index.html). There are also numerous Internet listserv groups where members will answer questions and share material; for example, the Society for Simulation in Healthcare (http://www.ssih.org) administers a listserv for its members.

Formal educational opportunities are also available for simulation faculty. For example, the Center for Medical Simulation at Harvard University (http://harvardmedsim.org/cms/) conducts a variety of faculty development courses that are applicable to all professions using simulation. The Harvard course entitled "Simulation as a Teaching Tool" helps faculty members understand the value of thoughtful preparation and high-quality debriefing through a series of presentations and practical exercises. The course also introduces human factors and organizational behavior concepts that will improve the quality of any simulation program. Although you could certainly read about these topics in a journal, actually going to the center and living the experience is a very worthwhile undertaking. If the simulation center is affiliated with a college or university, its faculty might take the opportunity to attend classes in social psychology and organizational behavior. As one digs deeper into the simulation and education literature, these two disciplines will be more appreciated and should play important roles in how you plan and execute the scenarios and debrief with the participants.

Several textbooks, or chapters within texts, also focus on simulation. The Society of Critical Care Medicine has an excellent introductory text that takes the reader through the history of simulation to high-stakes team training (Dunn, 2004). I highly recommend this book to anyone beginning their journey as a simulation educator. For journal readers, much of the simulation material can be found in discipline-specific journals and the excellent *Simulation in Healthcare: The Journal of the Society for Simulation in Healthcare*. For example, those searching for nursing-specific literature should consult Lupien's (2007) chapter on high-fidelity patient simulation.

CURRICULUM DEVELOPMENT

Although simulation can be an effective tool to drive an educational program, it cannot replace a thoughtful, well-designed curriculum. It is a mistake to believe that such a curriculum will materialize upon the acquisition of a high-fidelity patient simulator; in most cases, the curriculum should exist prior to the establishment of a simulation center. Let's examine two approaches to curriculum development to see which one works best.

Fakename University has a thriving allied health program with a school of nursing and a medical school. The nursing and medical schools follow the curriculum recommendations established by the respective state boards, and their faculty is generally regarded as the best in the region. Fakename is a first rate operation in most respects. Former student Agnes Deepockets recently gave

$50,000 to the university, exactly enough for one high-fidelity patient simulator and some video equipment. The university decided to use the funds to open a simulation lab. Within a few short weeks, the mannequin was delivered, the cameras installed, and signs hung announcing the arrival of the university's latest teaching tool. A select group of faculty attended training on the graphical user interface and hardware. Everyone was happy—until it became apparent there was no plan to integrate this great new tool into the existing curriculum. As a result, the mannequin sat unused except for occasional skills practice.

Bedrock University also has a medical and nursing school. Bedrock's dean of nursing is an innovator who monitors the educational journals and attends national conferences. Last year, the dean convened a committee to study high-fidelity patient simulation and make recommendations on its integration into the university's existing courses. The committee found that several courses in both schools could benefit from simulation; in particular, the committee planned to incorporate simulation into existing courses to create an environment of experiential learning (Dewey, 1994). Wholesale changes to the courses were not necessary to accommodate the new technology, just thoughtful revision of existing syllabi. In the nursing school, for example, faculty identified several disease processes not commonly seen in the clinical arena over the course of a semester. Clinical placement time was adjusted to permit caring for these "patients" in the simulation lab. As a result, the students benefited from experiences that otherwise would have been lost but for the addition of a high-fidelity patient simulator.

In the best-case scenario, the simulation curriculum should support an existing program of study. At my center, simulation is an integral part of three nurse fellowship programs and several physician education programs. Simulation is incorporated into existing syllabi at defined intervals to provide experiential learning in support of knowledge acquisition. When planning the simulation schedule, therefore, one must take into account the knowledge level of the participants.

The curriculum should create opportunities for critical thinking, experiential learning, and reflective practice (Gordon, Oriol, & Cooper, 2004). Begin by listing the learning objectives you hope to achieve. Bloom's taxonomy is a wonderful resource for identifying objectives within the cognitive and affective domains (Bloom, Mesia, & Krathwohl, 1964). A similar taxonomy is also available for the psychomotor domain (Simpson, 1972). Objectives should be tailored to the needs of the disciplines participating in the case. Bear in mind that these objectives will likely be similar for all disciplines but at some point they may diverge. A new graduate nurse, for example, will likely not have the same knowledge base relative to critical care pharmacology as a third-year resident physician; nevertheless, it is not unrealistic to have them work together as long as the learning objectives are adjusted accordingly. Desired outcomes should be observable or measurable to determine whether the students met the objectives. The objectives should not be secrets; share them with the students during the simulation briefing session.

Resist the temptation to incorporate too many objectives into one simulation. This is a common mistake, and one that proves frustrating to students. My first simulation cases were terribly complicated, including too many clinically based objectives and almost no behavioral objectives. I expected participants to accomplish a lot in a compressed time frame, with almost no attention paid to teamwork or communication skills. This rookie approach led to two types of responses from students: Some students quickly learned that the scenario was about accomplishing a checklist of tasks without regard to critical thinking, while others left frustrated because they could not meet all of the objectives. As you might imagine, my first simulation cases, packed with objectives, lasted 30 to 45 minutes each with barely any time remaining for debriefing.

Thankfully for my students, I progressed from my rookie phase and now devote considerable time to constructing reasonable objectives. Two or three clinical and behavioral objectives tend to be the happy medium for most of the students served by my center. Scenarios ordinarily conclude within 15 minutes unless something extraordinary is happening or the case was purposely designed to have a long duration. For students who are new to simulation, the objectives are usually very simple and are intended to familiarize them with the mannequin and introduce principles of teamwork—for example, recognize apnea, ventilate the patient, call for help, and communicate with the responding code team. On paper, this process looks simple, but it is surprising how many issues emerge during the debriefing.

Ample time should be allocated for a meaningful debriefing session. The purpose of simulation is to promote experiential learning. By comparison, the purpose of debriefing is to promote reflective practice, where the professional examines his or her own understanding of and response to the clinical situation (Rudolph, Simon, Dufresne, & Raemer, 2006). In this part of the program, the instructor seeks to determine, through careful inquiry, whether the students actually understood what was wrong with the patient and appreciate the implications of their actions. Once again, it is surprising what emerges from these sessions, including fundamental ignorance of basic physiology. For example, I am repeatedly told that it is an absolute contraindication to administer oxygen to a patient with chronic obstructive lung disease. This notion, of course, is based on old science and requires correction, but I would not have known the student was operating with outdated knowledge had I not asked,

"I noticed you did not apply oxygen to that hypoxic patient. Help me understand your decision." Depending on the complexity of your scenario, nonjudgmental debriefing can easily last twice as long as the case itself. Do not shortchange yourself or your students in this part of the curriculum.

If experiential learning is the primary goal, then the various disciplines should learn from and teach one another just as they would in the clinical setting. Although the learning objectives should be tailored to the learners' needs, it is acceptable to have overlapping objectives common to all disciplines. On a typical first day at the Patient Safety Institute, all disciplines are given instruction in hand hygiene, patient identification, and use of proper personal protective equipment. These three objectives are incorporated into every subsequent scenario. As the students' fund of knowledge increases, we encourage them to share their new understanding with their colleagues either at the bedside or in the debriefing session.

The curriculum should have an evaluative component of some sort. This sounds easy but often proves difficult in practice due to the nature of simulation and team education, where there may be many participants from different disciplines in the room. How does one know whether the intern understands the rationale for certain actions? Can one be sure that the nurse understands the pathophysiology? Even in situations where members of only one profession are present in the room, it may be impossible to evaluate each participant's knowledge absent a written test or direct inquiry of each participant. Placing an individual student in the room to care for the patient may be one way to evaluate understanding; conversely, it may prove nerve wracking and unproductive if the student is accustomed to practicing in a clinical environment where assistance is readily available. I do not pretend to have the answer to this dilemma but suggest you thoroughly review the literature when it comes time to design your evaluation process.

Routine programmatic evaluation in the form of pre- and post-course questionnaires can be very helpful. This review can take the form of a needs assessment at the beginning of a program, followed by an end-of-program survey to determine whether the students feel their needs were met. It is an excellent method to mine for feedback that might not otherwise emerge during the debriefing sessions, such as "I felt rushed" or "I felt like the instructor was picking on me during the debriefing." Feedback like this should result in a review of the curriculum and methods.

Any curriculum development process should be collaborative, involving teamwork among the various disciplines that patronize your center. If disciplines will practice in teams, the cases and objectives should be developed in teams. Each session should begin with a faculty briefing to assure that all members will follow the same plan, and conclude with a faculty debriefing to evaluate whether the plan was effective. At my center, we also have midday faculty meetings, usually during lunch, to fine-tune plans for the second half of the day.

GOING FORWARD

Innovation does not happen overnight. Establishing an interdisciplinary simulation program may take several months, but rest assured that the investment is worth it. Start modestly, build a track record of success, and publicize activities. Obtain regular feedback from students, faculty, and stakeholders. My center has run more than a dozen nurse fellowship programs over the past two years, and no two have ever looked exactly alike because we constantly refine the curriculum in response to changing educational needs.

Be alert for opportunities to get people out of their silos and practicing together in the simulation center. As word of the center's success spreads, new groups will express interest in using simulation as an educational tool. Although these groups may initially want to train individually, encourage them to embrace interdisciplinary team education as soon as they are comfortable in their new simulation environment, thereby meeting the recommendation for interdisciplinary team training put forth by the Institute of Medicine.

As the center grows, it may be useful to establish a formal steering committee consisting of your organization's leadership and members from the larger educational community in your region. There is great value in having high-quality input from a variety of sources both within and outside your organization. Explore ways to use the center for community outreach; for example, open the center to public school students to expose them to the various health sciences careers. The possibilities for an interdisciplinary simulation center are endless.

References

Bloom, B., Mesia, B., & Krathwohl, D. (1964). *Taxonomy of educational objectives* (Vols. 1–2). New York: David McKay.

Dewey, J. (1994). Thinking in education. In L. B. Barnes, C. R. Christensen, & A. J. Hansen (Eds.), *Teaching and the case method* (3rd ed., pp. 9–14) Boston: Harvard Business School Press.

Dunn, W. (Ed.). (2004). *Simulators in critical care and beyond.* Des Plaines, IL: Society of Critical Care Medicine.

Gordon, J., Oriol, N., & Cooper, J. (2004). Bringing good teaching cases "to life": A simulator-based medical education service. *Academic Medicine, 79,* 23–27.

Kohn, L., Corrigan, J., & Donaldson, M. (Eds.). (2000). *To err is human: Building a safer health system.* Washington, DC: National Academy Press.

Lupien, A. (2007). High fidelity patient simulation. In M. Bradshaw & A. Lowenstein (Eds.), *Innovative teaching strategies in nursing and related health professions* (4th ed., pp. 197–214). Sudbury, MA: Jones and Bartlett.

Rudolph, J., Simon, R., Dufresne, R., & Raemer, D. (2006). There's no such thing as "nonjudgmental" debriefing: A theory and method for debriefing with good judgment. *Simulation in Healthcare, 1*(1), 49–55.

Simpson, E. (1972). *The classification of educational objectives in the psychomotor domain* (Vol. 3). Washington, DC: Gryphon House.

Society for Simulation in Healthcare. (2008). [Sim center directory]. Unpublished. Retrieved July 3, 2008, from: http://www.ssih.org/public

An Interdisciplinary Simulation Training and Education Program for an All-Hazards Response

Joy Spellman

INTRODUCTION

In any disaster—whether natural, accidental, or intentionally delivered by the hand of someone who would choose to do us harm—the effects of the event can be significantly minimized by a well-trained response. Since the tragic events of September 11, 2001, discipline-specific education programs designed to increase competency levels have gone a long way toward improving categorical response skill sets. The Center for Public Health Preparedness at Burlington County College in New Jersey has established a simulation center that offers customized, multidisciplinary training for this purpose throughout the state. The establishment of this simulation center as a valid and effective training resource is discussed in this chapter.

CENTER FOR PUBLIC HEALTH PREPAREDNESS

State and local response systems have been in place since civic-minded citizens in colonial times joined forces when this country took its first halting steps as a nation. Local response teams—which are as varied as the communities they serve—have evolved with the times, improving their response times, providing continuing education, and employing new technology in the service of the general public. In the past, disaster response was often a narrowly focused event solely managed by the semblance of responders available. The devastating terrorist attacks on the United States on September 11 illustrated with chilling detail the pressing need to expand the focus of emergency response. Terrorism preparedness, encompassing chemical, biological, radiological, nuclear, and explosive (CBRNE) agents and appropriate responses to them, has been clearly identified as an area in which new skills must be developed (Spellman, 2007). Similarly, geographic isolation is no longer seen as an effective response approach. What happened on that beautiful day in

September in New York City, Washington, D.C., and the Pennsylvania country-side required a response from the entire country.

The Center for Public Health Preparedness (CPHP) program was initiated in 2000 to strengthen emergency preparedness by linking academic expertise with state and local agencies. The Centers for Disease Control and Prevention (CDC) has since provided funding to colleges and universities across the nation to establish a network of training and education resources. After the tragic events of September 11, 2001, this network took on the challenge of emergency preparedness in the face of terrorism. The CPHP has the following national goals:

- Strengthen public health workforce readiness through implementation of programs reflecting newly identified needs.
- Strengthen capacity at state and local levels for terrorism preparedness and emergency public health response (CDC, 2002).

The CDC has further outlined key priorities for funding agencies:

- Identify existing preparedness materials.
- Promote linkage between healthcare organizations and public health agencies across the country.
- Enhance the evidence base for effective preparedness (CDC, 2003).

Furthermore, CDC funding has strategically directed each CPHP to deliver competency-based training and education that meets the identified needs of the state and local agencies (Columbia University School of Nursing Center for Health Policy, 2002).

THE CENTER FOR PUBLIC HEALTH PREPAREDNESS
AT BURLINGTON COUNTY COLLEGE

Burlington County College, a comprehensive community college, is located in New Jersey's largest county and holds as one of its goals to provide state-of-the-art technologies in the education and training of all individuals through an appropriate mix of delivery systems.

Among its four campus locations, the Mount Laurel campus is the hub of science, mathematic, and technology studies. Recognizing its long tradition of community-based education, Burlington County College applied for and received designation as a Center for Public Health Preparedness Specialty Center.

A well-trained front-line response can reduce the impact of emergency incidents. In New Jersey, state and local responders and employers designated for emergency management duties are not always afforded the opportunity to train adequately to respond to large-scale incidents. Inherent in the nature of terrorist and natural threats to the public health is their comparatively infrequent occurrence. The randomness of such events does not afford responders the experience required to improve response to disaster. Indeed, many charged with responding may understand classroom and textbook response to a crisis situation, but they are often unsure of their role in an actual event. To address this situation, Burlington County College established the Center for Public Health Preparedness Simulation Center.

High-fidelity patient simulation is a rapidly growing educational modality that allows trainees to respond to scripted scenarios, with the goal of improving their critical-thinking and decision-making skills. Using simulation as a teaching tool can test and evaluate actual response—something a static classroom environment and a textbook can never provide. In addition, the use of simulation to identify training gaps and weaknesses is generally accepted more readily by the trainee.

The primary goal of the center is to increase the number of front-line public health workers at state and local levels who are competent and prepared to respond to terror-related incidents, infectious disease outbreaks, and other threats to public health. To meet this goal, our CPHP has assured the CDC that we will do the following:

- Develop and implement a simulation laboratory that will provide ongoing education and training to public health workers, first responders, clinicians, and civic business leaders utilizing scripted scenarios for high-fidelity human patient simulators and scripted scenario development for three-dimensional computer simulation.
- Install all major software related to emergency response, including pluming software, biological and chemical agent databases, and radiological detection and informational databases with demographic, topographic, and meteorological information.

With this program in place, the dedicated staff at the CPHP set out to establish Burlington County College as a valid effective training site with measurable outcomes.

PLANNING: THE ROAD TO PREPAREDNESS

Disaster planning must be an evolving document to be used to respond to and eventually recover from an emergency event. To craft such a plan, input from multidisciplinary responders is essential. Institutionally, Burlington County College set out to assess the training needs of not just the region, but the state.

The national network of CPHPs must accelerate availability and access to terrorism-specific training as a part of its public health workforce development plan. Furthermore, CDC-defined competencies for curricula development and evaluation of competency-based training validate the current approach (CDC, 2005). Auf der Heide (2006) has noted that disaster planning is only as good as the assumptions on which it is based. To establish a successful simulation site, Burlington County College examined several assumptions concerning the use of the center as a training venue. New Jersey is the most densely populated state in the union, home to more than 8 million citizens and 41,000 miles of roadway. Thus the first assumption to be altered was that trainees would travel to the simulation lab from a distance. Additionally, it is not reasonable to expect certain agencies to suspend operations or leave minimum staffing in place to travel for training. In promoting safe response for both the responder and potential victim through the use of simulation technology, reducing on-site staffing defeats the goal of the simulation experience. Quarantelli (1983) noted that those who may respond in a disaster may not be from the home community; therefore, to assure effective planning, responders out of jurisdiction must be included in planning and training events. Having observed principles of assumptions versus reality, the CPHP broadened its point of view to include statewide training in a variety of settings.

A multidisciplinary approach to emergency response training must be coordinated to be effective. In a state as diversified—both geographically and culturally—as New Jersey, the technical and/or clinical staff of the CPHP must meet to discuss the requesting agency's training needs. In utilizing a high-fidelity patient simulator, a rural area scenario may be developed, keeping in mind that a hospital may be a 20-minute drive from the planned training site. In an urban location, rush hour traffic may add to the complexity of the response. As these examples suggest, the training plan must be reflective of the culture of the region or the organization itself.

Training at our simulation center may be conducted in the 5000-square-foot, state-of-the-art laboratory; alternatively, arrangements may be made to drill and/or train in the requesting facility. The CPHP has also provided simulation during large-scale, multiagency field drills (see Figure 8-1). No matter what the setting, all simulation scenarios are custom designed. This approach assures that each training opportunity delivers the most realistic simulated experience possible. This point is significant in terms of simulation in a prehospital setting as opposed to an emergency room environment or hospital unit.

Competencies for public health emergency preparedness have been outlined elsewhere (Gebbie, 2002) and include analytic assessment skills, basic public health communications, and community-based practice. The CDC has endorsed training to increase competencies for public health emergency preparedness. In prehospital training, coordination and communication among multidisciplinary team members, including law enforcement and personnel at receiving hospitals, must be included as part of the program. Solid competency-based practices are not diminished or obscured by the inclusion of a multidisciplinary response force.

While exercising in a hospital setting, the simulation training tests clinical response, outcomes, and clinical skill sets. Evacuation, in-vacuation (moving occupants to a secure area within the same building), and the use of personal protective equipment may be added layers to the session. In one exercise conducted at a large hospital, the response to an accidental radiological release in the nuclear medicine department was tested using high-fidelity patient simulators as "patients" with varying degrees of morbidity who populated the area. Running such a scenario provides staff with ample opportunities to test and revise their response plan before an actual event presents itself.

Put simply, the simulation center's planning efforts take into consideration the needs of all training groups. This effort is time-consuming and labor-intensive to be sure. But is it effective? To date, more than 8000 responders have trained through this facility. In this sense, planning our program is indeed the path to preparedness.

Figure 8-1   Simulation Setup for a Field Drill

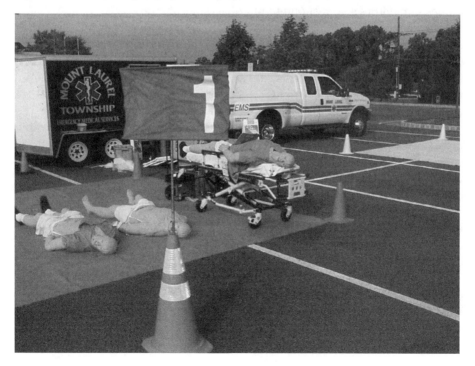

WHAT ARE SIMULATORS?

Simulation training has been utilized for decades in other educational settings, such as aviation, medical schools, and military operations. In the context of disaster response, the use of high-fidelity patient simulators is the only way to train, test, and learn from a real-time, all-hazards incident before an actual occurrence. Simulators, simply put, allow practitioners and responders to practice without harming real patients. During a large-scale drill, the presence of simulators allows the professional, for example, to intubate a patient, stem the arterial flow of blood from a wound, or stabilize a compound fracture.

We have purchased simulators that represent the three levels of fidelity: low, moderate, and high. The term *fidelity* refers to the complexity of the mannequin. Low-fidelity simulators allow the trainee to practice a specific skill on a one-on-one basis, such as immunization or changing a "patient"-occupied bed. Moderate-fidelity simulators are more realistic, although their clinical characteristics are not physiologically correct. Many of these simulators offer trainees the opportunity to listen to breath sounds; however, the chest does not rise. By contrast, high-fidelity simulators gently persuade students to suspend their disbelief and expand their imaginations. These mannequins blink, breathe, and have various and programmable breath, heart, and bowel sounds. They can be intubated, primed with fluids to bleed, cry, and urinate. High-fidelity simulators also respond to pharmacological interventions.

We use one type of fidelity simulator or a combination of types depending on the scenario we are running (Institute of Medicine and National Research Council, 1999). For example, in a field drill where the trainees wished to test their trauma intervention skills, physicians arriving on scene who ordered morphine, 1 mg, for their "patients" then watched as the simulators responded as actual victims would.

High-fidelity simulators are particularly effective when programmed within a particular time frame. For example, three of our four high-fidelity patient simulators "died" on a field after responders failed to intervene within 20 minutes of the call. Given this outcome, one might be inclined to think of the exercise as a failure. To the contrary: The responders encountered construction en route to the mock disaster site and formulated alternative routes after this exercise's debriefing, resulting in a successful drill the second time it was run. Through the simulation, we learned that disasters are chaotic, disorienting, and stressful. No form of preparation is a waste of time and effort.

The CPHP purchased a computer-based simulation system that covers emergency response incidents with a multidisciplinary approach because it was recognized that response to disasters requires a certain level of preparedness training for nonclinical professionals (i.e., administrators, managers, and in-house law enforcement officers). Today's computer platforms provide for

Figure 8-2   Simulation Setup for a Trauma-Based Field Drill (Plane Crash)

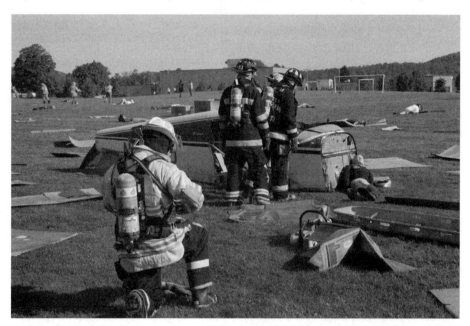

realistic and interactive synthetic environments for almost any training scenario (Advanced Interactive Systems, 2006). The computer's generated images can place the trainee in a variety of settings, including natural environments, urban areas, movable building interiors, airports, and schools. The desktop program in the simulation center can accommodate 25 trainees at a time, allowing for homogenous or multidisciplinary participants to test their role as responders among other responding groups.

The virtual environments are graphically robust, possessing high-resolution 3-D visualizations. High-fidelity sound and acoustics immerse the trainee in the setting. A joystick allows the learner to navigate through the unfolding incident.

Simulation technology may be used in a simple application such as testing an evacuation plan or in a multidimensional setting as illustrated in a trauma-based field exercise (see Figure 8-2). Whether low-fidelity simulators or the most complex models are used, training using simulation offers the learner several benefits:

- Simulation training is convenient and can be flexibly scheduled. The CPHP will train on weekends and on all shifts.
- Training reduces risk to victims while providing experience for students in a nonthreatening environment.

- Simulation training boosts confidence.
- Simulation provides realism on visual, physiological, and environmental levels.
- Simulation is an active form of learning.
- Simulation affords the student a comfortable degree of latitude during the learning process. The student can repeat a skill until proficiency is achieved.
- High-fidelity patient simulators record interventions as they occur, providing teacher and trainee alike with objective feedback.
- A variety of scenarios are available for training purposes, including uncommon ones (Gordon, Wrekerson, Shaffer, & Armstrong, 2001; Kobayashi, Shapero, Suner, & Williams, 2003; Nehring, Ellis, & Lashley, 2001).

As the risk of using simulation as a training modality may sound too good to be true, it is important to acknowledge that this learning system also has some drawbacks:

- Simulation is a relatively new technology. In terms of its use in disaster preparedness training, it is a cutting-edge development. There may be some reticence on the part of trainees to engage in the experience. To allay their fears, the CPHP does a 30-minute general assessment session where trainees can observe, touch, listen, and become comfortable with the technology.
- Simulation interactions are impersonal.
- Accessibility to simulation training is limited. Privately owned operations rarely open their doors to trainees.
- Skilled simulation technicians are a scarce resource. Formal training through the simulation companies is costly.
- High-fidelity patient simulators are expensive. They range in price from $20,000 to $200,000. Warranty coverage can also be expensive.
- To conduct in-house training, sufficient space is needed (Gordon et al., 2001; Nehring et al., 2001).

SIMULATION RESOURCE MANAGEMENT

The CDC award of $755,000 was a generous one, and it allows the CPHP at Burlington County College to operate one of the nation's largest civilian simulation centers. Like many institutions, Burlington County College originally had four simulators that were used exclusively in the nursing program:

- One top-of-the-line high-fidelity model that is not portable
- One pediatric high-fidelity simulator

Figure 8-3   Simulator Models at the Burlington County College CPHP Lab

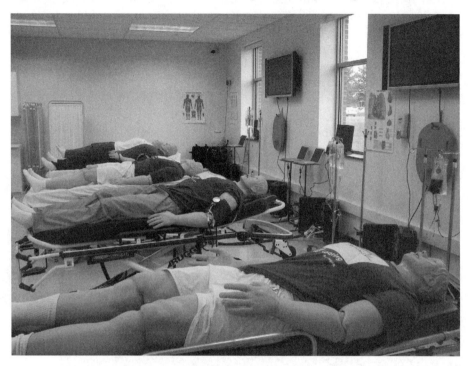

- One infant high-fidelity model
- One adult emergency care (ECS) high-fidelity portable simulator

In 2003, the state of New Jersey purchased 10 ECS models to use for training after the CDC designated Burlington County College as a CPHP lab (see Figure 8-3). This author proposed that the state-owned simulators be housed at the simulation center with assurance that all 21 counties would benefit from their use. The simulators arrived and within days were part of a multijurisdictional field drill. Simulators have been a part of emergency preparedness activities ever since.

Grant monies are a scarce resource, so they should be used judiciously. A 1500-square-foot classroom was identified as the laboratory for the CPHP. Desks in the room were left in place to hold desktop and laptop computers purchased with grant funds. The simulation software described earlier was acquired and downloaded onto all machines. Training for staff was provided by the software company. Accordingly, because the simulators were delivered to us by the New Jersey State Department of Health and Senior Services, the need to expend grant funds for simulators was replaced by the need to support these valuable machines by purchasing medical equipment and supplies to transform the classroom into a realistic clinical environment. Calls were placed to the region's hospitals to see if any old equipment could be donated. Several Strykers, two hospital beds, and some waiting room furniture found their way to the laboratory. Expired IV fluids, catheters, and airway management trays were donated. Through the magic of the Internet, used equipment—a crash cart, ER overhead lamp, EKG machine, pediatric cribs, and wheelchairs—were bought at deep discounts.

Burlington County College has a rich history of investing in technology. To make its simulation laboratory as immersive as possible, four large-screen plasma televisions were wall mounted and connected to each simulator's laptop, resulting in an easy-to-read means of visual affirmation for trainees. Two wireless simulators—perfect for field drills—were purchased by the center at the grant's end.

As the center was accumulating its equipment stock, feedback from statewide agencies suggested that traveling to the center for training might

Figure 8-4   Simulator Trailer

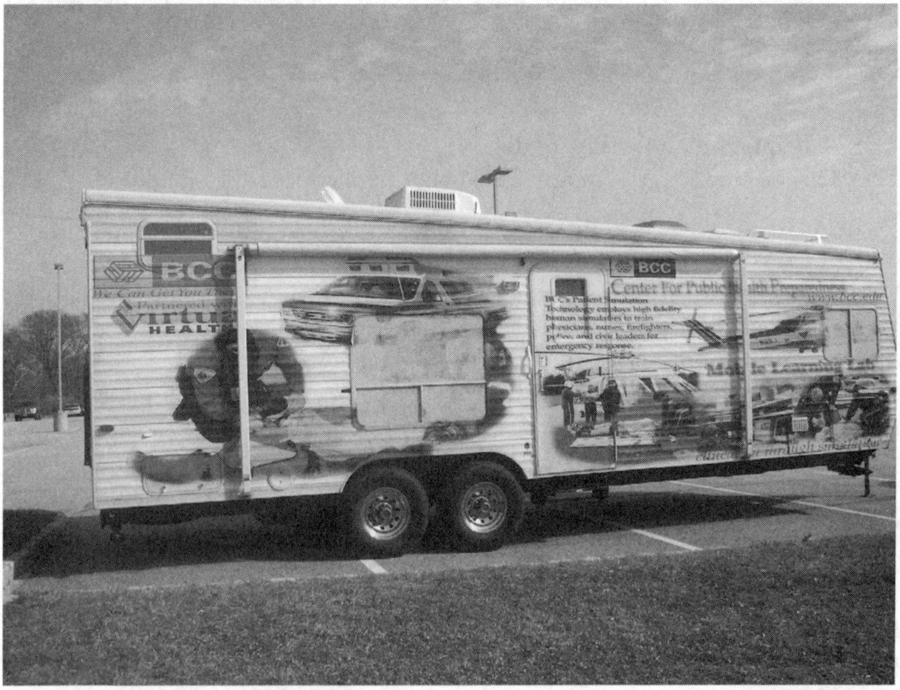

prove troublesome. An investigation into the possibility of purchasing a trailer to transport simulators to other parts of the state began. Fortunately, the college offered an existing pickup truck and a 30-foot trailer. The CPHP was now mobile (see Figure 8-4)!

Mobile capacity may be the single most significant innovation employed by the CPHP. As noted earlier, New Jersey is the most densely populated state in the country; however, the state is only 172 miles long. Although the process is labor intensive for CPHP staff, the benefit of having simulation drills on-site makes the effort worthwhile for all involved. With mobility comes expense, of course. Tolls, truck maintenance, and parking fees are budgeted under local travel.

Resource management also necessitates building, nurturing, and maintaining partnerships (Kyle, Via, Lowy, Madsen, Marty, & Mongan, 2004). Indeed, partnerships are the lifeblood of any organization. The continuation of these arrangements assures successful growth and quality improvement. Burlington County College's partnership with the state of New Jersey is an excellent example. More than $1 million in simulator equipment resides at the simulation center. In turn, more than 8000 responder groups representing each of the state's 21 counties have received training through the CPHP.

The simulation center recently accepted delivery of three new simulators from the state, two pediatric and one infant, bringing the total number of simulators at the CPHP to 19. This partnership is mutually beneficial to all involved. The CPHP and state continue to explore ways to strengthen the partnership and improve service delivery.

Burlington County College has leveraged the center's equipment, training, and space in innovative ways. Nevertheless, nothing gets done without reliable, technologically proficient staff. Finding such employees in 2005 proved a challenge in terms of obtaining the appropriate skills and finding interest in an emerging field. Through the college's well-established tradition of implementing technology on all levels of operations institutionally, employees and students from the science, mathematics, and technology traits were recruited to work at the center. State department funds were used to train employees over a five-day period by the simulation company representatives. This three-way partnership continues as the technologies expand.

SEE HOW IT RUNS

The New Jersey Commission in Science and Technology supports the development of technology-based business. For example, Burlington County College's High Technology Small Business and Life Science Incubator is an engine for economic growth in New Jersey, creating new jobs, products, and services. In May 2007, the CPHP moved into a new 5000-square-foot laboratory. Desktop computer classrooms and human patient simulation laboratory space occupy separate areas, but are joined architecturally by an administrative area. Burlington County College absorbs the cost of the highly sought-after space.

The evolving nature of simulation technology requires consistent assessment of training needs of the communities served (Institute of Medicine and National Research Council, 1999). The CPHP found that repeat requests for assistance with exercises required multilayered scenarios that will play out quickly with an experienced response team. For example, a preprogrammed chemical spill scenario may be revised to reflect preexisting cardiopulmonary disease or coexisting trauma related to the incident. The physiological benchmarks must also be accurate. The instruction book that accompanies each simulator serves as a great resource; however, to delve into the inner workings of the simulator, more intense training is needed. Technical training in such a distinct subspecialty is not routinely available; notwithstanding this constraint, the simulation center at Burlington County College utilizes these resources for staff development and to jump-start professional enthusiasm:

- Personalized training through the simulation manufacturer can provide staff members with invaluable insight into programming and maintenance of the simulator. Although it is certainly not inexpensive, this program of study lends itself to a train-the-trainer methodology and allows all employees to benefit from the one-on-one training.
- Larger, more established simulation companies host annual conferences that offer numerous break-out sessions to the attendees, many of which include hands-on experience. These symposiums also allow attendees to develop long-distance relationships with staff at other simulation centers.
- Joining professional associations can prove valuable. Many have an international membership, such as the International Society for Simulation in Health Care, and regional simulation groups are often supported by simulation-equipment vendors.
- Checking into CDC-funded CPHP networks and visiting the Web sites of CPHPs can uncover a treasure trove of information. Many offer free links for video conferencing, allowing staff to learn without leaving home base. Some CPHPs provide educational DVDs at no charge. While learning about how to operate its own system, the simulation laboratory will be able to add to its resource library.
- Local talent and expertise may be available. Ask law enforcement officials to provide in-service education to staff members about the importance of crime scene investigation or evidence preservation. Your team

may find the new information helpful in terms of programming and simulator placement.

- Network, network! Surely one of the best ways to build relationships and contacts, networking is also an effective means to disseminate information (Pittaway, Robertson, Munir, Denyer, & Neely, 2004). If you are shy, consider volunteering and connecting with people in a setting that is familiar and comfortable. Networking may lead to collaboration on projects and grant funding so always bring a supply of business cards.
- Allow staff "practice" time. At the Burlington County College simulation center, one practice day is blocked out each month to provide staff with time to practice their skills in an area of their choosing. Each staff member works with a simulator of his or her choosing and may run through scenarios, practice moulage techniques, or work on becoming more familiar with medical terminology.

Finding sufficient staff for such labor-intensive work might strain many a department's budget. Based on this author's experience, failure to recruit students to work in the center would be a serious oversight. Generally speaking, students are computer savvy and not intimidated by the constantly changing technology. Additionally, the work experience serves as an impressive addition to a resume. Students who worked in the CPHP at Burlington County College have become graduates of the Community Emergency Response Team (CERT) and have successfully completed free online Federal Emergency Management Administration (FEMA) coursework. Many students qualify for student financial aid, and their salaries are paid from federal monies.

Simulation exercises require a lot of time before, during, and after the event. To illustrate this point, consider this timeline for a field drill the CPHP conducted:

February 1: Inquiry received by the CPHP.

February 13: Follow-up call to set up a face-to-face meeting.

February 28: Meeting at the requesting agency is held. A formal request is made for an in-house drill and evacuation to be held May 15. Scenario: influenza outbreak at long-term care facility with transport to hospital.

March 15: Telephone conference to discuss clinical programming to be approved for clinical content by CPHP director.

April 1: CPHP member makes an on-site visit to assure that the power source is sufficient and access barriers are identified. Team member proceeds to the hospital to familiarize staff with the plan.

April–May: Scenario is constructed and revised.

May 10–13: Scenario run-through is conducted with all staff.

May 14: Trailer is loaded and equipment is secured and reviewed against the department checklist.

May 15: CPHP crew arrives 90 minutes before the start of the drill to unpack, set up, moulage, and power up. After exercise activities, the team participates in debriefings to improve CPHP performance.

May 16–17: Unpack, deprogram, clean, and flush the simulators.

Imagine a CPHP conducting two drills weekly. Welcome to the world of emergency preparedness using simulation technology!

Is simulation effective as a training tool? Without a doubt. Is it labor intensive? Absolutely. Is it expensive? You bet. In fact, anything termed "labor intensive" has a significant expenditure of labor in comparison to capital. Without grant funding, costs of simulation are significant, most particularly when mobile training is involved. The CPHP at Burlington County College is a public venture, and 13 of its simulators are owned by the state of New Jersey. Under the terms of the agreement forged between the partners, no training fees may be charged. Fees may be collected for training on Burlington County College equipment, however.

Mobile training, as illustrated by the timeline referenced earlier, almost always involves overtime for personnel. Tolls, gasoline, and simulation equipment, including carbon dioxide canisters and fabricated body fluids, must also be factored into the cost analysis. A breakdown of travel costs distributed to financial department personnel for review in 2007 suggests a cost of $1600 for the actual drill event. Factoring in the preparation and resolution phases, the true cost hovers around $5000. The CPHP staff, however, are committed to the philosophy that we will deliver more than is expected. To that end, Burlington County College continues to fund the operation of the CPHP as an exhaustive search for operational funding continues.

A NURSE IS A NURSE IS A NURSE . . . NOT!

Make no mistake about it: There will not be an effective response to a disaster without a nursing presence, starting with planning. Nursing leaders within institutions—both public and private—must insist on being included as key players in the planning process. Resource identification is an essential part of disaster planning (Veenema, 2003); because nurses practicing in all disciplines are recognized experts in resource allocation, their inclusion in all aspects of planning is crucial to the success of the plan. Likewise, assessment, intervention, and evaluation are skills nurses use daily. If simulation is to be used in exercise planning, nurses' input in the form of clinical knowledge is required. During pre-drill meetings between the CPHP at Burlington County College, a nurse must be present. Without his or her presence, the meeting will not be concluded. Before the scenario is approved for simulation planning, a nurse reviews clinical context to ensure the accuracy of the stages and transitions of the content.

In New Jersey, the importance of the roles played by nurses in disaster planning is evidenced by their inclusion on regional and state preparedness committees. Participation on committees enables nurses to share their abilities with the rest of the response team. This exchange becomes a two-way street for nurses: They have the opportunity to learn more about the roles of other responders. Given the nature of nursing practice, collaboration in all settings of practice lends itself to being a part of an interdisciplinary framework (Spellman, 2007). In building partnerships among nursing colleagues, public health nurses are well placed to bridge the gap that often separates prehospital intervention and hospital admission. All field drills using the CPHP simulators call upon nurse representatives of local and county health departments to act as on-site responders. These field nurses take on the role of direct communicators with ER participants, sharing their assessment skills from the disaster site with the receiving facilities.

Within a nursing practice framework, multiple-nursing-specialty simulation is an excellent way to foster collegiality among nurses who recognize the need to become proficient in disaster response-related skills. To repeat, there will not be a response without nurses.

FUTURE DIRECTIONS

A survey entitled "Ready and Willing" revealed that 80% of nurses and physicians polled were more than willing to respond to a disaster, but only 20% believed that they had the knowledge and skills to do so safely (Alexander & Wynia, 2003). Preparing nurses of varied backgrounds to respond to incidents that they have never seen before and may encounter very infrequently requires new and creative approaches to education and training (Spellman, 2007). Practice builds both competency and confidence, which explains why a basic all-hazards introduction to biological, chemical, radiological, and explosive events, along with response guidelines, should be routinely included in the undergraduate nursing curriculum. Ideally, this basic coursework will stress the importance of nursing assessment, infection control, proper use of personal protective equipment (PPE), interdisciplinary communication, and participation in all planning activities. General nursing programs in New Jersey already offer their students just such an introduction: a two-hour lecture followed by a two-hour simulation laboratory experience.

Continuing education credits for nursing in this field must be developed as well, with attention being given to content reflective of the practice setting: prehospital, school, hospital, or corporate. Efforts are under way in New Jersey to offer continuing education units (CEUs) in disaster preparedness. Through this coursework, nurses can increase their knowledge base and build their competency levels while meeting state licensing requirements. The challenge, however, is to find ways to offer programs to nurses that will interest, educate, and revitalize the nurses' sense of being an integral part of a response. Video conferencing, online offerings, and local conferences are all ways to meet the requirements for CEUs.

At the CPHP at Burlington County College, we are looking at ways in which nurses and physicians can use and benefit from the computer-based system presently used for nonclinical responders. This system would allow both clinical and administrative personnel to interact on screen within the context of a disaster event. For example, one can assemble all participants in the classroom together and have them respond as they would in an actual event. Each station operates independently. In this simulation modality, nurses exercise their roles within an agency along with other members of their institution's response team. Such an exercise can help identify weaknesses and strengths in the institution's emergency plan. Revisions to the plan can then assure that the emergency response document does not become static.

Reflecting the tumultuous time we live in, agencies, schools, and institutions must keep abreast of the many challenges that are constantly arising. Likewise, nurses must take their rightful place as a member of emergency response teams. The simulation center at Burlington County College will work with nurses in New Jersey to see that happen.

References

Advanced Interactive Systems. (2006). *Reality response software project.* Retrieved January 16, 2008, from http://www.ais-sim.com

Alexander, G. C., & Wynia, M. K. (2003). Ready and willing? Physicians' sense of preparedness for bioterrorism. *Health Affairs, 22,* 189–197.

Auf der Heide, E. (2006. The importance of evidence-based disaster planning. *Annals of Emergency Medicine, 47*(1), 34–49.

Centers for Disease Control and Prevention (CDC). (2002). *Centers for Public Health Preparedness: Goals.* Retrieved November 16, 2007, from http://www.cdc.gov

Centers for Disease Control and Prevention (CDC). (2003). *Centers for Public Health Preparedness: Guidance for public health emergency preparedness.* Retrieved November 16, 2007, from http://www.cdc.gov

Centers for Disease Control and Prevention (CDC). (2005). *Centers for Public Health Preparedness network activities: National public health emergency preparedness curriculum.* Retrieved November 16, 2007, from http://www.cdc.gov

Columbia University School of Nursing Center for Health Policy. (2002). *Bioterrorism and emergency readiness competencies for public health workers*. Atlanta: Centers for Disease Control and Prevention.

Gebbie, K. M. (2002). Emergency and disaster preparedness. Care competencies for nurses: What every nurse should and may not know. *American Journal of Nursing, 102*, 46.

Gordon, J. A., Wrekerson, W. M., Shaffer, D. W., & Armstrong, E. G. (2001). "Practicing" medicine without risk: Students and educators response to high fidelity patient simulation. *Academy of Medicine, 76*, 469–472.

Institute of Medicine and National Research Council. (1999). *Chemical and biological terrorism: Research and development to improve civilian medical response*. Washington, DC: National Academy Press.

Kobayashi, L., Shapero, M., Suner, S., & Williams, K. (2003). Disaster medicine: The potential role of high fidelity medical simulation for mass casualty incident training. *Medicine and Health Rhode Island, 86*, 196–200.

Kyle, R., Via, K. K., Lowy, R. J., Madsen, J. M., Marty, A. M., & Mongan, P. D. (2004). A multidisciplinary approach to teach responses to weapons of mass destruction and terrorism using combined modalities. *Journal of Clinical Anesthesia, 16*, 152–158.

Nehring, W. M., Ellis, W. E., & Lashley, F. R., (2001). Human patient simulation in nursing education: An overview. *Simulation and Gaming, 32*, 194–204.

Pittaway, L., Robertson, M., Munir, K., Denyer, D., & Neely, A. (2004). Networking and innovation: A systematic review of the evidence. *International Journal of Management Review, 5/6*(3 & 4), 137–168.

Quarantelli, E. L. (1983). *Delivery of emergency medical care in disasters: Assumptions and realities*. New York: Irvington.

Spellman, J. (2007). The role in preparation of the public health nurse in disaster response. In T. Veenema (Ed.), *Disaster nursing and emergency preparedness for chemical, biological and radiological terrorism and other hazards* (pp. 588–599). New York: Springer.

Veenema, T. G. (2003). Chemical and biological terrorism preparedness for staff development specialists. *Journal for Nurses in Staff Development, 19*, 218–225.

CHAPTER 9

Hospital-Based
Competency Development

Linda J. von Reyn

The current challenges faced by healthcare settings are well documented in the professional and lay literature. The scarcity of appropriately prepared nursing personnel, the aging of the population, and the cost of providing health care has created a situation that requires immediate and innovative solutions. Rovin and Formella (2004) describe the current issues in nursing as being "qualitative" rather than "quantitative" in nature. By this terminology, they mean that the issues faced by the nursing profession are not just a shortage of adequate numbers of nurses, but rather the dissatisfaction of nurses from working in a "system" that is designed neither to make the work easy nor to function as a system with well-coordinated components. Redesign of the healthcare system has been, to date, overwhelming or undesirable to the many vested parties, and the United States continues to struggle with a general shortage of many professional and allied healthcare resources. It was in response to staff nurse shortages and a changing demographic of nurse applicants that Dartmouth-Hitchcock Medical Center (DHMC) implemented a Nurse Residency Program that embedded high-fidelity human patient simulation into its efforts to develop competency in novice nurses.

PLANNING

One unique feature of DHMC is its rural and relatively remote location. While this environment is attractive to many, one must be satisfied with this type of social setting when seeking employment in the area. DHMC, an integrated academic medical center, provides inpatient care services at Mary Hitchcock Memorial Hospital, a 429-bed tertiary care hospital within the full-service tertiary care medical center. The average case mix index of 1.71 results in an inpatient population with high acuity that requires complex treatments and interventions, and has complex healthcare needs. In addition, DHMC is located within a federally designated area of underserved rural citizens. The lack of local healthcare resources causes rural citizens to delay seeking out health care until their situation has reached a level of significant need.

Creating a Nurse Residency Program

The unique features of a tertiary medical center in a rural setting with very high patient acuity created special challenges for attracting adequate numbers of qualified nurses. By 2003, it was clear that it would be impossible to maintain adequate staffing levels if DHMC continued to rely heavily on attracting experienced nurses. There were growing staffing shortages, limited experienced nurse applicants, and a seeming excess of recent-graduate applicants—that is, nurses who were newly graduated from their nursing program or who had been in practice for less than nine months. The Directors of Nursing Practice and Nursing Research, in partnership with an Education Associate, brainstormed solutions for integration of recent-graduate nurses into a highly complex, acute care setting.

The structure of a Nurse Residency Program was developed and a Health Resources and Services Administration (HRSA) grant application was submitted and awarded. The project had two overarching purposes:

- To implement and evaluate an innovative residency program with both theoretical and clinical components designed to assist recent-graduate registered nurses in their transition from novice to competent nursing practice in medical/surgical specialties
- To expand and strengthen critical care specialty practice using innovative educational experiences for recent graduates and registered nurses with experience at both DHMC and other rural hospitals that were members of an existing consortium, the Dartmouth-Hitchcock Alliance (DHA)

The existence of HRSA grant support was crucial in the early development of the program. It provided support to both personnel and equipment needed to establish the program.

Program Description

The responsibility for implementation of the program was incorporated into the work of the Office of Professional Nursing, a centralized nursing office designed to support the practice, education, and research interests of direct care nurses. The details of the Nurse Residency Program and Year 1 outcomes have been described by Beyea, von Reyn, and Slattery (2007). The program started in 2004, was 12 weeks in length, and had three distinct tracks: Medical/Surgical, Pediatric, and Adult and Pediatric Critical Care.

It subsequently expanded to include Intensive Care Nursery, Birthing Pavilion, and an Emergency Department Bridge Program. The Medical/Surgical tract consisted of 80 hours of didactic/skills/instruction and self-directed learning exercises, 40 hours of integrated simulated experiences using a high-fidelity patient simulator, and 380 hours of clinical experience with a preceptor delivered over the duration of the 12-week program. The Critical Care components of the program included 160 hours of didactic/skills/instruction, 80 hours of integrated simulation experiences, and more than 700 hours of clinical experience with a preceptor. Examples of didactic and simulated topics can be found in Table 9-1. For the purposes of this chapter, the focus of interest will

Table 9-1   Nurse Residency Program Didactic and Simulated Clinical Topics

Didactic Topics:	
Physical comfort management	Human factors: patient safety
Psychological comfort support	Communicating with the healthcare team
Activity/exercise management	Infection management
Elimination management	Medication safety
Nutrition support	Safe patient handling
Neurological management	Device and patient interface
Respiratory management	Age specific considerations
Skin and wound management	Latex allergy
Cardiac management	Health system/information management
Tissue perfusion management	Patient education
Coping assistance	
Simulated Topics:	
Respiratory: sedation, chest tubes, trach care	Peripheral vascular: deep vein thrombosis (DVT), blood product
Cardiac: shockable and non-shockable rhythms, acute coronary Syndrome, shock	Neurological: stroke, seizures, confusion and restraints
Nutrition/elimination: diabetes, renal failure	

be the development of the Immersive Leaning Lab (simulation lab) and the infrastructure to support the integrated simulation experiences.

Outcomes

Several qualitative and quantitative outcomes were selected for tracking. These included (1) nurse residents' perception of their clinical competence, confidence, and readiness for independent practice; (2) nurse residents' performance in the clinical and simulated environment; and (3) length of orientation. A more detailed explanation of outcomes is presented later in the chapter.

NUMBER AND TYPES OF PERSONNEL FOR STAFFING

General Resources

DHMC was fortunate to have significant resources available to develop and implement the integrated simulation scenarios and experiences. The anesthesia department had begun to use a high-fidelity patient simulator to enhance learning for sedation and resuscitation care. The physician champion of that program assisted the Nurse Residency Program personnel to understand the importance of the Immersive Learning Lab (simulation lab) structure and process and provided technical expertise for simulation resources. In addition, there were 15 clinical nursing specialists, 1 nursing education associate, 4 unit-based clinical educators, and the Directors of Nursing Practice, Nursing Education, and Nursing Research available to assist with development of the program. Additional centralized education associates and unit-based clinical educators were added as the numbers of nurse residents increased.

Integrated Simulation Scenarios

The simulated scenarios occurred within a four-hour block of time within the Immersive Learning Lab. In the first week of the Nurse Residency Program, nurse residents were assigned, based on their clinical specialty (i.e., surgery, medicine, neuroscience), to a team with three or four other nurse residents. This team remained intact throughout the program, ensuring that members of the team learned team dynamics, crew resource management, and closed-loop communication in addition to developing clinical competencies.

Each lab session was videotaped, and at the conclusion of every lab session, the nurse residents participated in reflective learning with their lab facilitator and teammates. This element of the lab experience was considered essential, as the ability to learn through reflection not only assists in the development of competency (Benner, 2000) but also in the development of critical thinking (Forneris, 2004). Finally, each nurse resident was evaluated for his or her behaviors, attitudes, and skill development at the completion of every lab session. The findings of these evaluations were shared with the unit-based educators and preceptors to enhance the ongoing competency development of the nurse resident.

Immersive Learning Lab Resources

To ensure the appropriate expertise was available for the integrated simulation experiences, DHMC hired a Nursing Simulation Specialist who was responsible for the development of curriculum and educational materials for different levels and types of training related to the Immersive Learning Lab. In addition, she coordinated all aspects of the operation, maintenance, support, and troubleshooting for the lab and associated equipment. She was also responsible for training scenario facilitators and bringing the concept of reflective learning into the simulated learning experience.

Because the Immersive Learning Lab was developed in the early days of nursing's use of high-fidelity patient simulators, the Simulation Specialist did not have particular expertise in this field. Rather, she was an individual who possessed the qualities of organization, critical thinking, technical competency, and curiosity. She learned about the technology alongside the directors and other educators, but continued to develop her own expertise in the learning method that exceeded the expertise of others, ultimately becoming an expert in the use of this methodology.

The early integrated simulation experiences were conducted with one educator acting as both the simulator operator and the facilitator of the scenario. After the Nursing Simulation Specialist was hired and additional education associates became available, the standard was to have two educators available for each simulated experience—one educator to operate the simulator and a second educator to facilitate the scenario and associated learning. This setup created the most realistic experience for the nurse resident.

The role of the simulator operator was straightforward—full concentration on the operation and function of the high-fidelity simulator. In contrast, the facilitator served in several roles within the lab, including being a partner to the primary nurse resident, a charge nurse "on the unit," a harried physician, or a distraught family member. Because of this varied role, it was important that the scenario facilitator stay current and be competent in various aspects of clinical practice. For the scenario to be realistic, the facilitator had to be aware of potential complications for the "patient" and real issues and problems that the nurse resident would face in their day-to-day clinical practice.

The role of facilitator was filled by either a centrally based education associate or the unit-based educator from the nurse resident's clinical area.

When education associates were hired, they were selected from a slate of direct care nurses who were interested in shifting their focus to education and orientation. Their current knowledge of clinical practice was considered a key qualification for the role.

Growth in the Nurse Residency Program created significant strain on the personnel responsible for the lab's functioning. During the second year of the program, more than 100 nurse residents participated in the program, which required DHMC to allocate additional resources to the lab. Factors considered in developing the appropriate level of personnel needed for optimal functioning of the Immersive Learning Lab are listed in Table 9-2. Once the needed level of resources was identified, the Senior Nurse Executive advocated for and obtained the requested level of resources from administration.

Of all the personnel resources available to implement the Immersive Learning Lab, the Nursing Simulation Specialist proved to be the most important in bringing the lab up to full function. The depth of knowledge and expertise required to understand the technical components of the lab, including high-fidelity patient simulators, complex audiovisual equipment, and the cognitive components of immersive learning using high-fidelity patient simulators, were such that it was essential to have at least one individual who possessed the full range of competencies in this field. Her ability to understand and schedule personnel, establish the necessary supplies, and support other educators to become accomplished in using the lab was critical to the success of the program.

Table 9-2   Assumptions Used to Determine FTE Resources

- Class preparation equals one-half hour of preparation time for every hour of class, then 25%
- Class time—actual time spent teaching in classroom
- Class up/down—time needed to set up and break down classroom, one hour setup and one hour breakdown
- Simulation prep—one-half hour of preparation time for every hour of simulation, then 25%
- Simulations—two instructors for lab time for each simulation
- Simulation up/down—time needed to set up and break down scenario, one hour setup and one hour breakdown
- Contact/communications—time needed to connect with nurse residents and their local directors and educators. Equals two hours per day per FTE
- Nurse Residency Program FTE Total—total FTE requirement for associate/ specialist working in nurse residents program

FACULTY EDUCATION

On-Site Education

Although the number of nurse residents who participated in the first year of the program was relatively modest ($n = 56$), it was anticipated that a minimum of 100 nurse residents would be educated through the program yearly. The program was designed to incorporate the Nursing Simulation Specialist and both the central and unit-based educators as faculty in the integrated simulation scenarios, working either as the operator or as the facilitator. This evolution led to a large group of nurses who needed first, education on the function of the high-fidelity patient simulator and second, education on the process of immersive learning using high-fidelity patient simulation.

To provide this education, several day-long, on-site sessions were provided by the equipment vendor. As part of these sessions, each faculty member had a computer for his or her own use so as to become familiar with the simulation software. The sessions also provided education on the assembly of the high-fidelity patient simulator. All of the clinical specialists and educators received their initial training at these early sessions. There was also an effort to invite other nurses throughout the medical center who might have an interest in this technology and who might be willing to provide support as needed to the Immersive Learning Lab. Some of the lab faculty were able to attend these sessions twice as a way to reinforce the information being presented.

In addition, nurse educators who regularly served as faculty had the opportunity to attend education sessions that were offered externally. The vendor sponsored a regular "user-group" education session that all of the educators attended at least once. The user-group meetings allowed faculty to become familiar with specific and more detailed elements of simulator operation, be introduced to experiential learning techniques, and network with others who were also learning about this teaching method. In addition, faculty members were able to attend random continuing education meetings offered by specialty organizations that focused on the use of high-fidelity patient simulators as a teaching tool. As possible, faculty were able to attend these various meeting and bring their learning back to the cadre of lab-advocate faculty that had emerged at DHMC.

Education for Academic and Healthcare Partners

After the first year of operations in the Immersive Learning Lab, DHMC received many queries from other healthcare sites that were interested in developing a simulation lab as well as from our academic affiliates whose nursing students did clinical rotations on the DHMC campus. Many were thinking about how they might establish a simulation lab on their own campuses to support students in their acquisition of skills and critical thinking.

Over the course of two years, DHMC offered four, day-long education sessions and invited all interested parties to come and learn about using a high-fidelity patient simulator as an education tool. The break-out sessions at these meetings included information on what was needed to set up a simulation lab, suggestions on how to create a good scenario, and demonstrations of integrated scenarios. Interestingly, some faculty members from academic programs were startled by the acuity of the patients in the various scenarios. They were not aware that recent graduates were asked to take on such intense assignments. This interchange highlighted the need for academic faculty to partner with clinical sites to clearly understand the environment in which recent graduate nurses were being asked to practice. These educational offerings also gave our education associates the opportunity to develop and present material to an audience. This alone was a professional development opportunity for many of the associates.

Early on, our academic partners voiced interest in establishing a simulation lab but often were uncertain about what content to cover in the lab. Through the work with nurse residents, DHMC had determined there were several aspects of practice for which recent graduate nurses needed significant support, regardless of their basic preparation. These items included intravenous (IV) medication administration, blood products administration, IV and patient-controlled analgesia (PCA) pump functions, and response to urgent and emergent health status changes originating from any major system dysfunction—cardiac, respiratory, or hemodynamic, for example. The reason for these areas of deficiency were easy to understand: Nursing students often get very little practice in performing these tasks and functions because they are either prohibited by the clinical site or because they occur so infrequently as to not happen during a particular student's clinical rotation. DHMC suggested that building simulation scenarios that allowed students to practice dealing with these types of events and situations would significantly improve the ability of the recent graduate nurse to enter into the healthcare setting.

Continuing Education

Even after becoming facile with the use of the high-fidelity patient simulator as an educational tool, it was necessary to provide continuing education for faculty to enable them to extend their expertise or to learn about new techniques and equipment. Faculty members had the opportunity every one to two years to attend a regional or national meeting that had a focus of using high-fidelity patient simulators for training. We also encouraged lab faculty to develop abstracts for submission to various specialty meetings. For several years, abstracts developed by DHMC faculty have been accepted for presentation at many national conferences related to simulation.

Inter-rater Reliability

Soon after establishment of the Immersive Learning Lab, it became obvious that work was needed on the development of inter-rater reliability for the integrated scenarios. At the completion of each lab session, the faculty facilitator rated each participant in four general areas: attitude, competency, intellectual skill, and interpersonal skills. These lab ratings were very important in helping faculty to advise the unit-based educator about particular needs for each nurse resident. Faculty understood that it was important to be consistent in how each nurse resident was rated from week to week, and how students were rated in comparison to other nurse residents.

The Nursing Simulation Specialist developed a set of case studies from the archive of scenarios. She then asked each faculty member to view the case study and complete the evaluation tool based on that case study. The variation in how each faculty member evaluated nurse residents could then be examined. Following this exercise, steps were taken to standardize elements of the evaluation. A glossary of terms was created to describe how a nurse resident might perform in the lab, and each faculty person began to evaluate the nurse resident using this standard glossary. As new faculty entered into the lab, they were taught this evaluation technique, which significantly increased consistency of evaluation for the nurse residents.

Maintaining Clinical Awareness

The effectiveness of the faculty facilitators was directly related to their knowledge and awareness of day-to-day clinical practice. This characteristic was important in the selection of faculty members to fill this position. Indeed, it became quite challenging to maintain for nursing associates who spent all of their time working on centralized nursing education and working in the lab. Some of the associates had PRN positions in their previous clinical units, which helped them to maintain their clinical competency. For others, there was an expectation that they would arrange to shadow colleagues in the various clinical areas or would return to their previous units to spend time working during "down" times in the Immersive Learning Lab. Although this expectation was clearly set for faculty, it was and still is consistently difficult for centralized education associates to make or find the time to spend in clinical areas.

DEVELOPING SCENARIOS

To assure consistency in the development of scenarios, a template was created to guide this activity. Initially, scenarios were created to match the Nurse Residency Program class content. Subsequently, scenarios were developed to address other high-risk, low-frequency events as well as events that were more common and that the nurse resident needed to manage frequently. A list of possible scenarios was developed based upon (1) clinical problems—for example, abdominal pain or acute intoxication and withdrawal; (2) skills, such as wound dehiscence and neuraxial analgesia; (3) processes, such as admission, discharge, and giving report; and (4) "typical patient scenarios" or emergency scenarios that might arise in specialty areas, such as neuroscience and hematology/oncology. This list was then used to develop the first set of scenarios and became the ongoing worklist for scenario development.

Each of the educators was asked to develop the case study that would become a scenario and that guided the programming of the high-fidelity simulator. The following format was used for case study development:

1. Scenario label/title
2. Learning objectives for the scenario
3. Case study detail:
   a. Patient history, presenting symptoms, initial lab values, initial plans for medication, initial outcomes
   b. Next phase of patient situation, response to initial plans, ongoing data on signs, symptoms, lab values, medications
   c. Final outcome, disposition

The case study was written as completely as possible to cover all elements of the patient trajectory and their treatment. These details were then used to develop the scenario that would be presented in the lab and to which the nurse resident would react. In addition, the case study was used to program the high-fidelity patient simulator and to develop action points within the simulation—that is, events that required some action by the nurse resident. The introduction of family members and other clinicians into the scenario was planned so as to make it as realistic as possible.

COSTS

There were many direct and indirect costs associated with establishing a simulation lab—for example, personnel costs, equipment costs, space costs, and supply costs. At the initiation of the Nurse Residency Program, the personnel costs and equipment costs were known. The cost for establishing the space was less certain, and the supply costs were an unknown.

Support of Senior Administrators

It was absolutely essential to have the support of the senior administrators when establishing a simulation lab. This point may sound obvious, but the extent to which the Senior Nurse Executive partnered with the project team and advocated for the project throughout the organization was significant. Her support was essential to secure both the necessary space and the fiscal resources for the program. She committed the initial fiscal resources for the purchase of a high-fidelity patient simulator from her departmental budget and secured the remainder of the needed funds by soliciting her colleagues to contribute funds from their respective non-operating, special funds. She was able to garner this support because her ideas for how the simulation lab would support patients and all direct care providers were realistic and compelling. She elicited the support of another senior administrator to assist with price negotiation, as this was his area of particular expertise.

After securing the necessary funds for purchase of the high-fidelity patient simulator, the Senior Nurse Executive advocated for the program with the Executive Vice President to gain his approval for the additional personnel needed to make the project successful. Her initial requests for personnel related to staff that would work directly within the Nurse Residency Program and in the Immersive Learning Lab. Subsequently, however, she requested the addition of unit-based educators needed to support the large number of recent-graduate nurses who, due to the success of the program, were introduced to the clinical setting.

Personnel Costs

Because the Immersive Learning Lab was a component of the Nurse Residency Program, the cost of personnel included the total full-time equivalent (FTE) support needed for the program. One could determine the cost of personnel needed for a simulation lab alone from Table 9-2. The Directors of Nursing Practice and Nursing Research were existing resources. Additional personnel added to staff the lab included the Nursing Simulation Specialist and three nursing education associates; their number was based on the original plan to educate 100 nurse residents yearly. Although the actual resource needs varied greatly throughout the year, with maximum resource needs of 10 FTEs weekly and minimum needs of 1.7 FTEs weekly, the initial request was established at 3 FTEs with a plan to incorporate unit-based educators as necessary. The Nursing Simulation Specialist required master's degree preparation; a baccalaureate degree in nursing was the minimum educational requirement for the education associates.

Understanding that personnel costs have increased over time and vary by region, the initial investment of personnel approximated $344,000 annually, including the cost of benefits. In subsequent years, more nursing associates were added with expansion of the Nurse Residency Program and the Immersive Learning Lab. The return on this investment was great, however: Retention rates for recent-graduate nurses at our hospital increase to 45% over their first three years of employment.

In the first year of the program, DHMC budgeted $6000 to be used toward education of personnel who would be working in the lab. This expense has remained fairly constant through the subsequent years of the program.

Equipment

The initial equipment secured for the Immersive Learning Lab and for integrated scenario simulations consisted of two Universal Patient Simulators (SimMan), manufactured by Laerdal. These high-fidelity patient simulators were the cornerstone of the proposed lab and were equipped with programmed scenarios and responded realistically to clinical situations. The cost of these two items included a Nursing Wound Module and Trauma Module ($31,702 each). Each also came with a compressor and regulator. Each simulator was attached to a dedicated laptop computer that held all the necessary software for case-based scenarios and physiologic responses; each of these two Dell laptop computers cost $3250. A high-fidelity pediatric patient simulator was located in a simulation lab maintained by the anesthesia department. The nurse residents in the Pediatric Track were able to use this pediatric simulator to make their integrated simulation scenarios more realistic.

A key component of the Immersive Learning Lab was the post-scenario reflective learning that occurred in a group setting. To capture the simulation experience and critical thinking, DHMC purchased a digital video equipment package ($4985). This equipment was necessary to load the videos on the computer, thereby augmenting the learning experience and assisting in the evaluation of individual competencies and programmatic outcomes.

In the second year of the program, DHMC was able to purchase a high-fidelity infant simulator to enhance the simulation experiences in both the Pediatric and Intensive Care Nursery tracks of the program. The center also purchased microsimulation software, which meant that the nurse residents could use interactive computer learning to enhance their competency development. The cost of the microsimulation software purchase was approximately $20,000.

Supplies

In addition to the equipment outlined earlier, the DHMC had to purchase books and additional learning modules, and to plan for the ongoing cost of medical supplies and forms used in the Immersive Learning Lab. The initial cost of books was approximately $1000. These resource books were the same as those utilized on the clinical units; that is, they were comprehensive and current resources that provided guidelines and evidence-based practice for day-to-day nursing practice. It was essential to have these resources readily available in the lab to help develop, in each nurse resident, the practice of understanding and using all available resources.

DHMC also purchased seven computer learning modules at a cost of $1200 each. These computer-based modules were used by the nurse residents as part of their independent learning experiences to prepare for simulation experiences.

To assure that the integrated scenarios were realistic, the lab had to be equipped with the same forms and supplies that would be found in clinical areas. DHMC spent approximately $700 and $7500, respectively, for these items. This amount covered approximately 300 integrated scenarios yearly.

ENVIRONMENTAL/SPACE CONCERNS

At DHMC, space was a scarce commodity, because clinical services and faculty numbers had expanded dramatically since the current structure was built in 1991. For this reason, the initial space allocated for the Immersive Learning Lab was a modest space of approximately 350 square feet with an attached closet.

The lab was remodeled to include a nurse's station and a fully functional head wall. Although the spatial relationship was not realistic relative to a clinical unit, the bed space area was realistic. In particular, it was deemed important to have a head wall with functional oxygen and suction. These elements are essential for the nurse resident to experience a realistic development of competencies and an understanding of how equipment (e.g., a ventilator) is set up and functions. The cost of remodeling the space approximated $15,000.

In Year 2 of the program, the space was realigned slightly to have the simulator operator located in the closet of the lab. The educators quickly learned that the nurse residents became attuned to when the simulator operator began to manipulate the situation. The lab experience was found to be more effective if changes in the scenario were not forecasted by the activity of the operator. The operator was able to see activity occurring in the lab through the use of a video camera installed into the patient area of the lab.

Because the formal simulation space was limited, integrated simulation scenarios were also conducted in clinical areas. As the program grew in terms of both numbers of nurse residents and complexity, it became necessary on occasion to bring the high-fidelity simulator to the nurse residents in their local areas. These simulations were quite effective, as the nurse resident used their familiar teammates, equipment, and processes to complete the scenario.

Three years into the program, DHMC was able to allocate an additional area for development of simulation space. The second lab, which was slightly larger than the original site, incorporated a designated space for infant simulation. The cost of remodeling this space was approximately $20,000.

In November 2008, DHMC opened the Patient Safety and Training Center, which serves as a centralized location for all low- and high-fidelity simulators. The simulations labs for the Nurse Residency Program will occur within this center beginning in 2009.

The experience at DHMC demonstrated that it was possible to have a highly successful simulation lab and learning experience in a modest space. The outcomes of the program were exceptional and the satisfaction of the nurse residents was high, despite the space limitations.

MAINTENANCE

Because of the complexity of the high-fidelity patient simulators and the audiovisual equipment, the nurse educators who worked in the lab partnered with members of the Biomedical Department to support the program. They were included in the educational sessions dealing with equipment design and function, and they purchased and installed the audiovisual equipment. These personnel also advised the educators on warranty issues and worked with the vendors on behalf of the educator staff to assure the best maintenance agreements and contracts. Given the cost and complexity of the high-fidelity patient simulators, it was important to protect the resource with appropriate warranty and replacement plans.

It is also important to consider how simulator upgrades will occur. Vendors routinely upgrade and improve their equipment and supplies. Assuring that these upgrades are considered as a part of the initial equipment purchase is important.

In an effort to support DHMC's academic partners in their attempts to establish simulation labs, members of the Biomedical Department offered to provide consultation with those partners regarding the purchase, maintenance, and warranty of equipment. Seeking out this assistance from the Biomedical Departments of local clinical sites may be a step that is often overlooked when one is developing simulation laboratory space.

INVOLVING LEARNERS

Nurse Residents

Nurse residents were asked to evaluate the didactic content of the Nurse Residency Program as well as the Immersive Learning Lab experiences in terms of both their effectiveness and their clinical pertinence. An overwhelming majority—95% or more of nurse residents—enjoyed the simulated experiences and believed these experiences should be part of the residency program. Ninety-eight percent rated the integrated simulation scenario and related content as helpful, while 95% reported that the simulated scenarios helped to develop their confidence. Qualitative comments from the nurse residents included remarks such as this:

> At the moment when the scenario begins to deteriorate, the simulation feels much like an actual crisis on the floors. There is confusion, most of which is related to my own inexperience. Repeated simulations will help build confidence as well as competency.

Other comments included "What we learn is what we do," "Great fun learning," "Very cool," "Puts the pieces together," and "Extremely helpful." Each year, the comments and suggestions of the nurse residents are considered, and appropriate changes are made to scenario structure and content as well as class structure and content.

Clinical Leadership

The nurse educators and clinical leadership are also asked to give feedback on the program and on the competency of the nurse residents. They tend to ask for modifications in the scheduling of simulation labs and for advanced notification of simulation lab dates. They report that because of the simulated lab experiences, there has been early detection of performance concerns, which allows them to support the learning of the nurse resident earlier and more effectively. They are highly satisfied with the caliber of the nurse residents at the completion of the residency program and indicate they (1) can more predictably take full patient assignments, (2) come prepared with skills that were previously missing in the recent-graduate orientee, and (3) are more poised and secure in their practice at one year.

CONTINUING EDUCATION

At the conclusion of the second year of the Nurse Residency Program, nurse educators at DHMC learned of Ebright's (2003) work on the concept of adding complexity to the work of the registered nurse and the factors influencing near-miss and adverse events experienced by new graduate nurses (Ebright, Urden, Patterson, & Chalko, 2004). Her ideas about how to assist novice nurses in adjusting to the interruptions and complexity of the acute care environment were incorporated into the integrated simulated scenario. In addition, techniques for overcoming the effects of interruption were added to the reflective discussion segments of the scenarios.

The nurse educators who work consistently within the simulation lab attend continuing education conferences on a regular basis to assure they stay current with technologies and educational theories relative to using high-fidelity patient simulators. In addition, nurse educators and other faculty are encouraged to present materials at regional and national meetings and to publish on topics related to using high-fidelity patient simulators as an education tool.

EVOLUTION AND FUTURE PLANS

Evaluation and Outcomes

Several outcomes have been evaluated in the Nurse Residency Program. Although these outcomes are considered relative to the entire program, the effect of the integrated simulated scenarios upon the outcomes is significant. Outcomes that have been measured include (1) level of confidence, (2) level of competence, (3) readiness for practice, (4) satisfaction, and (5) length of orientation. In levels of competence, confidence, and readiness to practice, statistically significant improvement has been noted to occur over the 12 weeks of the Nurse Residency Program. High levels of nurse resident satisfaction have been reported, and standardization was achieved in the length of orientation. The medical/surgical orientation was standardized to 12 weeks and the critical care orientation was standardized to 24 weeks. Previously, there had been wide variations in these time periods. Table 9-3 summarizes the measurement schedule and findings for each outcome.

One of the more difficult elements to develop was an assessment tool that allowed the nurse educator to evaluate all elements of nurse resident performance during the integrated simulated scenarios. To meet this need, lab faculty developed the *Simulated Structured Clinical Scenario Performance Evaluation* (SSCS), a tool that evaluates four elements: attitudes/behaviors, technical skills/competency, intellectual skills, and interpersonal skills. Use of

Table 9-3 Outcomes of the DHMC Residency Program: Interim Evaluation ($n = 108$)

Instrument	Baseline mean (SD)	Final mean (SD)	t	df	*Significance (2 tailed)
Self-efficacy for practice	71.72 (11.0)	85.18 (8.2)	-12.66	99	< .001
Confidence (global)	3.30 (2.0)	7.12 (1.4)	-15.41	100	< .001
Competence (global)	3.75 (1.8)	7.11 (1.4)	-14.89	100	< .001
Readiness for practice (global)	3.68 (2.3)	7.25 (1.5)	-12.70	100	< .001

*Based on a paired t-test

this tool revealed that over the course of the 12-week residency program, nurse residents demonstrated a consistent pattern of increased proficiency and confidence, an ability to "think on the fly," and consistent utilization of resources to problem-solve complex or difficult clinical situations. Early evaluations indicated that the impressions of our nurse residents by lab faculty coincided with the nurse residents' self-appraisal of their confidence, competency, and readiness to practice.

Extension of the Residency Program

DHMC now has five years of experience using the initial Nurse Residency Program design. Current literature supports the notion that new graduation orientation programs effectively support the novice nurse over a longer period of time (Krugman, Bretschneider, Horn, Krsek, Moutafis, & Smith, 2006; Pine & Tart, 2007; Poynton, Madden, Bowers, & Keefe, 2007). Beginning in 2009, the Nurse Residency Program will become one year in length and will add regular support and advanced learning opportunities for the nurse resident. As indicated earlier, the opening of the Patient Safety and Training Center will require some changes and adjustments in the program. These changes, however, are expected to increase the resources available to, and the efficiency of, the program.

Variable Needs of Resources

A consistent challenge for the Nurse Residency Program—and one for which no easy or satisfactory solution has been found—is the variable need for resources in the Immersive Learning Lab. Because new-graduate nurses seek employment after graduation in December and May, the Nurse Residency Program sees moderate resource needs in winter and very high resource needs in the months of July, August, and September. The educators are consistently challenged to provide the necessary resources during these periods, which are inevitably a time of high stress for program faculty. There have been efforts to solicit the support of nursing faculty from local academic partners for residencies that occur during the summer months. There has been limited success in this regard, as many school of nursing faculty do not have the clinical experience to support the integrated simulation scenario to the extent needed. Partnerships between healthcare settings and academic institutions to provide clinical experiences for faculty could provide nursing faculty with valuable experience to participate in simulated scenarios that might occur in their local school of nursing simulation laboratory or within the clinical affiliate labs.

Successful Recruitment and Integration of Recent-Graduate Nurses

It is because of the development of the Nurse Residency Program, including the experiences encountered within the Immersive Learning Lab, that DHMC has become a preferred employer for recent-graduate nurses. For the past three years, there have been three recent-graduate applicants for every available nurse resident position. Employment within the DHMC is highly sought after and has encouraged nursing students to seek nurse extern experiences and senior practicum experiences at DHMC. Although it is more difficult to evaluate the effect of the Nurse Residency Program at the point of care, nurse residents who go through this program are highly prepared to care for patients with complex needs and often perform more capably during crisis situations than more seasoned staff. There continues to be a high degree of satisfaction with the program, and it enjoys the ongoing support of nursing, medical, and administrative leaders alike.

References

Benner, P. (2000). *From novice to expert: Excellence and power in clinical nursing practice* (commemorative ed.). Upper Saddle River, NJ: Prentice Hall.

Beyea, S., (Kobokovich) von Reyn, L., & Slattery, M. J. (2007). A nurse residency program for competency development using human patient simulation. *Journal for Nurses in Staff Development*, *23*(2), 77–82.

Ebright, P. (2003). Understanding the complexity of registered nurse work in acute care settings. *Journal of Nursing Administration, 33,* 630–638.

Ebright, P. R., Urden, L., Patterson, E., & Chalko, B. (2004). Themes surrounding novice nurse near-miss and adverse-event situations. *Journal of Nursing Administration, 34,* 531–538.

Forneris, S. G. (2004). Exploring the attributes of critical thinking: A conceptual basis. *International Journal of Nursing Education Scholarship, 1*(9), 16.

Krugman, M., Bretschneider, J., Horn, P. B., Krsek, C. A., Moutafis, R. A., & Smith, M. O. (2006). The national post-baccalaureate graduate nurse residency program: A model for excellence in transition to practice. *Journal for Nurses in Staff Development, 22,* 196–205.

Pine, R., & Tart, K. (2007). Return on investment: benefits and challenges of baccalaureate nurse residency program. *Nursing Economics, 25*(1), 13–18, 39.

Poynton, M. R., Madden, C., Bowers, R., & Keefe, M. (2007). Nurse residency program implementation: The Utah experience. *Journal of Healthcare Management, 52,* 385–396.

Rovin, S., & Formella, N. (2004). Creating a desirable future for nursing. Part 1: The nursing shortage is a lack of creative and systemic thinking. *Journal of Nursing Administration, 34,* 163–166.

ACKNOWLEDGMENTS

This project was supported from funds from the DHHS HRSA, the Bureau of Health Professions (BHPr), Division of Nursing (DN) under grant number ID64HP03100-01-00, with the title *A Nurse Residency Program for Competency Development* ($471,444). The information, content, and conclusions are those of the authors and should not be construed as the official position or policy of, nor should any endorsements be inferred by, the U.S. government, DHHS, BHPr, or the DN.

A special thanks is extended to the team that makes the Nurse Residency Program so successful: Suzanne Beyea, Mary Jo Slattery, Fran Todd, and Carmeleta Beidler.

Unit 3

Developing and Implementing Scenarios

CHAPTER 10

Baccalaureate Nursing Education

Deatrah Dubose, Laurie D. Sellinger-Karmel,
and Robert L. Scoloveno

Currently, baccalaureate nursing education is confronting many major challenges, not the least of which is a nursing shortage. As a result of this shortfall in the number of professional nurses, there has been increased interest in the nursing profession by a more diverse student population, especially in the wake of a critical faculty shortage. Added to these challenges are the reductions in hospital admissions and patient lengths of stay, which often produce inconsistent practice experiences for students and greater competition among nursing programs for clinical sites (Lasater, 2007). Nurses today must also deal with rapidly changing technology, the need to manage complex health problems, and an increase in patient acuity (Ravert, 2002). These factors, coupled with the higher expectations of patients for quality care, inevitably influence the education of nursing students (Alinier, Hunt, Gordon, & Hardwood, 2006).

Confronting theses challenges demands that nursing faculty think about new teaching and learning strategies to prepare professional nurses to assume increasingly complex roles that require a high level of critical thinking and judgment if they are to provide safe quality care to patients (Lasater, 2007). The Committee on Quality of Health Care in America of the Institute of Medicine (2001), in its report titled *Crossing the Quality Chasm*, recommends a restructuring of clinical education and the creation of a culture of patient safety for all clinicians, including nurses, who care for patients. Nurse employers are also requesting that nursing faculty do a better job of preparing students because they can no longer provide lengthy and costly orientation programs (Jeffries, 2005). Clearly, innovative strategies are needed to provide nursing students with cost-effective, high-quality clinical experiences (Jeffries, 2006).

High-fidelity patient simulation provides an opportunity for innovative augmentation of clinical teaching. Clinical scenarios and specialized mannequins, simulating such patient responses as heart sounds, lung sounds, and patient reactions, allow students the ability to practice clinical skills in an education-ally controlled environment (Comer, 2005). High-fidelity patient simulation experiences in the baccalaureate nursing curriculum have been used as a learning strategy to improve nursing students' critical-thinking, decision-making, and assessment and intervention skills in a safe environment in which experiential learning can take place (Alinier et al., 2006; Medley & Horne, 2005; Rhodes & Curran, 2005). Implementing high-fidelity patient simulation into the baccalaureate curriculum also assists students in developing higher-level clinical judgment skills and confidence in clinical situations (Rhodes & Curran, 2005).

This chapter focuses on incorporation of high-fidelity patient simulators in the baccalaureate curriculum. The inclusion of simulation depends on the particular program's objectives, conceptual framework content, placement of the experiences within the baccalaureate curriculum, and philosophy re-garding evaluation. The development of scenarios is also discussed, including objectives for the simulation experience, content, and programming of the simulator. The faculty's role in implementation of simulation in the curriculum is discussed relative to selection of content, placement in the curriculum, and faculty orientation.

INCORPORATING SIMULATION INTO THE CURRICULUM

Simulation can be incorporated into the curriculum via didactic courses, clinical courses, physical assessment courses, and skills courses. However, the inclusion of simulation cannot be done in isolation from the total baccalaure-ate nursing curriculum, including learning objectives, content, and student outcomes. Rather, inclusion of simulation as part of the total curriculum plan validates the role of simulation for students and faculty. Faculty development is also integral to the incorporation of simulation into the curriculum.

Jeffries (2008) describes a faculty simulation-preparation program entitled *Simulations Take Education Preparation (S.T.E.P.)*. This program aims at providing faculty with easily accessible educational resources, training by fac-ulty members who are simulation champions and who have expertise in simu-lation, encouragement of the development of an implementation team for the development and implementation of simulations, and a coordination plan for implementation of the simulation experience. To obtain faculty support, teach-ers must feel prepared to used the simulations and be provided with assistance in simulation design and implementation (Jeffries, 2005). Simulation champi-ons can conduct faculty development seminars, build a scenario repository, and develop educational materials so that faculty members will be knowledge-able about operating the simulators and conducting the simulation experience.

The simulation learning experience is part of the undergraduate curriculum and, as such, is based on the conceptual framework of the curriculum, its objectives, and the evaluation methods identified by the nursing faculty. Learning experiences, including simulation, need to be identified relative to the curriculum map, which may vary according to the student served. For example, a generic baccalaureate nursing program's curriculum may be set up to offer certain classes in a certain sequential order. Other programs—accelerated baccalaureate programs, for example—may change the sequence in which the classes are offered. The principle of simple to complex student-centered experiences cannot be overlooked when developing and implementing the simulation experience. Some basic simulated experiences are better offered early in the curriculum, whereas other, more complex patient care scenarios should appear later in the curriculum.

Faculty preparing to lead students through simulated clinical experiences should be familiar with the design and content of the nursing curriculum and the placement of simulation within the curriculum. Students' previous and concurrent learning should be emphasized. Embedding the content in specific courses may help students tie together information being presented and skills being learned and practiced. Course syllabi should include simulation as a method of meeting the objectives of the course. In turn, measurable objectives identified for simulation should be related to the outcome measures of the nursing curriculum, as well as to the specific course in which simulation is offered.

It is beneficial to begin simulation experiences early in the students' nursing program. In this way, students can become familiar and comfortable with providing care for a variety of patients and their family members, comprehensively assessing patients with a variety of conditions, making decisions, taking appropriate action, evaluating care and revising the plan of care as necessary, and working as a part of a team. Early learning experiences become more complex as the student progresses through the curriculum; in particular, the number of patients can increase as more high-fidelity patient simulators become available.

Simulated clinical scenarios assist the students to think critically, use the nursing process, and learn skills in a nonthreatening environment. To ensure that these goals are met, faculty need to meet to determine how they want to incorporate simulation in the entire curriculum (Seropian, Brown, Gavilanes, & Driggers, 2004). This collaborative effort of the faculty should identify critical learning needs that can be assessed and evaluated through the use of high-fidelity patient simulation.

At the same time, course faculty should be integrally involved with the direction of the simulation experience. For example, they may suggest changes that should be made in the experience to reflect the objectives of the particular course. Changes can be implemented in both the simulation experiences and the course content in an effort to make the student learning experiences more relevant to professional nursing practice. Ultimately, the didactic, clinical, and simulation experiences should work together in a symbiotic manner.

High-fidelity patient simulators provide realism and interactivity that enable learners to problem-solve in patient situations. Other computer-based, low-fidelity simulators also assist students in performing skills and learning to problem-solve effectively (Jeffries, 2006). Research has shown that although both methods are educationally sound, high-fidelity simulation gives students more opportunity to have active involvement in a realistic situation where they can synthesize knowledge and problem-solve relative to patient care (National League for Nursing & Laerdal, 2006). Because of the cost of high-fidelity patient simulators, however, a combination of approaches may be used.

Jeffries (2008) points out that successful implementations of simulation share the following elements: objectives that match the content of the simulation, a set time limit for the simulation and debriefing encounter, limitations on the number of students and assignment of student roles during simulation. As the student progresses through the curriculum, the simulation experience should progress from more teacher-driven scenarios to more student-driven experiences. The level of student is clearly important, but the teacher in all situations needs to explain the ground rules of the simulation activity (Jeffries, 2008).

Simulation experiences can be offered during a clinical rotation, lab time, or didactic class time. Time allocated for each simulated experience will depend on where in the curriculum simulation is to be offered. The number of students who will be in attendance during each simulated experience will also be controlled by this decision. These decisions should be made as part of the blueprint for the simulation within the curriculum.

DEVELOPMENT OF CLINICAL SCENARIOS

Development of a clinical scenario takes planning and time. What is important is the class with which the scenario will be placed (i.e., health assessment, skills course, or clinical course). At our institution, Rutgers College of Nursing, simulation is placed in clinical courses. Simulation is run in conjunction with the simulation team and clinical faculty. The simulation team members are "super-users" of the simulator and are responsible for the creation of scenarios. Every effort is made to ensure that the scenarios match the patient population that is seen during the nursing students' clinical rotation. Our focus is on nursing skills and critical thinking.

Lower-division students who experience simulation early in their clinical rotation are exposed to scenarios that are more basic and simple. The goal in this case is to help them communicate effectively with the patient and to become more comfortable with performing a health assessment. The idea was to create a scenario where the patient has a problem that can be easily fixed so the focus could remain on health assessment.

Those lower-division students who participate in simulation later in their clinical rotation are exposed to scenarios that focus on clinical nursing skills and critical thinking. For lower-division students in the adult medical–surgical rotation, the scenario that students experience is a patient who has chest pain. The same process in creating the scenario is again repeated. Thus, for one semester, there are two scenarios available.

The idea of an asthma attack with continuous nebulizer treatments and the assessment and reassessment of the pulmonary system was created for the junior-level nursing student in adult medical–surgical nursing. Time was taken to create the scenario based on current evidence-based nursing practice. The pathophysiology of the disease process was also reviewed to ensure that the simulator was programmed correctly to act like a patient having an asthma attack. Clinical objectives for the scenario were created and cross-referenced with the clinical course objectives to ensure consistency.

Identifying the Topic

Movement toward creating the scenario can proceed once the decision has been made concerning the course in which the scenario will be placed. The first step for the faculty or the simulation team would be to choose a topic for the scenario. Topics should be related to the clinical focus of the students working where the clinical scenario will be used. For example, if the scenario will be placed in a clinical course, then the scenario should be related to the clinical rotation. If the students will be in a medical–surgical rotation, then the clinical scenario should be related to any disease process that the students may experience during that rotation. If the scenario will be placed in a health assessment course, then the scenario should be related to the body system being taught. An alternative idea is to include a head-to-toe assessment for test-out purposes.

The health assessment scenario illustrated in this chapter is a focused assessment of the cardiac system for test-out purposes. The health assessment course at Rutgers is given in the first semester of the junior year, concurrent with the student's first theory and clinical course dealing with childbearing women and neonates.

Determining Objectives

Once a topic is selected, the next step is to determine the objectives for the scenario. Knowledge of the course, level, and terminal objectives is also important. The objectives must also be consistent with the objectives listed in the syllabus for whatever course of which the scenario will be a part. Objectives should be created using Bloom's taxonomy (Bloom, 1956). For example, the objectives for the Care of the Cardiac Patient scenario illustrated in this chapter are profiled here:

By the end of the simulated experience, the student will be able to do the following:

- Demonstrate a focused cardiac assessment
- Identify the normal and abnormal assessment findings of the cardiac system

These objectives are then compared to the following objectives for our health assessment course. These objectives can also be included as additional objectives for the scenario:

- Recognize variations in the health states of well individuals
- Demonstrate clinical reasoning/judgment in developing appropriate nursing diagnoses from an assessment of human behaviors in the well individual and family
- Identify social and cultural dimensions in assessing the health of diverse populations
- Communicate effectively in basic health assessment

Creating the Scenario

The next step is to create the scenario. The faculty or simulation team needs to determine which signs and symptoms the high-fidelity patient simulator will role-play during the scenario. The use of a current pathophysiology textbook is useful to ensure that the simulator is exhibiting the proper symptoms that relate to the disease process it is trying to simulate. It is also critical that the faculty or team members decide which critical knowledge and behaviors are expected of the student during the scenario. Current evidenced-based nursing practice is the basis on which expected student outcomes are decided. All resources used to create the scenario should be listed as a reference for the students as well as for the faculty.

For the health assessment scenario, the students are expected to introduce themselves, measure vital signs, and perform a focused cardiac assessment. Students are expected to have completed preparatory work prior to coming to the simulation experience. As part of their preparation, they receive a history of the patient's present illness as well as a health history of the patient. A number of questions to answer about the scenario are also provided. These questions, which relate to the disease process that will be covered in the scenario, give the students an idea of what to focus on while they prepare for the scenario. Faculty and staff also have access to the student preparatory material. Box 10-1 provides an example of the health history and preparatory questions for the students.

At this point, the course faculty or simulation team must build and create the actual scenario. Thoughts should be given to how the high-fidelity patient simulator should look for the scenario. The scenario used as an example in this chapter involves a 59-year-old male patient. Props can be used to increase the realism of the scenario. Props can be obtained from stores selling costumes or Halloween supplies. Department stores, such as Target, Wal-Mart, Marshalls, and Kohl's, are other great places to shop for props for the high-fidelity patient simulator. Male wigs and beards can be used to make the simulator appear more convincing as the male patient that has been constructed for the particular scenario. In addition, clothes, such as a male shirt and pants with shoes, can round out the appearance of the patient in a particular environment used in the scenario. The patient in the example is short of breath and is in congestive heart failure. To simulate pitting lower-extremity

---

Box 10-1   Preparatory Materials for a Scenario on Health Assessment for a Patient with a Cardiac Condition

History: Mr. S is a 59-year-old male that presents to the outpatient cardiology clinic for routine follow-up. He has a past medical history significant for hypertension, diabetes mellitus, coronary artery disease, congestive heart failure, and dilated cardiomyopathy. He has had several coronary stents placed in the past. He is relieved to have this appointment because he has run out of furosemide a week ago and is starting to have some shortness of breath.

Prep Questions:
1. What physical assessments are important for a cardiac examination?
2. What are the normal and abnormal findings related to the heart?
3. What are some of the expected findings for a person with heart disease?

Box 10-2   List of Supplies for Health Assessment Scenario

Office chart
Male shirt
Male pants
Shoes
4 ice packs
2 Ace wraps
Male wig
Beard

---

edema, ice packs can be placed around the simulator's calves and secured by covering them with Ace wraps. A list of these supplies should be created so that it will be easier for the staff to set up the scenario before the students arrive (see Box 10-2).

Programming the Scenario

Programming the high-fidelity patient simulator follows the development of the scenario on paper. The high-fidelity patient simulator should be programmed to mimic a person in heart failure. The heart rate should be between 90 and 110 beats per minute. The blood pressure should be elevated at 160–170/90. Heart sounds can also be programmed to include an S_4 heart murmur. The respiratory rate should reflect a person with shortness of breath and should be in the vicinity of 28 breaths per minute. The breath sounds should be programmed to reflect crackles. The bowel sounds should be programmed to be normoactive. The brachial and radial pulses should be programmed to be +3 and the pedal pulses should be programmed to be +1, if possible. Because students will not be able to weigh and measure the height of the high-fidelity patient simulator, they will have to be told the patient's height and weight when they ask. An alternative idea is to have this information listed in the office chart when they bring it to examine the patient. It is also impossible for students to check the simulator's temperature and the capillary refill rate, so they must be told the patient's temperature (98.6°F) and capillary refill rate (< 3 seconds) when they inquire.

The staff or the faculty member testing the students should have both this information and questions in place to guide the students during their health assessment. The entire scenario is found in Appendix A (for students) and Appendix B (for faculty). For example, the nurse educator should ask the following questions of the student while the physical examination is being performed:

1. Which heart sounds coincide with the pulse?
2. Where is the apex of the heart?
3. Why does this patient have pitting edema?
4. Why does this patient have an extra heart sound? What is the significance of the heart murmur?

The desired student actions for successful completion of this scenario include the following steps:

- Introduces self to the patient
- Performs and documents patient history appropriately
- Performs and documents physical assessment based on the patient's history and presentation
- Performs cardiac assessment accurately
- Recognizes and describes abnormal heart sounds
- Scores edema based on a four-point scale

ORIENTATION TO HIGH-FIDELITY PATIENT SIMULATION

Once the students arrive, prior to beginning the scenario, it is best to provide an orientation to the use and purpose of simulation in nursing education and to explain how it will be used for the particular course, including the expectations for the student. Orientation includes an explanation of the objectives of simulation in general. These objectives include the fact that much of the learning can be done by watching a video before coming to simulation or it can be done in person as a discussion before beginning the simulated experience. In addition, faculty members should emphasize to the students that although the scenario is patient centered, it does not always depict a "real" patient situation. For example, although some clinical findings can be simulated, such as pale skin color and edema, jugular venous distention (JVD) and jaundiced sclera cannot yet be simulated. Therefore, as the patient is assessed, students may need to make assumptions and "pretend" that these conditions are noted. In addition, some expensive equipment (e.g., a pulse oximeter, a portable oxygen tank, and a ventilator at our college) may need to be "simulated." It is important to cue students so that they are aware of what is "made up" during orientation so that when they are actually participating in simulation, reality can be the focus. Orientation helps the students "plan," strategize, and ready themselves for a "live" experience.

Once the overall orientation to simulation is complete, discussion of the need for a plan for each patient is reviewed. Students are reminded that without a short-term plan, they might do simply what they are comfortable doing—for example, introducing themselves, washing hands, and checking a name band. However, without a plan or the establishment of priorities, when students step out of their comfort zones, they may find themselves looking down at the patient, with the patient looking up wondering why the student doesn't know what to do next! Orientation provides students with a chance to work together to formulate that plan of care.

Making mistakes as a part of learning is an element of the learning experience. The simulated experience assists students in recognizing errors and identifying plans that foster safe patient care. Performance anxieties are addressed in orientation as a means of decreasing apprehension. If students believe they will be graded on this experience, their anxiety levels will likely be somewhat higher. However, if the simulated experience is used purely as a learning tool, their level of anxiety may be lessened.

Finally, students are socialized to their upcoming new role as a registered professional nurse. In some cases, students will be exposed to several skills that they, as students, may not be permitted to perform in the hospital setting. Examples include taking verbal or phone orders, giving intravenous push (IVP) medications, and, in some cases, gathering information and actually communicating those facts to the healthcare provider! The skill of accepting and writing legal orders can be reviewed in orientation so that when this skill presents itself in the simulation, interruption to the scenario is avoided. Students are not reminded to review pending laboratory values, but instead are told to seek their own laboratory results when they feel they can safely leave the patient's bedside. Finally, delegation of responsibilities is reviewed and the roles of other healthcare disciplines are discussed. Although different scenarios involve various combinations of healthcare disciplines, a general discussion is encouraged concerning the necessity of delegation.

METHODS OF PRESENTING THE SCENARIO

There are several ways to interact with students during a simulated experience, with these possibilities ranging across a continuum from mostly instructor-driven simulation to mostly student-driven simulation. At the beginning of the curriculum, the instructor typically controls the amount of information and the speed at which the scenario is run. As the students gain more experience with the high-fidelity patient simulator and increased theoretical knowledge, procedural skills, and clinical judgment, the scenarios can become completely student driven by the end of the curriculum. As always, the objectives of the course and the goals of the faculty for the students will direct the method used. The time for each method can vary and is largely based on the time available. Each method is discussed in more detail in this section.

Instructor-Driven Simulation

Simulation can be led with prompting and guidance by the faculty member. This style keeps students focused with guidance and instruction throughout the decision-making process. Roles are assigned or chosen after orientation. Each student begins the first state and continues until he or she has completed all of the states. Prompting is done at the bedside as needed to guide students in their prioritization of assessment, collection of data, interventions, and evaluation.

This style assures that students will progress in the direction intended by the faculty for the simulated experience. It offers moderate cueing or prompting to accomplish immediate redirection. Learning opportunities are addressed at the actual time of occurrence. Despite moderate intervention by the faculty member, morale is higher at the end of the simulated experience. This style of simulation can, however, lead to "spoon-fed" students. Although frequent direction is offered, the educator's input comes after the students have been encouraged to make decisions as a group. Discussions at the bedside lengthen the amount of time required for this style of simulation instruction.

Partial Instructor-Driven Simulation

A moderate method of facilitation involves either assigning roles for each student or having each student identify a role he or she would like to experience. It is important to encourage students to take on different roles with each simulated experience. The instructor can treat simulation as scenes from a play (referred to as a "state"). When state 1 begins, the students enter the room (with a plan) and carry out their plan without interruption. This approach gives the students time to carry out their intended plan and offers them the opportunity for self-corrections. Group decisions and discussions are employed to assist in the recognition of problems presented. If the students venture off track, as often happens, the simulated experience is taken in that new direction. Redirection can be introduced in the form of verbal cues by the "patient," incoming lab results, or healthcare provider phone calls. Otherwise, redirection will not occur until the students themselves change the direction of the experience or until the students reach a time when they need to leave the bedside to either obtain labs or call the healthcare provider. That ends the state and begins a debriefing session with the facilitator.

During the debriefing period, the faculty member can ask prompting questions, tie together students' assessment findings, and discuss how the students perceive they addressed their plan. This period of reflection gives students time away from the stress of hands-on care to regroup and assess their decisions. They may choose to alter their plan or recognize that they drifted from their intended plan. Being away from the bedside also offers students a chance to reorganize their thoughts without the simulation progressing so that further responses are required.

Once questions are answered and a new plan of care formulated, the students return to the bedside to continue what has now become state 2. This state continues until the simulated experience is completed. A debriefing session is then held at the end to summarize the totality of the simulation.

The benefits of this style include the fact that students are allowed to reorganize their thoughts without further simulated conditions altering their decisions. It promotes an opportunity for the student to self-correct or to correct one another as opposed to receiving instruction from a faculty member. This simulation approach also allows a new plan to be formulated before the next state is presented. Of course, regrouping after each state is very time-consuming. This point must be addressed when considering time restraints in each individual nursing program.

Student-Driven Simulation

The third type of facilitation again begins with an appropriate orientation. During this phase, roles are assigned or picked, and a plan is initiated. When the students go to the bedside, however, there is no interruption between states. The students continue with simulation until the scenario is complete.

At the conclusion of the simulated experience, the students exit to a conference room and a faculty member asks prompting questions and begins debriefing. The flow of the simulated experience and transition from state to state tends to be smoother with this approach, which offers the students the opportunity to self-correct and redirect themselves. However, the simulation may also take a turn in the wrong direction: Often students don't know what they don't know. In this situation, redirection can be introduced in the form of verbal cues by the "patient," incoming lab results, or healthcare provider phone calls.

This instruction method may not be the optimal choice for new students, as they may go for too long a period of time without a facilitator *pulling* together the knowledge behind the decision-making process. There is no guarantee that students will ever realize that they have not addressed a situation safely or correctly. This outcome may, in turn, lead to poor morale at debriefing.

EVALUATION OF CLINICAL SCENARIOS

Simulation and course faculty need to become familiar with a variety of scenarios as well as the learning needs of the students attending the simulation experiences. The simulation faculty can then choose an appropriate simulated experience that will strengthen or support the needs identified by the course faculty. Choosing a scenario that requires a head-to-toe assessment initially, for example, may be an appropriate choice for students who are taking a physical assessment class or who are just beginning to work in the clinical setting for the first time. Choosing the right "mix" is very important.

In evaluating the success of a specific experience or a particular clinical scenario, faculty members must assess several factors. Was the chosen simulated experience successful in meeting the identified needs of the students? Did it address the critical thinking intended and was it presented at a level appropriate for the students? If psychomotor skills were part of the simulated experience, did they enhance the experience or take away from the critical thinking intended? At first, simulation may identify learning needs and weaknesses within the curriculum.

Combining the simulation faculty's evaluation with the students' evaluations of their experience in simulation can provide a process evaluation for the course and the overall curriculum, which can then be reviewed by the faculty. In addition, student evaluations of their experiences serve as feedback for the course. Again, one must ask the following questions: Was the chosen simulated experience successful in meeting the identified needs of the students? Were the students able to identify the actual and potential problems? Was the simulated experience appropriate for the level of the students? Were students able to think critically so as to identify and care for the simulated problems presented? Finally, was the style of presenting this individual simulated experience most effective in attaining the desired outcomes? (For further information on evaluation, see Chapter 19.)

FACULTY DEVELOPMENT

Faculty development will be an important aspect in the success of any simulation program, no matter which simulation method the nursing program or faculty decides to use. It is important to review learning outcomes, the nursing curriculum, and expected student performances so that each new faculty member can be correctly oriented to the use of the high-fidelity patient simulator. Faculty shadowing is often encouraged, because it allows the faculty to see how students' responses and actions can change the direction of the simulated experience. Becoming aware that different learning outcomes are possible for different scenarios makes shadowing especially helpful, as the faculty can see how styles of facilitation can be changed based on the desired learning outcome.

SUMMARY

Baccalaureate nursing education faces a number of major challenges today, including the nursing shortage, the nursing faculty shortage, and competition for clinical experiences for students. Confronting theses challenges demands that nursing faculty use innovative, cost-effective, and high-quality clinical learning experiences. High-fidelity patient simulation experiences can be placed in the nursing curriculum to increase baccalaureate nursing students' critical-thinking and decision-making abilities and to improve their assessment and intervention skills in a safe environment.

The incorporation of simulation in the curriculum is based on the conceptual framework, objectives, and content of the curriculum. The S.T.E.P. preparation program described by Jeffries (2008) assists baccalaureate nursing faculty in turning simulation into an integral part of the curriculum. Once the plan for simulation is designed, scenarios are developed based on the level of student, and placed appropriately in the curriculum. Each scenario should include objectives, defined roles for faculty and students, a debriefing session, and a method of evaluation. The integration of simulation into the baccalaureate nursing program can enhance student learning in a challenging nursing and educational environment.

References

Alinier G., Hunt, B., Gordon, R., & Harwood C. (2006). Effectiveness of intermediate-fidelity simulation training technology in undergraduate education. *Journal of Advances in Nursing, 54,* 359–369.

Bloom, B.S. (1956). *Taxonomy of educational objectives. Handbook I: The cognitive domain.* New York: David McKay.

Comer, S. K. (2005). Patient care simulations: Role playing to enhance clinical understanding, *Nursing Education Perspectives, 26,* 357–361.

Committee on Quality of Health Care in America, Institute of Medicine. (2001). *Crossing the quality chasm: A new health system for the 21st century.* Washington, DC: National Academy Press.

Jeffries, P. R. (2005). A framework for designing, implementing, and evaluating simulations used as teaching strategies in nursing. *Nursing Education Perspectives, 26,* 96–103.

Jeffries, P. R. (2006). Technology trends in nursing education: Next steps. *Journal of Nursing Education, 44*(1), 3–4.

Jeffries, P. R. (2008). Getting in S.T.E.P. with simulations: Simulations take educator preparation. *Nursing Education Perspectives, 29,* 70–73.

Lasater, K. (2007). High-fidelity simulation and the development of clinical judgment: Students' experiences. *Journal of Nursing Education, 46*, 269–276.

Medley, C. F., & Horne, C. (2005). Using simulation technology for undergraduate nursing education. *Journal of Nursing Education, 44*, 31–34.

National League for Nursing (NLN) and Laerdal. (2006). *Designing and implementing models for the innovative use of simulation to teach nursing care of ill adults and children: A national, multi-site, multi-method study.* New York: NLN.

Ravert, P. (2002). An integrative review of computer-based simulation in the education process. *CIN: Computer, Informatics, Nursing, 20*, 203–208.

Rhodes, M. L., & Curran, C. (2005). Use of the human patient simulator to teach clinical judgment skills in a baccalaureate nursing program. *CIN: Computers, Informatics, Nursing, 23*, 256–262.

Seropian, M. A., Brown, K., Gavilanes, J. S., & Driggers, B. (2004). An approach to simulation development. *Journal of Nursing Education, 43*, 170–174.

Student Version of the Scenario of the Patient with a Cardiac Condition

OBJECTIVES

- By the end of the simulated experience, the student will be able to demonstrate a focused cardiac assessment.
- The student will be able to identify the normal and abnormal assessment findings of the cardiac system.

CARE OF THE PATIENT WITH A CARDIAC CONDITION

History of Present Illness

Mr. S is a 59-year-old male who presents to the outpatient cardiology clinic for routine follow-up. He has a past medical history significant for hypertension, diabetes mellitus, coronary artery disease, congestive heart failure, and dilated cardiomyopathy. He has had several coronary stents placed in the past. He is relieved to have this appointment because he ran out of his furosemide a week ago and is starting to have some shortness of breath.

Prep Questions

1. Which physical assessments are important for a cardiac examination?
2. What are the normal and abnormal findings related to the heart?
3. What are some of the expected findings for a person with heart disease?

References

Copstead-Kirkhorn, L., & Banasik, J. (2005). *Pathophysiology* (3rd ed). St. Louis: Elsevier.

Jarvis, C. (2004). *Physical examination and health assessment* (4th ed.). St. Louis: Saunders.

McKenry, L. N., Tessier, E., & Hogan, M. A. (2006) *Mosby's pharmacology in nursing* (22nd ed.). St. Louis: Mosby.

Faculty Version of the Scenario of the Patient with a Cardiac Condition

OBJECTIVES

- By the end of the simulated experience, the student will be able to demonstrate a focused cardiac assessment.
- The student will be able to identify the normal and abnormal assessment findings of the cardiac system.

CARE OF THE PATIENT WITH A CARDIAC CONDITION

History of Present Illness

Mr. S is a 59-year-old male who presents to the outpatient cardiology clinic for routine follow-up. He has a past medical history significant for hypertension, diabetes mellitus, coronary artery disease, congestive heart failure, and dilated cardiomyopathy. He has had several coronary stents placed in the past. He is relieved to have this appointment because he ran out of his furosemide a week ago and is starting to have some shortness of breath.

Prep Questions

1. Which physical assessments are important for a cardiac examination?
2. What are the normal and abnormal findings related to the heart?
3. What are some of the expected findings for a person with heart disease?

Supplies

Office chart

Male shirt

Male pants

Shoes

4 ice packs

2 Ace wraps

Male wig

Beard

Instructions

Place two ice packs around the simulator's calves and cover with Ace wraps. Dress the simulator with the shirt, pants, and shoes. Put on the wig and beard. Prepare the patient's chart. Tell students when they inquire about the simulator's temperature. Ask critical-thinking questions while the students are performing the cardiac assessment.

Turn the simulator on and click on the Patient with a Cardiac Condition scenario.

Simulator Actions

Temperature: 98.6°F

Heart rate: 98

Blood pressure: 165/90

Respiratory rate: 28

Heart sounds: S_1, S_2, S_4

Breath sounds: with bilateral crackles

Bowel sounds: normoactive

Brachial and radial pulses: +3

Pedal pulses: +1

Table 10-APP_B1

Student Actions:	Critical Thinking Questions
• Introduces self to the patient • Performs and documents patient history appropriately	1. Which heart sounds coincide with the pulse? 2. Where is the apex of the heart?

Table 10-APP_B1 (*continued*)

Student Actions:	Critical Thinking Questions
• Performs and documents physical assessment based on the patient's history and presentation • Performs cardiac assessment accurately • Recognizes and describes abnormal heart sounds • Scores edema based on a four point scale • Notifies healthcare provider of the assessment findings	**3.** Why does this patient have pitting edema? **4.** Why does this patient have an extra heart sound? What is the significance of the heart murmur?

References

Copstead-Kirkhorn, L., & Banasik, J. (2005). *Pathophysiology* (3rd ed). St. Louis: Elsevier.

Jarvis, C. (2004). *Physical examination and health assessment* (4th ed.). St. Louis: Saunders.

McKenry, L. N., Tessier, E., & Hogan, M. A. (2006) *Mosby's pharmacology in nursing* (22nd ed.). St. Louis: Mosby.

CHAPTER 11

Associate Degree Nursing Education

Kathy Carver and Penny L. Marshall

Simulation in associate degree nursing programs is a perfect fit to blend classroom didactic and clinical teaching. The active learning style of simulation allows for reinforcement of both psychomotor and communication skills, in addition to encouraging critical thinking and allowing for hands-on management of patient problems. Incorporating simulation prior to the actual patient experience provides an optimal opportunity to prepare the student for "the real world." Simulation provides a safe, nonthreatening platform for instructor guidance and individual coaching. Having students work in small groups of three to four at the bedside is an essential component of the simulation experience.

Simulation is not just clinical, lab, or classroom time, but rather a unique combination of all three. It blends the best of those settings by integrating content, skills, patient problems, and role development within the patient scenario. This chapter discusses the place of simulation in the curriculum of an associate degree program in nursing and describes the methods of evaluation used for this teaching methodology. It concludes with a discussion of the development of a scenario involving an end-of-life situation used in the second semester of the program.

PLACE OF SIMULATION IN THE CURRICULUM

Simulation has the potential to allow students to experience patient care from the actual eyes of the health practitioner. Even students with previous experience often do not realize the scope of the registered nurse's role and responsibilities for patient safety. Simulation provides students with a point from which to assume their beginning role. It fosters critical thinking by incorporating opportunities for students to pause the scenario to address questions and resolve patient care problems. Simulation gives students the extra time needed to develop confidence and master beginning-level skills.

The use of simulation in programs is driven by the curriculum content and level of objectives to be covered in it. Specifically, the scenario objectives should correlate with the course objectives. Scenario development, in turn, incorporates new skills and, knowledge so that students are constantly challenged to use their critical-thinking and decision-making skills. Challenging the students with each scenario promotes growth and progress toward program outcomes.

First-semester simulations focus on basic assessment, communication, and documentation. Skills and nursing interventions are added as they relate to the curriculum content. Simulations should be offered frequently to provide students with ample opportunities for reinforcement and repetition. Second-semester content and expectations focus on further developing the skills from fundamental levels, but often a specialty area is introduced to expand those skills' applications into new settings. During the last two semesters, simulations increase in complexity and individual students assume the primary nurse role and delegate tasks to the other group members. This greater complexity within the simulations gives students opportunities to use their management skills to direct patient care and delegate responsibilities to the other group members.

It is important to communicate the purpose of simulation and its potential benefits to the students. Students should be advised if the simulation experience will be used for learning purposes, evaluation purposes, or a combination of the two. Creating a safe environment means that faculty members need to clearly identify expectations for student preparation, behavior, and student performance during the simulation.

EVALUATING THE STUDENT USING SIMULATION

If simulation is done to evaluate objectives, the evaluation tools need to be shared with all parties—for example, as a clinical evaluation form or a skills checklist. Ideally, students will have previous simulation experience before they are evaluated via this means. If simulation is being used as a teaching strategy, students should still be held accountable for having adequate preparation for the event. The group experience will be dependent on each student being able to assume the role he or she is assigned.

Evaluation using simulation provides an excellent platform through which to compare student performance. Because the patient scenario is the same for each student, faculty have an opportunity to see all students on a level playing field and identify those students who need remediation. Many faculty members struggle with the task of evaluating students' clinical performance in non-simulation environments because of the wide range of student learning needs and the uniqueness of each patient situation. In such situations, the presence of multiple variables may interfere with the evaluator's ability to gain a true picture of the students and to evaluate them adequately. Many faculty members tend to verbalize one of two viewpoints when evaluating students: (1) They think students should perform a skill perfectly every time, or (2) they rationalize minimal performance by saying that the student needs more time or has dealt with a difficult patient. Either way, identification of the lack of progress at the end of the semester minimizes chances for the student to be successful.

Simulation can benefit both faculty and students when it is used in conjunction with clinical assignments. Performance—and evaluation of that performance—during simulation typically correlates with the student's clinical performance. Identifying a student's lack of progress early in the semester allows for devoting additional resources and selecting other options to improve the student's ability to meet course objectives. The scenario described in this chapter, for example, provides an opportunity for the faculty member to evaluate the student's skills in communication, patient advocacy, and role assumption.

IDENTIFYING THE TOPIC OF THE SCENARIO

Trends in contemporary health care include an aging population, increasing levels of chronic illness, and an overburdened healthcare system. In response to these trends, there has been a surge in interest in the quality of care offered to individuals with advanced disease and terminal illness. Competent end-of-life (EOL) care is essential in the face of the increased proliferation of hospice and palliative care programs, and with an aging society that faces ethical challenges such as withdrawal from life-sustaining treatments.

Because nurses spend more time at the bedside caring for patients at the end of life than members of any other professional group, it is vital that they be prepared to manage the complex needs of terminally ill patients and that they receive up-to-date education in palliative care. Unfortunately, the education of healthcare professionals in EOL care was essentially nonexistent in years past (American Association of Colleges of Nursing, 1997; Ferrell & Coyne, 2002; Ferrell, Virani, & Grant, 1999b). Both the medical and nursing education communities have failed to sufficiently educate health professionals about how to provide competent care to dying patients (Ferrell & Coyne, 2002; Ferrell, Virani, & Grant, 1999b; Field, Cassel, & Committee on Care at the End of Life, 1997). Furthermore, many physicians and nurses report how inadequately prepared they were as students to care for dying patients and their families. Medical and nursing curricula have been conspicuously lacking in educational materials that focus on end stages of most diseases, palliative care strategies, and clinical experiences that encompass care of dying patients and their loved ones (Ferrell, Virani, & Grant, 1999a, 1999b; Field et al., 1997; Matzo & Sherman, 2001).

A pivotal milestone in the movement toward quality EOL care was a project supported by the Robert Wood Johnson Foundation that was designed to strengthen nursing education to improve EOL care by accomplishing three goals:

- To improve EOL care content included in major nursing textbooks
- To increase content in EOL care tested by the national nursing examination
- To support key nursing organizations in their efforts to improve nursing education and practice in EOL care (American Association of Colleges of Nursing, 1997)

The scenario described in this chapter addresses many physiological issues, but the emphasis is on communication skills, and more specifically on communication skills used in EOL care. The older adult depicted in this scenario has been chronically ill for more than 20 years with diagnoses of chronic obstructive pulmonary disease, diabetes mellitus, congestive heart failure, and end-stage renal disease. The patient is now hospitalized for congestive failure, but refuses care and requests to be discharged home. Family members are divided about the patient's request, and students must handle the ensuing conflict.

As part of the scenario, the student must assume the role of patient advocate and provide information about options for the patient, family, and healthcare providers to be discussed openly. A family conference occurs to discuss the patient's request and the need for completing an advance directive. Nurses from a home care hospice agency are included in the conference to inform the family about the goals and implementation of hospice care. At the end of the conference, the simulation continues back at the bedside, but the patient is home with hospice nursing. The family is present, and the hospice nurses arrive to assess and manage the patient's needs.

WHY AND HOW THE SCENARIO WAS DEVELOPED

This scenario was developed to blend the specialties of gerontology and mental health/communication during the second semester of an associate degree nursing program. In this course, the students care for the same patient in previous scenarios during the semester. The first scenario of the semester focuses on a gerontological assessment and profile of the health needs of a 65-year-old patient who has underlying chronic health issues. Subsequent simulations focus on two health complications, a stroke and chronic renal failure.

The latter scenario occurs when the patient is 85 years old (20 years after the initial assessment) and represents the progression of his life, including how his illnesses have decreased his quality of life. It was a logical progression for students to then be confronted with EOL issues. As part of the course, students had developed a nurse–patient relationship with the patient prior to this final scenario.

The EOL focus provides a context in which discussion of family values and sensitivity to cultural and spiritual beliefs can take place and which students can assess. In particular, the scenario focuses on communication skills instead of placing a heavy emphasis on the psychomotor and disease process highlighted in earlier scenarios. Ethical dilemmas occur as a result of the patient's refusal of care and the lack of a completed advance directive. Students have to process the role of a patient advocate when family members have conflicting opinions.

Another major factor addressed by this scenario is the issue of death and dying. Reenacting this emotional time allows students to respond based on previous personal experiences and to gain confidence that they can handle difficult communications. In addition, students come to appreciate the importance of the nursing role as part of the healthcare team while assisting the patient and family as they transition from traditional health care to palliative/hospice nursing care.

THE IMPLEMENTATION PROCESS

The timing of this scenario (i.e., the point at which students undertake it) in relation to the curriculum content structure is important. Its content—basic communication skills, ethical dilemmas, gerontology assessment, and death and dying with EOL care nursing care—is essential for students to discuss prior to engaging in the simulation. These concepts require time to process and are difficult to fully grasp. If this scenario is used without adequately preparing the students for it, students likely will not be able to assume the RN role independently. Faculty members portray the patient and family members, including espousing their values and beliefs. Conflict is present in that one family member does not want the patient to go home, whereas the other family member supports the patient's request. Faculty can coach the students if needed by giving cues through their dialogue as the patient or family member.

Faculty from different specialties and/or teaching teams will need to be included in the design and implementation of the simulation. Depending on a particular program's structure, faculty review of the scenario and planning may need to be done outside the normal teaching groups. This scenario is faculty and time intensive, but having a larger simulation teaching team involved provides for a richer, truly unique experience for the student.

Three faculty members are needed per student group. One faculty member serves as the voice of the patient, and the other two faculty members serve as family members. Nonfaculty personnel have also been used as family members because of logistical and faculty availability issues. Each simulation group includes four students. The time needed for each simulation group is 90 minutes, which includes time in the hospital, family conference, home setting, and debriefing. If that amount of time is not available, the scenario can be divided so that only time at the hospital bedside or home setting is included, with the family conference being added if possible. Time for students to process the conversation and to practice their communication skills is an essential element of the scenario, so that part of the simulation should not be compromised (i.e., truncated) if a shorter time period is allocated for the simulation.

Adequate time must be given for the debriefing process. Previous death experiences will likely surface as topics of conversation, and faculty need to be prepared for emotional responses by the students. Additional follow-up with students may be necessary. Students become acutely aware of the potential for conflict with their values or beliefs as they intervene in the nurse role, and their awareness of their personal biases and judgments can serve as a starting point for excellent discussion threads during the debriefing. Debriefing usually lasts at least 30 minutes.

Faculty should discuss and define expectations and roles clearly. Our personal experience indicates that it is a good idea for students to share the primary role or decision-making role, for several reasons:

- Students need to know how to prioritize, and this experience allows faculty members to hear their analysis of their assessment and the rationale for their decisions.
- If the students do not agree initially, the discussion and analysis are often stronger because the student cannot simply react and see what happens. That is, students have an opportunity to discuss what are the best steps to take and why.
- Students share the responsibility with other students in case an error or decision is not effective and a positive patient outcome is not achieved.

For this scenario, all students will assume a primary role at some point, with two students being in charge while the patient is in the hospital and the other two students being in charge in the patient's home as hospice nurses. When not in the primary nurse role, students will act as student nurses. Documentation is always an expectation, and the primary nurses will be held accountable for documentation and communication to other healthcare professionals if needed.

The dual setting of the scenario—in the hospital and in the patient's home—is intended to reflect the patient's transition from the traditional healthcare setting to hospice care. Cues from the environment are important for the students to assess and make inferences about the patient's and family members' spiritual beliefs and cultural background. Use of family pictures, religious objects, books, and items with sentimental value allow students to see the patient as a unique individual. The reason the scenario was developed with the multiple settings was twofold. First, most students will be in acute care nursing positions when this dilemma is presented. Second, the use of a family conference and home setting helps to define the family and patient concerns using a healthcare team approach. Although this approach is labor intensive for faculty, it allows for presentation of a broader spectrum of the nursing care experience.

SUCCESSES AND CHALLENGES

The overwhelming success of this scenario derives from its focus on student communication skills; psychosocial, cultural, and spiritual assessments; and exposure to an ethical dilemma. Most simulations emphasize psychomotor skills and medical–surgical nursing care, so this scenario represents a clear change of pace. During the traditional scenarios, students with strong psychomotor skills enjoy the leadership or primary role. With the change in emphasis in the EOL care scenario, however, those same students quickly identify at the beginning of the simulation that the critical physical needs are present but the scenario quickly stalls because of the patient's refusal of care. Students with strong communication skills then become instrumental to the group. New student leaders emerge because of their communication strengths, which might not have been previously recognized. This scenario offers an opportunity for those students to be assertive and to demonstrate their strengths to their peers. Those students who are not comfortable talking to the patient about death or emotional issues become aware of their individual needs. Some students, for example, have discovered that they were not comfortable communicating unless they were administering physical care or interventions.

A second success of this scenario is its ability to bring to the fore the issue of end of life. Death is the "elephant in the room" that no one talks about, and students confront their fears about death and experiencing death as healthcare professionals during this simulation. Students enter nursing with a caring and giving attitude toward the suffering of others, and they know they can manage the stress and hard work from previous life experiences. Confronting a patient who is dying is an experience that students verbalize they are anxious about and have an uncertainty about their personal responses. This simulation allows students to confront those feelings and to experience them prior to a Code Blue or unexpected event in which death is the outcome. Students walk away from this scenario with a new perspective on the nurse's role and responsibilities, and the confidence that they can deal with EOL issues.

Another reason for the success of this scenario is that it crosses all disciplines. Faculty members inevitably have experiences that they draw upon when fulfilling their roles in the simulation. Faculty from mental health, gerontology, and medical–surgical disciplines, for example, all have the necessary expertise and experience to assist in the success of this scenario.

Numerous challenges are also associated with this simulation. Much time is needed to plan and organize the number of faculty involved. The time frame to run the actual scenario is a large obstacle that must be overcome. To keep the student group size small, repetition is needed. Teaching with each group is emotionally draining for faculty members, especially if they must handle multiple scenarios in one day. The emotional distress displayed by the faculty greatly enhances the realism, however, and the students cannot anticipate this fact in advance because each faculty group provides its own interpretation of the situation.

USE OF SIMULATION USING DIFFERENT LEVELS OF FIDELITY

A major advantage of this scenario is that high-fidelity simulators are not integral to its implementation. The critical element is to have a mannequin (patient) that communicates. This capability can be created by use of a wireless microphone with the speaker located under the bed frame to reflect the patient's voice. Most static mannequins do not have eyes that are open. Although this characteristic may distract students at first, as the scenario unfolds, they will not even recognize the lack of eye movement. During the home setting, it is very reasonable that a patient would not open his eyes even as he is speaking because of his delusions and EOL experience.

Any vital signs that students may want to assess can be placed on the mannequin to reflect the assessment data if you have a low-fidelity mannequin. For example, the blood pressure can be placed on the actual blood pressure cuff for the students to record. Heart and lung sounds can be identified by the use of sticky notes or labels on different chest wall locations. It is important for students to perform each skill or assessment and to obtain the information themselves instead of just having a faculty member verbalize the information. The effectiveness of all simulations relates to the fact that students must discover or ask for relevant information appropriately.

STUDENT EVALUATIONS FOR THE SIMULATION EXPERIENCE

Simulation experiences should be evaluated by students at the end of the scenario. Use of a simple tool with a rating scale should be completed after the debriefing session. Some students verbalize their evaluation during the debriefing, but written forms allow for students to reflect more fully on the experience and give them greater time to respond. Faculty members set the tone for the simulation, and they should emphasize both the importance of evaluations and the confidentiality of the information prior to the scenario.

Other forms of feedback can include a review of the scenario during a class or large-group time to discuss the highlights of the simulation and clarify any outstanding issues. Feedback by faculty members that takes the form of a general, overview perspective of how all the groups performed is also helpful. Faculty can accomplish a review of content and highlight common threads shared by all groups without breaking the student–faculty confidentiality bond as it relates to the individual simulation groups. This follow-up also allows students time to review the content and further reflect upon their simulation experience. This type of feedback has been well received by students.

At our institution, actual student feedback about the simulation written on evaluation forms included the following comments:

- Very emotional but very needed. I really feel like I may be more qualified to help a patient and their family through this time in their life. This scenario reinforced what I have considered my calling as a nurse—to work with the elderly and the end of life.
- The conference was probably the most helpful because the questions the son and daughter asked helped me think about how I can be better prepared to answer them.
- This scenario is very challenging and emotional draining and requires thought about emotional concerns as well as physical concerns.
- This was helpful trying to talk with a grieving family.
- This scenario gave me a better understanding of the dying process and how to support the family.

Of the 60 students who participated in our simulation, all students evaluated the scenario positively and considered it to be relevant to their learning per their written evaluations.

FUTURE CHANGES

Future changes might include a multidisciplinary approach and the addition of various cultures to the patient profile. Portraying a patient/family from a different ethnic, cultural, or religious background would add another dimension to the complexity of the situation. As mentioned earlier, this simulation focuses on communication skills instead of placing a heavy emphasis on the psychomotor and disease process covered by earlier scenarios. Students who are in social services classes might potentially participate in the simulation by engaging in their professional roles during the family conferences and arranging for hospice care as part of the scenario. Students from different cultures might portray the family members, thereby adding a new cultural component to the simulation and increasing the realism of the interaction. To include language barriers as part of the scenario, students from foreign language courses might speak for the patient or act as hospital interpreters. Clearly, simulation is a great platform for students from a variety of programs to interact in very realistic settings.

ADVICE FOR FACULTY WHO WANT TO REPLICATE THE END-OF-LIFE SCENARIO

Even though the EOL simulation is not an actual clinical experience, students' ability to recognize the EOL event and perform effectively the first time is critical for their transference of knowledge to real-world settings. The use of evidenced-based scenarios is essential to ensure a close correlation between simulations and real life. The actual patient history and health concerns can be changed easily to mesh more closely with the current topics of your program and curriculum without distracting from the intent and design of this scenario. The essential components to be included are the communication skills, EOL care, and patient advocacy role. Actual pamphlets and information from a local hospice nursing group may be made available for students to use as a resource during the family conference and in the home setting. The students in the hospice nursing role appreciate being able to use it during the family conference to validate their role.

References

American Association of Colleges of Nursing (AACN). (1997). *A peaceful death: Recommended competencies and curricular guidelines for end of life care. Report from the Robert Wood Johnson End of Life Roundtable.* Washington, DC: Author.

Ferrell, B. R., & Coyle, N. (2002). An overview of palliative nursing care. *American Journal of Nursing, 102*(5), 26–31.

Ferrell, B. R., Virani, R., & Grant, M. (1999a). Analysis of end-of-life content in nursing textbooks. *Oncology Nursing Forum, 26,* 869–876.

Ferrell, B. R., Virani, R., & Grant, M. (1999b). Strengthening nursing education to improve end of life care. *Nursing Outlook, 47,* 252–256.

Field, M. J., Cassel, C. K., & Committee on Care at the End of Life. (1997). *Approaching death: Improving care at the end of life.* Washington, DC: National Academies Press.

Matzo, M. L., & Sherman, D. W. (Eds.). (2001). *Palliative care nursing: Quality care to the end of life.* New York: Springer.

End-of-Life Scenario

Title of Scenario: End-of-Life Scenario
Student Level: Second semester or with gerontology/mental health concepts
Category of NCLEX-RN Blueprint:
Guides to Learning: Gerontology book—end of life; nursing drug handbook of choice; references listed at end of scenario

---

———— OBJECTIVES ————

1. Assess the physical, psychosocial, cultural, and spiritual needs of the patient and family during the end-of-life phase.
2. Differentiate pain management from acute care to the home setting using principles of analgesia to control pain, delirium, and prevention of toxicity.
3. Compare and contrast different types of cultural expectations and values as they relate to end-of-life passage.
4. Assess the patient's and family's need for teaching about palliative and hospice care.
5. Apply ethical principles and concepts as they relate to end-of-life care, decision making, and conflict resolution.
6. Analyze common barriers to providing effective communication throughout end-of-life care.
7. Describe the use of therapeutic communication—presence, active listening, reminiscence therapy, forgiveness facilitation, and family support.
8. Evaluate the patient's response to nursing care and management of patient symptoms.
9. Describe the mechanisms of action, indications for use, contraindications, drug interactions, and nursing care for the following drug classifications:
   Analgesic medications for acute and palliative care
   Antianxiety medications
   Anticholinergics
   Antiemetics
   Diuretics

PREPARATION FOR PATIENT SCENARIO

1. Which assessment data are important to collect for signs of neurological/respiratory/circulatory/renal function?
2. Which nursing interventions are altered because of the patient's end-stage renal disease and the location of an arterial–venous shunt used for dialysis?
3. What are the principles of pain management during the end-of-life process, and how are they different from the principles used when managing acute pain?
4. Which fluid/electrolyte changes would you anticipate with this patient? When would oral fluids/food not be indicated?
5. Why is positioning important for patients? What is the physiologic rationale for nursing care?
6. Why are the medications indicated for this patient? Which considerations would be important when planning nursing care and administration of medications?
7. What is the role of the nurse with the patient and family as they make decisions regarding healthcare interventions? What is an advance directive?
8. Which information would be helpful to the patient and family about palliative and/or end-of-life care?
9. Which ethical principles should the nurse keep in mind when assisting with the advance directive and planning for the patient's end of life?
10. Which communication skills are important to facilitate the nurse–patient relationship?

SKILLS REQUIRED TO PREPARE FOR THE SCENARIO

Vital signs and physical assessment
Identification of possible abnormal heart and lung assessments
Blood glucose monitoring
Monitoring intravenous fluids and use of pump
Administration of medication: oral, sublingual, transdermal, subcutaneous, intravenous
Foley catheter placement and maintenance
Communication skills: presence, active listening, reminiscence therapy, forgiveness facilitation

SCENARIO OUTLINE

Student Role

Two students will be primary nurses at the hospital. The other two students will be role-play as nursing students during the hospital setting. During the last segment, the groups will reverse their positions, and the nursing students will become the hospice nurses.

Instructor Notes

The scenario starts in the hospital 24 hours after the patient's admission. The students will be able to review the acute care of pulmonary edema. The patient continues to have difficulty breathing, but is alert and verbalizes a request to go home. The patient refuses to have morning care and dialysis, and insists that he be discharged. The patient states that he has pain, but the medication is not effective. He refuses to take more pain medication until he is discharged. The hospital nurses should assess the patient for level of consciousness and alertness, and should chart when the advance directive is signed and witnessed.

(Time at the bedside: 25 minutes)

Patient Vital Signs and Assessment

Temperature: 37.5°C
Pulse: 124, irregular; atrial fibrillation rhythm
Respiration: 30—shallow, crackles bilaterally in lower lobes, nonproductive cough
Blood pressure: 148/92
Oxygen saturation: 90%
Blood glucose: 210; done 0700
Urine output: 100 past 12 hours, tea colored; Foley catheter in place

Programming for METI HPS or ECS

Patient: Truck driver

Respiration:
- Shunt fraction: 25
- Oxygen consumption: 375
- Tidal volume factor: 0.75
- Breath sounds: abnormal
- Respiratory rate factor: 1.25

Cardiac:
- Ischemic sensitivity: 0.22
- Cardiac override: atrial fibrillation
- Heart rate factor: 1.25

Family are either present at the bedside or come in while the students are talking with the patient about his refusal of care. The inclusion of two family members (a son and a daughter may be used to highlight gender differences when communicating about end of life) is helpful to portray conflicting responses. One family member accepts the patient's feelings and request to go home; the other family member is against the patient's refusal of care.

The students may need to have the family members leave the room if they are upset.

The students should look for the advance directive: The patient has not completed it.

The hospital nurse may need to call the physician to notify him or her about the patient's refusal of dialysis and medication. The physician will concur that the patient has talked to him or her before about stopping dialysis and advise that the patient complete the advance directive. The physician then orders the patient's discharge after a decision is made regarding his request.

A **family conference** is scheduled in a separate room away from the bedside. The following roles are present at this meeting:

- Primary nurse: assumed by the assigned students
- Hospice nurse: assumed by the assigned students
- Family: son/daughter or two children assumed by the faculty

(Time at the conference: 20–30 minutes)

The agenda for the conference is for the students (primary hospital nurse role) to discuss advance directives, and then for the students (hospice nurse role) to discuss hospice nursing. The students should identify the options in terms of the decision-making process:

- Advance directive: used first
- Substitute judgment: the family decides based on what they think the patient wants
- Best interest decision: the physician/family decide based on society's values or healthcare recommendations

The faculty members portraying the family members continue their conflict and have heightened emotions while disagreeing with each other. Students need to redirect the family verbalizations to focus on the patient's request. The family members may verbalize the following points:

- Why did you not arrive sooner to the hospital?
- Dad just needs to have his dialysis so he can get better.
- Why are you telling Dad it is okay to stop dialysis?
- How can you control pain at home when the medication is not helping now?

The conference concludes that the family will have hospice care.

The scenario switches back to the **home,** where the setting change has occurred. The patient will complain of pain, moan, be restless, and have episodes of delirium. The patient may verbalize the following points:

- I will be with you [deceased family members] soon.
- I caught that fish.
- I am hurrying.
- The train is coming.
- It feels warm.
- It is so light, peaceful.

Patient Vital Signs and Assessment

Temperature: 36.0°C

Pulse: 56, irregular; atrial fibrillation rhythm

Respiration: 12—shallow, crackles bilaterally in lower lobes, nonproductive cough

- Audible gurgling sound with respirations
- Cheyne-Stokes respiratory pattern can be present

Blood pressure: 80/50

Oxygen saturation: 80%

Urine output: none for the past 12 hours; Foley catheter in place or can be removed

Programming for METI HPS or ECS

Patient: standard man

Respiration:
- Shunt fraction: 30
- Oxygen consumption: 400
- Tidal volume factor: 0.60
- Breath sounds: abnormal
- Respiratory rate factor: 0.75

Cardiac:
- Ischemic sensitivity: 0.22
- Cardiac override: atrial fibrillation
- Heart rate factor: 0.6
- Systemic vascular resistance: 0.7
- Venous capacity: 1.25

Cheyne-Stokes pattern: respiratory override 6/min, then turn override to 18/min

Two Points for Students to Manage

- The patient will experience some out-of-body behavior and verbalizations. Students should not try to reorient the patient, and should encourage his spiritual release and emotions. Have the students focus on effective communication.
- The patient will experience breakthrough pain. Students should realize that the Roxinal is not dosed correctly. The patient should be able to have 10% of the long-term morphine sulfate dose of MS Contin. His dose is 180 mg per day, and 10% would be 18 mg per dose.

Students should assess the family members' needs for emotional and spiritual support.

To assist with stopping the simulation, the family thanks the nurses for coming to the home and walks them to the door. It is very awkward to try to interrupt the scenario, and this step allows for a more natural break in the action.

DEBRIEFING

Potential Statements to Facilitate Emotional/Values Clarification

- Tell me about how you are feeling.
- What was difficult for you when you were in the hospital room? At the conference? At the home?
- Which communication skills did you use? How did you assess the family's nonverbal communication?
- How did this experience compare to your thoughts about death?
- How would you validate that the patient understood what would happen when he went home?
- Did you find it difficult to say the word "death" within the context of the conversations?
- Why did the family have conflict?
- How did you assess the stages of the grieving process for the patient and the family?

- What did the patient value at this time of his life? Which values did the family have?

EQUIPMENT SETUP

Hospital

- The location of IV access is important because students need to be aware of AV fistula.
- The IV site can be either peripheral on the opposite hand or a jugular/ subclavian site can be used as an alternate site, depending on the level of the students.
- The IV catheter is located on the back of the left hand.
- The dialysis shunt is in the right forearm. Use a small endotracheal tube, and place it in a looped position, under the skin or wrapped using Coban.
- IV fluid and pump (optional).
- Oxygen: nasal cannula and oxygen flow meter if available.
- Foley catheter.
- Blood pressure cuff.
- Temperature monitor.
- Cardiac monitor (optional).
- Blood glucose monitor and supplies.
- Medication per medication administration record. Students will not have time to administer the medications, or you can have the medications already administered for the morning.
- Patient gown, ID bracelet, and Ted Hose.
- Peripheral edema: use of memory foam covered with Ted Hose.
- Moulage: clubbing and cyanotic nail beds, cyanosis/dusky facial coloring. The coloring can be obtained by mixing white grease paint with hand cream, applying it over the mannequin's face, and letting it dry. It should give a light coloring; add blue coloring as needed.
- Advance directive form. Download a form from an area hospital or state Web site.
- Hospice pamphlets from agencies in your area.
- Hospital chart with history of past 24 hours/MAR.

Home

- The patient's home address is on the entrance into the simulation area.
- The patient does not have IV access or a cardiac monitor. The Foley catheter can be removed.

- The patient can be in bed or a recliner chair.
- Put up drapes and fabric to cover up the hospital headboard. You can use a moveable screen that can be rolled behind the head of the bed.
- Table lamp.
- Personalize the environment by adding family pictures, favorite candy, a quilt/comforter, and other items.
- Spiritual cues: Bible, cross, pictures, books.
- Hospice literature and books from local organization.
- Home log book of medication administration, with family notes.

SCENARIO BACKGROUND

The patient is an 85-year-old male who was admitted with an acute episode of congestive heart failure. He has a history of end-stage renal disease, diabetes, hypertension, anemia, and chronic congestive heart failure with atrial fibrillation. He goes to dialysis three times a week.

Psychosocial

The patient's wife died 3 years ago. He has one son and one daughter, both of whom live out of town. The patient has been in an assisted-living apartment for the past 3 years. However, he has been living with his daughter for the past 3 months because of his declining independence and inability to perform activities of daily living.

Patient Home Medication

Acetylsalicylic acid (ASA): 81 mg po tablets daily
Alprazolam (Xanax): 0.25 mg po three times a day prn
Nitroglycerin patch: 7.5 mg transdermal patch every day, remove at bedtime
Hydrochlorothiazide (Hydrodiuril): 50 mg po daily
Carvedilol (Coreg): 12 mg po daily
Sertraline hydrochloride (Zoloft): 150 mg po daily
Potassium: 10 mEq po daily every other day
Calcium carbonate: one tablet with meals
Multivitamin with iron: one tablet po daily
Vitamin B_{12} injections: at the doctor's office
Epogen: injections once a week, 50–100 unit/kg subq

Spirolactone (Aldactone): 25 mg po daily
Furosemide: 60 mg po daily
Lantus insulin: 15 units at bedtime
Insulin: NPH 15 units and regular insulin 12 units A.M. dose; regular insulin
    10 units before dinner
Coumadin: 5 mg po daily
Digoxin: 0.125 mg daily

Physician Orders for Admission

Diet: 2 g Na, 1800 cal, diabetic, renal diet
Intravenous fluids: 0.45% normal saline at 50 cc/h
Vital signs with oxygen saturation q 4 hours
Neuro/circulation checks every 2 hours
Accucheck AC and HS
Oxygen saturation ≤ 92%; titrate oxygen per nasal cannula
Nitroglycerin patch: 7.5 mg transdermal patch
Hydrochlorothiazide (Hydrodiuril): 50 mg po daily
Carvedilol (Coreg): 12 mg po daily
Sertraline hydrochloride (Zoloft): 150 mg po daily
Calcium carbonate: one tablet with meals
Multivitamin with iron: one tablet po daily
Enoxaparin (Lovenox): 15 mg subq every 12 hours
Morphine sulfate: 1–2 mg IV every 2–3 hours prn for pain
Lantus insulin: 10 units HS
Insulin: NPH 15 units and regular insulin 12 units A.M. dose; regular insulin
    10 units before dinner
Sliding scale:
    Accucheck > 150–200: 2 units
    201–225: 4 units
    226–250: 6 units
Spirolactone (Aldactone): 25 mg po daily
Digoxin: 0.125 mg IV daily
Furosemide: 60 mg IV daily
Foley catheter
Colace: 100 mg po twice a day
Alprazolam (Xanax): 0.25 mg po three times a day prn for anxiety
Respiratory treatments: albuterol q 4 hours and prn for s/s respiratory
    distress
Consult for dialysis: Monday/Wednesday/Friday

Home Care Orders

Roxanol: 10 mg every 2 hours prn
MS: continuous 90 mg po every 12 hours
Duragesic: 75 mcg patch every 3 days
Ativan: 2 mg sublingual liquid every 4 hours prn anxiety
Haloperidol: 0.5–2.0 sublingual liquid every 4 hours prn delirium
Decadron: 4 mg po with food prn for severe pain/dyspnea
Acetaminophen: 650 mg suppository every 4 hours prn for elevated temper-
    ature
Compazine: 25 mg every 12 hours suppository prn for nausea
Scopolamine: 1.5 mg transdermal patch; can titrate up to 3 patches apply-
    ing every 12 hours

Laboratory Data

CBC

Red blood cell count: 4.2 m/mm^3
Hemoglobin: 9.0 g/dL
Hematocrit: 28%
Reticulocyte count: 0.75% of RBC
MCV: 100 mm^3
MCHC: 39%
Platelets: 100,000/mm^3
White blood cell, total: 6.0 × 10^3/L

Chemistry/Metabolic Profile

Sodium: 130 mEq/L
Chloride: 94 mEq/L
Potassium: 4.0 mcg/L
Blood urea nitrogen (BUN): 140 mg/dL
Creatinine: 15.6 mg/dL
GFR: 5 L/day
Albumin: 2.7 g/dL
Glucose: 180 mg/dL
Calcium: 8.2 mg/dL
Phosphorus: 5.5 mg/dL
Magnesium: 2.0 mg/dL
ALT: 38 μ/L
AST: 45 μ/L

Cholesterol: 260 mg/dL
BNP: 600 mg/dL

Coagulation Profile

Prothrombin time (PT): 18.0 seconds
Partial thromboplastin time (PTT): 30 seconds
INR: 2.4

Urinalysis

Specific gravity: 1.008
Protein: 8 mg/dL
No WBC, RBC, ketones

Arterial Blood Gases

pH: 7.34
PaO_2: 75
$PaCO_2$: 46
Bicarbonate: 18

Digoxin

Level: 1.8 ng/mL

References

Casarett, D. J., & Quill, T. E. (2007). "I'm not ready for hospice": Strategies for timely and effective hospice discussions. *Annals of Internal Medicine, 146,* 443–449.

Chu, J. (2007). Communication at end-of-life for family members. *American Journal of Nursing, 107,* 72DD–72FF.

Lofmark, R. (2007). From cure to palliation: Concept, decision, and acceptance. *Journal of Medical Ethics, 33,* 685–688.

London, M. R., & Lundstedt, J. (2007). Families speak about inpatient end-of-life care. *Journal of Nursing Care Quality, 22,* 152–158.

Miller, J. F. (2007). Hope: A construct central to nursing. *Nursing Forum, 42*(1), 12–19.

Noble, H., Kelly, D., Rawlings-Anderson, K., & Meyer, J. (2007). A concept analysis of renal supportive care: The changing world of nephrology. *Journal of Advanced Nursing, 59,* 644–653.

Roscoe, L. A., & Schonwetter, R. S. (2006). Improving access to hospice and palliative care for patients near the end of life: Present status and future direction. *Journal of Palliative Care, 22*(1), 46–50.

CHAPTER 12

Acute Care for Advanced Practice Nurses

Karen S. Kesten, Helen F. Brown,
Stephen Hurst, and Linda A. Briggs

Programs that prepare and educate advance practice nurses (APN), including acute care nurse practitioners (ACNP), certified registered nurse anesthetists (CRNA), and acute and critical care clinical nurse specialists (CCNS), are challenged to determine the degree to which technical skills unique to the care of critically ill patients should be integrated with cognitive skills. Faculties endeavor to provide the best methods to integrate didactic content, technical skills, and clinical practice into the curriculum. Developing proficiency in assessment, diagnosis, and management of acute, urgent, and emergent situations for critically ill patients is a primary goal of instruction. Education methodologies strive to ensure synthesis of knowledge and retention of skills in a nonthreatening environment so as to ensure patient safety.

This chapter describes the use of a high-fidelity human simulation laboratory in a university school of nursing, where the goal is to provide the best opportunity for synthesis of these skills for the ACNP and CNS student. It addresses decision making by personnel ranging from novices to experts, selection of an appropriate learning scenario, development of the scenario content, the actual implementation process, the successes and challenges of the implementation, use of diverse simulation tools, student evaluation, and future challenges for educators.

Traditionally, the integration of didactic content and clinical skills occurs in the clinical arena, under the supervision of faculty members and preceptors. However, the clinical environment may not be able to provide adequate exposure for students to diagnose and manage certain patient situations owing to time constraints or unavailability of clinical sites. Additionally, limited time frames, variable settings, inconsistent skill sets of preceptors, and competition for clinical placement sites may create barriers to effective synthesis of knowledge and skills. Further, student participation in the management and direction of emergency measures could potentially place the real-world patient at risk. In contrast, the simulation lab provides an opportunity for students to practice critical decision making in both low-frequency and high-stakes situations, without any party experiencing a penalty for mistakes. Subsequent debriefing by faculty and students then creates an opportunity to review and reinforce appropriate behaviors and to discuss areas for improvement. This feedback mechanism facilitates the retention of the materials discussed, as they relate to the student's experiences. Prior to implementing the learning scenario, educators need to determine which specific skills APNs need to safely assess, manage, and treat acute and critically ill patients.

SELECTING A LEARNING SCENARIO

In preparation for each semester, faculty members meet to review the course objectives and identify the course content and skills to teach in the simulation laboratory. From this list, ideas for scenarios may emerge. The initial step in selecting a learning scenario is to identify the purpose, goals, and expected outcomes of the simulated experience (see Figure 12-1). An example of goals for a scenario might include mastery of psychomotor skills, demonstration of diagnostic reasoning, and coordination of interventions and management during a simulated patient situation. While both the ACNP and the CCNS are responsible for managing the care of critically ill patients, a review of the scope of practice for each role and an analysis of the likelihood of application of those skills are incorporated into the decision-making process (Scherer, Bruce, Graves, & Erdley, 2003). Sources such as APN practice surveys, suggested or mandated competencies, potential employers, professional organizations, individual state Nurse Practice Acts, and advisory boards may be used to determine which skills are likely to be needed by the various advance practice roles (see Table 12-1). Nurse practitioners spend the majority of their time providing direct patient care, whereas clinical nurse specialists divide their time more evenly between expert care at the bedside, education, consultation, and research (Kleinpell-Nowell, 2001). Practice surveys of APNs report that while technical skills may be used by either the ACNP or the CCNS, the ACNP is more likely to need invasive procedure technical skills practice (Kleinpell-Nowell, 2001). Skills training may be offered to both the CCNS and the ACNP, with more emphasis being placed on these technical skills for the ACNP. An annual review, revisions, and updates to those skills also occur.

Frequently encountered clinical problems that significantly influence patient outcomes are also considered. For example, faculty members in advanced practice programs frequently focus on respiratory failure and hemodynamic instability as part of patient scenarios. The exemplar scenario in this chapter is the patient in shock: This scenario illustrates the application and

Figure 12-1   Simulation Preparation

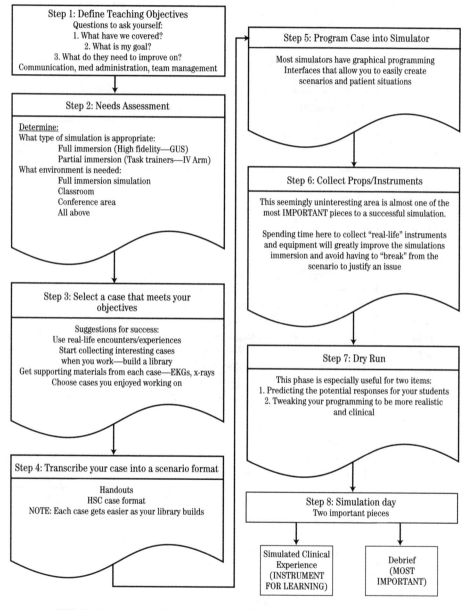

Step 1: Define Teaching Objectives
Questions to ask yourself:
1. What have we covered?
2. What is my goal?
3. What do they need to improve on?
Communication, med administration, team management

Step 2: Needs Assessment

Determine:
What type of simulation is appropriate:
    Full immersion (High fidelity—GUS)
    Partial immersion (Task trainers—IV Arm)
What environment is needed:
    Full immersion simulation
    Classroom
    Conference area
    All above

Step 3: Select a case that meets your objectives

Suggestions for success:
Use real-life encounters/experiences
Start collecting interesting cases
    when you work—build a library
Get supporting materials from each case—EKGs, x-rays
Choose cases you enjoyed working on

Step 4: Transcribe your case into a scenario format

Handouts
HSC case format
NOTE: Each case gets easier as your library builds

Step 5: Program Case into Simulator

Most simulators have graphical programming
Interfaces that allow you to easily create
scenarios and patient situations

Step 6: Collect Props/Instruments

This seemingly uninteresting area is almost one of the
most IMPORTANT pieces to a successful simulation.

Spending time here to collect "real-life" instruments
and equipment will greatly improve the simulations
immersion and avoid having to "break" from the
scenario to justify an issue

Step 7: Dry Run

This phase is especially useful for two items:
1. Predicting the potential responses for your students
2. Tweaking your programming to be more realistic
    and clinical

Step 8: Simulation day
Two important pieces

Simulated Clinical
Experience
(INSTRUMENT
FOR LEARNING)

Debrief
(MOST
IMPORTANT)

NOTE: Time to create a simulation can vary, as a rule of thumb add 25% to your estimated time—this allows for any unforeseen issues—i.e, equipment procurement problems, programming issues, etc.

Table 12-1   Selected Skills for the Acute Care Advanced Practice Nurse

Cognitive	Assessment, diagnosis, and management of fluid and electrolytes
	Assessment, diagnosis, and management of hypovolemic, cardiogenic, distributive, and obstructive shock.
	Implementation of sedation and analgesic concepts
	BLS and ACLS algorithms
	Initiation of invasive and noninvasive hemodynamic monitoring, continuous ECG monitoring
	AHA ACS algorithms
	12 lead ECG interpretation
	Chest X-ray interpretation
	Titration of vasoactive medications
Psychomotor	Airway management, rapid sequence intubation, oxygen therapies
	Arterial line and central line insertion
	CPR, defibrillation, synchronized cardioversion, transcutaneous pacing
	Auscultation of breath, heart, and bowel sounds
	Pericardiocentesis, thoracentesis
Affective	Palliative care End-of-life care
	Emotional family outbursts, interruptions

synthesis of skills and knowledge related to the management of a complex patient situation with severe consequences. The optimal outcome for this activity is for the APN student to demonstrate complex critical-thinking skills, such as prioritizing multiple interventions that need to occur simultaneously. In the simulation, the APN student utilizes the technical skills necessary to intervene and direct care for a patient experiencing cardiopulmonary instability.

During the student's first experience with simulation, simple straightforward scenarios are chosen to facilitate learning. Initially, students are adjusting to the new learning environment and attempting to dispel their disbelief while participating in the simulation. During this phase, the student is adjusting to the patient simulator as a responsive mannequin, who can answer questions, blink his or her eyes, and has a pulse. As the student progresses and becomes more familiar with simulation, more complex layers are added to the scenario development. For example, single-system problems may be presented initially, but these scenarios may evolve into multisystem problems over the course of the program, building on the knowledge and skills that students have acquired.

DETERMINING A FRAMEWORK FOR PROBLEM SOLVING

Novice to Expert Decision Making

Clinical competence has been identified by Benner, Hooper-Kyriakidis, and Stannard (1999) as being acquired through formal knowledge, clinical experience, and clinical performance. According to these authors, in nursing, clinical proficiency is achieved initially through formal knowledge acquired via the educational process, but is then further advanced through clinical experience. This process requires the development of cognitive, psychomotor, and affective skills. Because clinical competence entails more than simply decision making, psychomotor skill acquisition is imperative. Novice, advanced beginner, competent, proficient, and expert stages are linked with critical-thinking skills, pattern recognition, intuitive thought processes, and experiential knowing, all of which are key elements to progressing through the stages.

According to Benner, Hooper-Kyriakidis, and Stannard's (1999) "novice to expert" model, new APN students generally function at the advanced beginner level with graduate nursing skills. Occasionally, one may encounter a novice student who has met the minimum clinical experience criteria and who is adjusting to the role of graduate nurse. According to Benner et al., the novice tends to focus on tasks and checklists, striving to accomplish the tasks in a timely fashion. This learner thrives on rote memory learning. In preparation for the simulation experience, the novice APN critical care student is asked to focus on memorization of the sequence of a physical examination, remembering the OLDCARTS acronym (onset, location, duration, characteristics, associated symptoms, relieving factors, timing, severity) during history taking, and memorizing treatment algorithms for selected urgent and emergent situations.

In contrast, the advanced beginner is able to assess and collect data and possibly perform a basic analysis (Benner et al., 1999), but is unable to accomplish more complex data analyses. The advanced beginner APN is able to collect the pertinent findings for a simulated patient and pinpoint which system is at risk. Often, he or she is not yet able to list all possible differential diagnoses, but can attempt to do so with guidance from faculty members. It is at this point in the simulation experience that faculty members may elect to use the "timeout" approach. Such a break in the action, which occurs when the student has retrieved all pertinent findings from the history, physical exam, and diagnostic testing, provides a learning opportunity for the student and a teachable moment for the faculty. The advanced beginner benefits from greater faculty interface and the opportunity to reflect on the patient scenario.

Typically, according to Benner et al. (1999), the competent nurse makes sound decisions in routine situations. This APN student manages both high-frequency and low-acuity situations with greater confidence. If a situation appears out of the ordinary, the competent nurse consults his or her resources to solve the problem. The APN student consults his or her colleagues with confidence, recognizing a deviation from the norm. The competent APN student also turns to his or her PDA, medication resource, handbook, and/or patient's chart and validates any findings.

During the next stage, a proficient nurse is able to recognize uncommon situations and to problem-solve early in the situation. Proficient nurses learn best from case studies and group thought processes (Benner et al., 1999). Proficient APN students recognize urgent or emergent problems early in their assessments. Typically the complexity of patient learning situations increases with each subsequent semester, building on the skill levels of students as they progress through the curriculum. Students demonstrate proficiency, for example, when initiating the ACLS algorithm appropriately for a patient with a life-threatening dysrhythmia. Although the faculty may allow students at this level to proceed down the algorithmic arm of their choice, the learning scenario is driven to accomplish a prescribed goal for the student. Proficient students learn quickly from their errors.

According to Benner et al. (1999), an expert is able to assess the situation by seeing the whole picture and seamlessly providing interventions. Students may not reach the expert role during their program of study; however, faculty have devised interesting ways of challenging even those students who appear to be experts. One method of doing so is to add a layer of complexity to the multisystem failure scenario by introducing interruptions from simulated family members who attempt to disrupt the flow of interventions. An alternative way to add complexity is to plan scripts in which team members do not want to follow established guidelines and pathways. Their recalcitrance challenges the student to think critically and to practice collaboration and assertive communication. Another approach to increasing scenario complexity is to introduce the opportunity for palliative care or end-of-life supportive care.

The goal of the faculty is to facilitate the progress of the advanced beginner/competent nurse along the continuum toward expert nurse by using clinical scenarios, problem-based learning, and simulation with repeated exposure. Initially simulation assists in establishing strong foundational habits of thorough history taking and physical assessment skills on which to build further development. Each semester progresses to more complex decision making and skill sets for caring for critically ill patients in the simulation lab. This evolution occurs in a nonthreatening environment in which students can learn from their mistakes. This knowledge is, in turn, transferred to actual patient care and fosters improved patient outcomes (Hravnak, Tuite, & Baldisseri, 2005).

Many techniques for problem solving are incorporated in high-fidelity simulation for advanced practice nursing students. Beginning with familiar content and processes, and then moving on to new and unfamiliar content, allows students to build confidence. As experienced nurses, students are encouraged to employ the nursing process as a framework for proceeding with their scenarios, as they should already be familiar and comfortable with this process. Newly acquired skills related to taking an in-depth history and physical assessment are then overlaid with the nursing process to build students' confidence and ability. For example, didactic and practical introductions to patient interviewing and physical examination are first presented in the Advanced Physical Assessment Course, a prerequisite for all clinical courses. Students then utilize their expanded skill sets in history taking and physical assessment in the simulation lab at the onset of their problem-based learning experience.

The clinical decision making emphasized in the simulation lab draws from current practice guidelines and evidenced-based practice that is introduced in the classroom and then implemented in the simulation laboratory. For example, appropriate guidelines for algorithms such as Basic Life Support (BLS) and Advanced Cardiac Life Support (ACLS) are reinforced in the didactic component of the course. Students are also required to have BLS and ACLS certification prior to enrolling in clinical courses. Application of these algorithms, as well as the American Heart Association's acute coronary syndrome and stroke algorithms, occurs during the simulation experience as well (Field, Hazinski, & Gilmore, 2006). For example, when making a differential diagnosis, students are expected to differentiate between ST-segment elevation myocardial infarction and non-ST-segment elevation myocardial infarction by following the nationally accepted guidelines (Field et al., 2006).

Determining the Skills to Be Practiced and Evaluated

As mentioned previously, numerous sources including practice surveys and suggested national competencies are considered when determining skills to be incorporated in learning scenarios. Following Benner, Hooper-Kyriakidis, and Stannard's novice to expert model (1999), skills practiced in the first clinical semester are more basic, such as advanced physical assessment techniques and patient interviewing. These skills build on the assessment skills of a graduate nurse, but introduce newly acquired advanced assessment skills. While diagnostic reasoning is introduced and evaluated in the first clinical semester, the level of critical thinking increases with progressive experiences across semesters. Scenario and skill selection also closely follows the lecture schedule for the clinical courses. For example, to reinforce the content delivered in lectures related to heart failure and pulmonary embolism, a scenario related to diagnostic reasoning and the patient complaint of dyspnea might be scheduled. In this scenario, the advanced practice student nurse learns to apply assessment skills and diagnostic differentials to a scenario in the simulation center to determine whether the cause of dyspnea in the patient is related to congestive heart failure or to pulmonary embolism.

Establishing Performance Criteria

Assessing students' progress and providing feedback are important summary functions following all simulation experiences. Initially feedback is provided primarily through post-simulation debriefing sessions. This approach is in keeping with the philosophy of providing a nonthreatening environment for learning. As students progress through the program, however, they both need and desire more detailed feedback. Recording observations while assisting with other tasks during simulation can prove challenging for faculty. Reviewing recordings can improve the detail of the evaluations, but can be a very time-consuming task.

A performance evaluation tool is typically used to assess performance of the APN student. The same tool can be used by students to perform self-evaluations (see Table 12-2). During the first semester, when many of the simulation experiences involve assessment and diagnostic reasoning, only the Phase 1 portion of the tool is completed as a self-evaluation. In the second and final semesters, the entire tool is completed as a self-evaluation. The faculty member completes the tool without assigning any grades for the simulations during the second and third semesters. Only the final comprehensive exam simulation experience is graded. Students who are in the debriefing room observing simulations either use the form or answer questions evaluating the

Table 12-2 APN Simulation Evaluation Form

Name: _____ Date: _____ Reviewer: _____
Scenario: _____

Phase I - Assessment

Student Action	Performed		Comment
	Yes	No	
Introduces self to patient			
Maintains realism—treating simulator as "real patient"			
Utilizes universal precautions			
Subjective Data Collection			
Efficiently collects subjective data within stated timeframe			
Subjective data collection appropriate for setting *(complete vs. focused)*			
HPI *(obtains minimum of 5 of 8 characteristics)* ☐ Onset ☐ Location ☐ Duration ☐ Description ☐ Characteristics ☐ Aggravating/Alleviating Factors ☐ Temporal Features ☐ Severity			
Past Medical History			
☐ Medications ☐ Allergies			

Table 12-2   APN Simulation Evaluation Form (continued)

Student Action	Performed		Comment
	Yes	No	
Past Surgical History			
Social History ☐ Tobacco ☐ Alcohol ☐ Drugs ☐ Occupation ☐ Marital Status			
Family History			
Review of Systems (*Complete history elicits minimum 9 systems,* *Focused history reviews minimum 4 systems*) ☐ General ☐ HEENT ☐ CV ☐ Resp ☐ GI ☐ GU ☐ MS ☐ Neuro ☐ Skin ☐ Endo ☐ Heme ☐ Psychosocial			
Utilizes other sources to collect subjective data (patient's chart, flow sheets, medication list, family member)			
Objective Data Collection			
Performs physical examination appropriate for scenario within stated timeframe			
Confirms findings with validator			

Table 12-2 APN Simulation Evaluation Form (continued)

	Yes	No			
Requests current lab data and radiographic data					
Remains vigilant to patient's clinical status including rhythm, heart rate, blood pressure, oxygen saturation, and pain level					
Interprets subjective and objective data developing and discussing the differential diagnosis for problem					
Identifies most likely cause of patient's problem					
Initiates interventions as subjective and objective data is collected					

Phase II - Intervention

Student Action	Performed		Comment
	Yes	No	
Orders diagnostic studies based on assessment of patient's problem			
Initiates medical interventions to resolve/stabilize the patient's problem ☐ Medications ☐ Intravenous fluids ☐ Oxygen ☐ Cardioversion ☐ Defibrillation ☐ Central line insertion ☐ Chest tube insertion ☐ Rapid sequence intubation			

Table 12-2   APN Simulation Evaluation Form (continued)

Student Action	Performed		Comment
	Yes	No	
Recognizes deterioration in patient's condition, initiates appropriate intervention			
Demonstrates appropriate use of			
☐ ACLS protocol			
☐ National standards/guidelines to manage the clinical situation			
Analyzes laboratory and radiographic data, comparing to prior studies			
Reevaluates assessment/diagnosis based on patient's response to treatment and additional diagnostic data			

Phase III - Stabilization

Student Action	Performed		Comment
	Yes	No	
Identifies endpoints indicating adequate resuscitation (*HR, MAP, O₂ Sat*)			
Demonstrates continued surveillance of patient while consulting with physician or arranging for admission or transfer			
When speaking with the consultant:			

Table 12-2   APN Simulation Evaluation Form *(continued)*

a. identifies himself/herself, the patient, the problem							
b. concisely relates the patient's problem and pertinent medical history							
c. relates the current status of the patient and treatment initiated including medications, intravenous fluids, procedures, such as cardioversion, defibrillation, or intubation							
d. reviews significant laboratory and radiographic findings							
e. states the proposed medical diagnoses with rationale							
f. describes current treatment plan							
g. requests admission or transfer of the patient							
Appropriately documents the encounter in SOAP note or H&P format							

Table 12-2 APN Simulation Evaluation Form *(continued)*

Phase IV - Leadership

Student Action	Performed		Comment
	Yes	No	
Demonstrates leadership in the management of the clinical situation as evidenced by: ☐ Collaboration with team members ☐ Delegation ☐ Consultation with peers ☐ Effective communication			
Demonstrates the ability to handle problem situations ☐ Technical *(equipment failure, inability to perform procedure)* ☐ Performance problem of team member ☐ Communication with family members *(distraught family member)* ☐ Physiologic *(termination of resuscitative efforts, end-of-life issues)*			
Remains professional throughout clinical situation			

leadership and communication skills of the team leader and team, as well as providing patient care according to guidelines or evidence-based practice. This format is used by the students over all semesters to assist the students and faculty in providing feedback during debriefing sessions.

SCENARIO DEVELOPMENT

As stated previously, the main objective of patient simulation is to allow students to combine didactic learning with clinical practice. To implement this type of educational experience for students the following fundamental questions should be considered (Lighthall et al., 2003):

- Does the envisioned scenario provide a reasonable replica of the human characteristics of the clinical situation?
- Does it present challenging problems that require critical thinking, and interpretation of both subjective and objective data?
- Does it provide opportunities for interventions requiring use of important psychomotor skills?
- Does it allow the student to manage the case with minimal assistance from the instructor?
- Does it provide an opportunity for a detailed appraisal of the student's performance and an opportunity for self-evaluation?

Developing a Roadmap

Scenario development is based on both the current course content and the expected clinical outcomes. When writing a patient scenario, taking advantage of faculty or clinical expert experience is often possible. Sources for the simulations may include student case presentations, journals, a faculty member's clinical practice, or a contrived situation.

Using a flowchart to map out critical events, key decision points, and alternative outcomes may be helpful to serve as a framework on which to add salient details. This chart or algorithm would incorporate the expected outcomes for successful completion of the human simulated scenario but also includes alternative pathways, which would lead back to the ultimate goal of the scenario (see Figure 12-2). For example, if the purpose of the scenario is management of a patient with atrial fibrillation with rapid ventricular response and hypotension, one arm of the algorithm would consist of identification of unstable tachycardia treated with cardioversion. An alternative treatment—for example, a drug intervention—would not be successful in this case and could potentially cause further deterioration of the patient. This deterioration would

Figure 12-2 Hypovolemia Algorithm

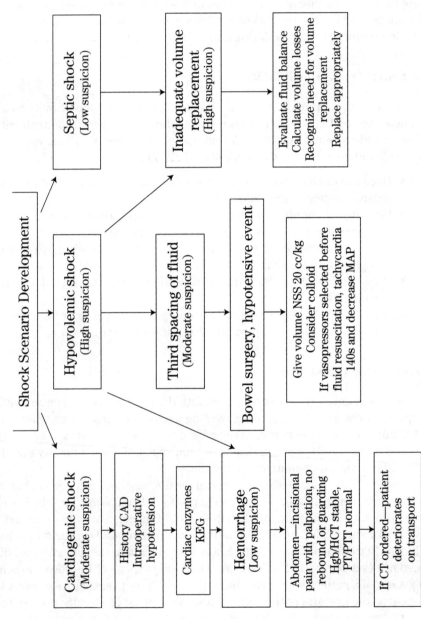

then loop back to the decision point for cardioversion of the patient. Although it is impossible to predict all actions students might take, anticipating the most likely responses helps to make the simulation unfold in a smooth, logical manner. Similarly, developing an algorithmic schema gives faculty members and technical staff a guideline to follow when implementing the scenario with the students. Notably, one resource for published algorithms (Field, Hazinski, & Gilmore, 2006) includes evidence-based guidelines.

Writing the Scenario Script

Once the flowchart, algorithm, or decision tree is completed, a script can be written for the scenario. This script includes the setting or scene, the types of participants, the patient details, and the props necessary to foster realism. Important teaching points and listings of pertinent references can also be included in the script to prevent omission during the simulation and to decrease future preparation time. Developing a standardized script format assists both participating faculty and the software engineer to unfold the scenario in an organized and logical manner (see Table 12-3).

It is a good idea to consider using a template that is divided into phases. In the first phase, the location of the patient is identified and the problem elucidated. As an example, suppose Mr. Ivan Trouble Breathing is a 58-year-old male who was admitted to the ICU 12 hours ago with bilateral lower-lobe pneumonia. The bedside nurse calls and states that the patient continues to desaturate despite being on a 100% non-rebreather mask. The lead-in to this scenario might be a page from the nurse, a change-of-shift report from a colleague, a call from the emergency department (ED) to admit the patient, or the arrival of the patient in the ED. Each of these situations requires the student to use a different skill set to obtain the data necessary to care for the patient. The patient presenting to the ED, for example, requires the student to obtain a full history, including the history of present illness, past medical history, past surgical history, social history, and family history; review of systems; and a physical examination. In this case, the skill set needed is the ability to efficiently obtain the necessary data while directing the bedside nurse to initiate interventions to stabilize and manage the patient's problem. For a patient located in the ICU or medical unit, the APN student will need to access currently available data in the medical record, evaluate vital sign patterns, determine fluid balance, evaluate laboratory data, and physically examine the patient.

Phase 1 of the simulation should include the subjective data collected from the patient, physical assessment findings, and ongoing physiological changes. Patient demographics, such as gender, age, race, and ethnicity, are recorded in

**Table 12-3   APN Scenario: Acute Care Advance Practice Nurse
Scenario #1–Hypovolemic Shock**

1. Purpose: To provide ACNP and CCNS students with a clinical situation requiring the recognition, diagnosis, and management of hypovolemic shock
2. Objectives: At the end of this simulation the APN student will be able to:
   a. Synthesize the patient's subjective and objective data to identify the potential causes of hemodynamic instability
   b. Develop a list of differential diagnoses selecting the most likely cause of the patient's hypotension
   c. Articulate the causes of hypovolemic shock
   d. Apply the principles of volume replacement to appropriately perform volume resuscitation of the patient
   e. Compare and contrast the risks and benefits of crystalloid versus colloid volume replacement
   f. Order appropriate diagnostic tests to evaluate the patient
   g. Recognize when the use of hemodynamic monitor would contribute to diagnosis and management of the patient
   h. Recognize appropriate situations for use of vasoactive agents
   i. Determine the endpoint in resuscitation, with stabilization of the patient or recognition of the futility of continued care
   j. Effectively communicate the clinical presentation, interventions, diagnostic studies, diagnosis, and plan to provider assuming care of the patient
   k. Document the clinical scenario using a SOAP format
3. Student Preparation: Review class lecture and assigned readings
4. Scenario Setting: Intensive Care Unit
5. Simulator setup-props: Intubated—#8 oral endotracheal tube, ventilator, A-line, central line, CVP, orogastric tube, Foley, IV fluid infusing—D_5 $^1/_2$ NSS at 150 cc/hr, Critical Care Flow Sheet, chart with H&P, lab data
6. Roles: Team Leader—APN student, Bedside RN—APN student, Scribe—APN student, Others by faculty
7. Scenario: You are paged by the bedside nurse who states, "Could you please come see Mr. Smith, a 58-year-old, 80 kg Caucasian male. He is tachycardic with low blood pressure." If APN student requests more information the bedside nurse states "He is 2 hours post colectomy for transverse colon cancer, intraoperative complication with 900 cc blood loss, hypotensive episode lasting 30 minutes, total operative time 4.5 hours. Problem: Tachycardia—125 b/m—outside parameter to notify practitioner."

Table 12-3 APN Scenario: Acute Care Advance Practice Nurse Scenario #1–Hypovolemic Shock (continued)

Subjective (Simulator Voice)	Objective (Validator—Faculty)	Physiologic Parameters	Expected Outcome (Student)	Teaching Points (Faculty)
Responds with + head nod to pain—indicates abdomen "points to 9 on liner scale" and endotracheal tube	**Neuro:** Awakens to calling name/light touch becomes restless, MAE =, appropriate nod to questions	Monitor: S. Tach. 126 w PVC's – 10%	*Time— 15 minutes*	Differential Diagnosis for Hypotension
	HEENT: PERRL, tracks with eyes, conjunctive pale # 14 OGT, # 8 OTT, MMM moist	A-line: 88/50	1. Collaborates with nurse—reviews vital signs, fluid balance, and oxygenation status	**VINDICATE**
		MAP:		**V—Vascular** (MI), **Volume**
	CV: RRR—tachycardia, S¹S², no M/R/G, peripheral pulses weak— +2/+4 carotid and femoral, R/PT/P others +1/+4, + facial and sacral edema	CVP: 3	2. Introduces self to patient	**I—Infection**
		RR: 16		**N—Neoplasm**
		Temp: 36⁰ C.	3. Obtain subjective data—Pain, SOB	(especially CNS—Ca)
		Vent: A/C 12		**D—Degeneration**
		TV: 700 cc, FIO₂: 0.4, PEEP 5 cm, Peak airway pressure: 12	4. Notes current status of vital signs, CVP	(ANS, Shy-Dragger, decreased baroreceptor response)
	Resp: Regular, Cleat on percussion, crackles bases	SpO₂: 98%	5. Performs focus exam of CV, Resp, and Abdomen	**I—Intoxication/ Iatrogenic**
		CV: normal		(narcotics/diuresis, vasodilators)
		Resp: crackles bases	6. Requests current lab data from nurse	**C—Congenital**
		GI: hypoactive bowel sounds		(Adrenal insufficiency, heart disease)
		OGT: bile		
		GU: Foley 20 cc		

Phase I—Assessment

**Table 12-3   APN Scenario: Acute Care Advance Practice Nurse
Scenario #1—Hypovolemic Shock (continued)**

Subjective (Simulator Voice)	Objective (Validator—Faculty)	Physiologic Parameters	Expected Outcome (Student)	Teaching Points (Faculty)
	GI: Midline abd. Incision dry, ND, hypoactive BS, incisional/generalized tenderness with guarding, OGT—bile **GU:** Foley—post op average 30 cc/hr Fluid balance—I: 3800 cc O: 1365 cc + 2435 cc **Skin:** Cool, dry, cap refill > 5 sec. Incision noted above		7. Request Chart—limited review 8. States differential diagnosis—minimum of 4 9. Identifies most likely cause of tachycardia and hypotension 10. Initiates fluid resuscitation as collecting subjective/objective data	**A—Allergic/ Autoimmune** **T—Trauma** **E—Endocrine** (DKA, HHC, Adrenal insufficiency, thyrotoxicosis)

Phase I—Assessment

Table 12-3   APN Scenario: Acute Care Advance Practice Nurse Scenario #1–Hypovolemic Shock (continued)

Phase II—Intervention				
Hypovolemic Shock S/P transverse colectomy due to • Third spacing from • Bowel surgery and ischemic episode (high suspicion) • Hemorrhage (moderate suspicion) • Inadequate volume replacement (high suspicion) **Coagulopathy** • Blood loss/transfusion (low suspicion)	**1. Fluid resuscitation** • Fluid deficit = 3200 cc • Give 1700 cc bolus over 20 minutes. • Reassess hemodynamics and UO • Consider changing to PA catheter if cause of hypotension remains unclear • 1 unit PRBC for continued hypotension **Diagnostic studies** • Hgb and HCT • Lactate • PT/PTT • CK/MB, Troponin • ABG • EKG	**If Fluid Bolus** minimum 20 cc/kg NSS or LR Heart rate 120s, BP 90/60, MAP 69–72 mmHg, SpO$_2$ 98% **If no fluids initiated during Phase I** • Incr. heart rate 130s • MAP 60s, SpO$_2$ 94% **If vasoactive drugs initiated prior to giving fluids** • Patient deteriorates • Heart rate 140s • MAP 60 mmHG • SpO$_2$ 90%	***Timeframe: 15 minutes*** 1. Recognizes hypovolemic shock Initial volume—20 cc/kg. 2. Considers crystalloid vs. colloid resuscitation 3. Calculates volume losses intraoperatively—determines that patient inadequately resuscitated intraoperatively 4. Orders appropriate diagnostics studies	1. Review differential Dx for hypovolemic shock 2. Discuss potential for other forms of shock in this patient • Cardiac—hx of CAD, check enzymes and EKG to R/O MI Cardiogenic shock • Septic—complicated intraoperative course 3. Calculates patient's volume loss from surgery (refer to handout) 4. Crystalloid vs. colloid replacement (refer to handout)

Table 12-3 APN Scenario: Acute Care Advance Practice Nurse Scenario #1–Hypovolemic Shock (continued)

	Subjective (Simulator Voice)	Objective (Validator—Faculty)	Physiologic Parameters	Expected Outcome (Student)	Teaching Points (Faculty)
Phase II—Intervention	**Metabolic acidosis** • Lactic acidosis due to intra- and postoperative hypotension— anion gap = 19	**Start Inotrope for MAP < 65 after adequate volume resuscitation** • Dopamine/ norepinephrine	• **If CT abd/pelvis ordered** • Patient deteriorates during transport and codes **With volume resuscitation** • Fluid = 2 L or 500 cc colloid • Heart rate decreases 100s, SpO$_2$ 98% • MAP increase to 68–70 mmHg indicating adequate volume resuscitation **If vasopressor added at this time** • Effective increase MAP to 70 mmHg	Hgb/ HCT, PT/INR, PTT, Troponin, CK/MB, EKG, ABG 5. Reevaluates patient after each intervention 6. Considers use of PA catheter for persistent hypotension not responsive to fluid resuscitation 7. After adequate volume resuscitation—considers vasoactive infusion to maintain MAP ≥ 65 mmHg norepinephrine or dopamine 8. Evaluates lab data	5. Acidosis – metabolic – • + anion gap • Low pH • Serum lactate 6. Oxygenation • P/F ratio 7. Is PA catheter necessary? 8. Diagnostic test • Hemorrhage • CT abd/pelvis • Ultrasound • OR for re-exploration.

Table 12-3 APN Scenario: Acute Care Advance Practice Nurse Scenario #1–Hypovolemic Shock (*continued*)

Phase III—Stabilization			

• Primary cause hypovolemic shock due to inadequate intra-operative volume replacement
 	
• Metabolic acidosis due to hypovolemia and hypotension
	• Continue IV fluids at 200 cc/hr × 6 hrs
	
	• Norepinephrine gtt to maintain MAP ≥ 65 mmHg
	
	• Collaborate with RN re goals for stabilized patient
	
	• Consult with surgeon
		Heart rate decreases to 100s
		BP 100/80
		MAP: 70–75 mmHg.
		SpO_2 98%
			Timeframe: 5 minutes
			1. Identifies endpoints indicating adequate resuscitation
			2. Continued surveillance of patient while consulting with surgeon/intensivist
			3. While speaking with the consultant: identifies himself/herself, the patient, the problem
			  • Concisely relates patient's problem, pertinent history, medical, and HPI
			  • Relates the current status of the patient and treatment
			  • Reviews significant lab/radiographic findings
			  • States the proposed medical diagnoses with rationale
			  • Describes current treatment plan
			4. Succinctly documents episode (*SOAP note*)
				Succinct skilled communication technique utilized

**Table 12-3   APN Scenario: Acute Care Advance Practice Nurse
Scenario #1–Hypovolemic Shock (continued)**

	Debriefing Questions	Student's Assessment of Performance	Faculty Tips
Phase VI—Debriefing	What went well during the care of this patient? Phase I? Phase II? Phase III ?	Team leader requested to critique performance—how the assessment, resuscitation, and stabilization phases evolved	**Guidelines**—Foster a mentoring nonjudgmental environment, **emphasis on performance not the performer**
	Was there an area which presented more difficulty—such as the differential for hypotension? Or identifying the most likely cause of the hypovolemia? Or calculating the volume deficit?	Team discusses strengths of performance and areas of weakness—Where could things have been improved? How?	Use open-ended questions to facilitate student discussion (i.e., debate and peer-to-peer learning)
	How could you be more effective in your assigned role?		Avoid using debriefing as a didactic session
	How was communication with the patient/family/team members?		

this section, as well as the patient's presenting history and other interview information. Essential data, such as vital signs, cardiac rhythm, respiratory pattern, oxygenation status, and abnormal physical assessment findings, should be delineated for the technical staff. This facilitates the programming of the simulator. Incorporating diagnostic data, such as laboratory and radiographic findings, increases the realism of the scenario. Analyzing these data in the context of the patient simulation will enhance the diagnostic reasoning experience for the student. It is imperative to review any real patient laboratory findings and radiographs being included in the script prior to presenting the scenario to the students so as to identify all metabolic derangements and radiographic findings. If a contrived patient scenario is being developed, it is important to scrutinize the laboratory data for realism. For example, if the student calculates the anion gap, and the simulated patient has an anion gap acidosis, the scenario should include a logical reason for the patient's acidosis. This careful attention to detail during scenario development helps avoid unexpected identification of impossible or unintended abnormalities during the student's simulation experience.

Desired student outcomes should be quantified, so that successful data collection and decision making in phase 1 move the scenario progression into phase 2, the intervention phase. As part of scenario development, the developer must establish how the physiologic parameters will change if the student does not accomplish specific core actions; the technical staff can then program the simulator with the appropriate parameter responses for both successful and unsuccessful achievement of expected goals.

Phase 2 occurs when the student has successfully achieved the diagnostic/critical-thinking tasks and/or psychomotor skills required in phase 1. Typically phase 2 comprises an intervention or resuscitation phase. At the conclusion of phase 1, the student should have identified a list of differential diagnoses for the patient. In phase 2, the student focuses on the most likely diagnosis for the patient's problem and initiates therapy. The scenario script should reflect the standard of care for a patient with this problem, the anticipated therapy, and the physiologic parameter settings for the simulator. If a flowchart was developed earlier, it can be used as a guide for delineating student actions and decision-making consequences. Expected student outcomes are clearly stated—for example, to establish intravenous access with two large-bore catheters, central line access, volume resuscitation, intubation, adjustment of ventilator settings, cardioversion or defibrillation, and interpretation of laboratory, radiographic, and electrocardiogram data. Analysis of ordered diagnostic studies by the APN student will either support the diagnosis or provide further clues as to the nature of the problem. This exercise provides the APN student with valuable diagnostic reasoning experience. Conclusion of this phase occurs when the patient is successfully stabilized.

Phase 3—stabilization—includes the transfer of care to a colleague or consulting physician, or transfer to a higher level of care. In this phase, the APN student is required to continue managing the patient to maintain a stable situation and comprehensively and concisely hand off care to a colleague. Communication and continued vigilance as the patient transitions to a different level of care are key student outcomes. Again, expected student behaviors and patient physiologic parameters are recorded in the script format. Demonstration of the expected behaviors signals the conclusion of the decision-making portion of the simulation. Activity is then directed to shift to the debriefing room.

Phase 4 consists of critical examination or debriefing of the simulated scenario. The simulation room should have the capability for recording the student–simulator interaction for performance review and self-critique purposes. The debriefing is conducted by a faculty member, who leads the participants in a detailed discussion of their simulated patient experience. The focus of the debriefing is on the performance, rather than the performer. Using open-ended questions encourages participants to examine the care provided to the simulated patient by identifying what went well, how management could be improved, and which alternative therapies or interventions might be employed. The atmosphere for debriefing should be one of constructive feedback, provided in a supportive and nonjudgmental environment. The debriefing should occur immediately following completion of the scenario. At this time, reviewing the recording of the experience may be beneficial to the students.

An alternative debriefing method is to have students review their performances and rate them according to the overall goal of the simulated scenario and expected student goals, noting both successes and areas for improvement. The benefits of debriefing include the reinforcement of a good performance and the opportunity to use a poor performance as a learning tool. The scenario developer should prepare a list of open-ended questions that are specific to the scenario, as well as broader questions that are appropriate to all patient simulation scenarios (see Table 12-3).

Setting the Stage

An environment that duplicates the workplace permits the APN student to evaluate and manage the high-fidelity patient simulator in a familiar clinical setting with appropriate monitoring and equipment. The high-fidelity patient simulator should be maintained in a room that can be adapted to the needs of various advanced practice nurse students: acute and critical care nurse practitioners, clinical nurse specialists, adult nurse practitioners, and family nurse practitioners. For example, when utilizing the high-fidelity patient simulator for acute and critical care APN students, the simulated environment would be an ICU or emergency department room equipped with noninvasive and invasive monitoring, a defibrillator, a pacemaker, a ventilator, vasoactive drugs, analgesics, sedatives, muscle relaxants, intubation equipment, various oxygen delivery devices, emergency drugs, and equipment carts.

As the amount and complexity of the equipment listed make clear, the simulation center requirements for APN student experiences may be considerably more involved than those for undergraduate students. Similarly, APN scenario development and implementation require more faculty and technical staff involvement and planning time. Further, the depth and variety of faculty clinical experience and the instructors' comfort level with simulators and technology are important to the success of the entire endeavor.

A close working relationship between nursing faculty and the technical staff of the simulation lab is essential for the development and maintenance of this type of educational experience for APN students. When faculty members have less experience or comfort with simulator use, the guidance and support of the center's technical staff become critical to the venture's success. Choosing an APN program faculty member to spearhead high-fidelity patient simulation experiences is a strategy that fosters continuity and progressive development of the program's efforts. Prior to the students' scheduled simulation experience, the lead instructor should meet with the simulation staff to identify which clinical scenarios will be utilized, discuss the purpose of the experience for the students, and program the simulator to have appropriate responses. When developing new clinical scenarios, it is helpful for the nursing facilitator and simulation staff to act out the scenario. This walk-through enables the scenario developer and simulation staff to identify any problems with the flow of the scenario or with programming the simulator. Such a pre-simulation meeting has great value, in that it will decrease the likelihood of technical problems that might otherwise diminish the quality of the simulation experience for the student.

STUDENT PREPARATION FOR SIMULATION

Introduction to patient simulation should occur in the first clinical course, with initial interactions consisting of more straightforward scenarios. During students' initial exposure to patient simulation, it is essential to establish rules of behavioral conduct that reflect the practice habits expected of students when delivering direct patient care. Students should be encouraged to approach the simulated situation as if they are caring for a "real" patient.

Methods that can be employed to enhance realism and help students to suspend disbelief include props, such as medication bottles, and familiar patient care equipment. In addition, an unseen faculty member in the control room can provide the "voice" of the simulator by speaking to the students in a conversational manner and asking them questions. For example, the faculty facilitator who is the "voice" of the simulator can encourage acceptable behaviors by asking questions such as "What are you talking about?" and "Is there something bad going on?" If a student leans inappropriately over or on the simulator, the voice may announce, "Ouch! You are leaning on my leg." If students address questions to faculty in the control room rather than to the simulated "patient," the faculty facilitator should redirect these questions to the simulated "patient." The goal is for the interaction between the student and the simulator to replicate a real student–patient encounter.

Having students dress as they would for their clinical rotation also encourages them to interface with the simulator as they would with a real-world patient. Students should be encouraged to bring equipment such as a stethoscope, reflex hammer, tuning fork, and pen light, as well as a calculator, handheld computer, and pocket reference materials.

Students frequently find high-fidelity patient simulation intimidating and anxiety provoking. Providing an orientation to high-fidelity patient simulation may decrease their apprehension. Having students watch former students or instructors caring for the simulated patient can provide the current students with an understanding of what is expected. Prior to the first simulation experience, students should review a recording of a high-fidelity patient simulation performed by instructors or former students. Faculty members should also review the purpose and goals of the simulated experience with the students at the beginning of each semester. The simulation director should orient the group to the room, equipment, means of interacting with the simulator (i.e., what it can and cannot do), computers available to review laboratory and radiographic data, and monitors where additional data such as facial appearance, skin color, and skin texture may be observed.

During this orientation session, both the instructor and the simulation director should emphasize that the focus of the experience is on learning. In addition, they should stress faculty expectations that the students will still be developing their proficiency in interviewing and management skills. Some mistakes are anticipated, and these errors should be viewed as additional opportunities for learning. Establishing how students will interact with the high-fidelity patient simulator, keeping the student-group size small, developing realistic scenarios, keeping the initial exposure simple, and providing for nonjudgmental, constructive post-simulation debriefing ensure that students will become comfortable with this interactive form of learning.

As each student progresses through the clinical courses of the APN program, he or she should become more competent at subjective and objective data collection. The simulation scenarios should, in turn, shift focus to the assessment of the patient condition and consideration of treatment options. Such scenarios should incorporate more complex decision making and utilize advanced skill sets, such as rapid-sequence intubation, central-line placement, and chest tube insertion. The student should also be expected to function more confidently as a team leader and should be prepared to assign roles and tasks to other team members.

IMPLEMENTING THE SIMULATION

The logistics of implementing patient simulation include the following steps:

1. Reviewing the scenario to ensure that it meets current standards and guidelines.

2. Ensuring that all involved faculty have current scenario materials.

3. Assigning the roles for faculty members, such as the voice of the simulator, the validator of physical findings, the in-room supervisor, and the debriefing facilitator, so that faculty may review their roles prior to coming to the lab. If students are used as cast members, such as family members, the expectations for those persons also need to be defined.

4. Coordinating with the simulation lab to ensure that the scenario is set up in the simulator and that all necessary equipment is available.

5. Arriving prior to the first scheduled scenario to set up the simulator with necessary props, such as an endotracheal tube, an orogastric tube, or intravenous lines.

6. Preparing flow sheets, the patient chart, an EKG, a medication record, pill bottles, and other props that increase the realism of the scenario.

Students should be assigned to complete the simulation in small groups; three students per group works well. This setup permits learners to play the roles of team leader, bedside nurse, and scribe. The role of scribe is to assist the team leader with recall of data acquired from the patient, physical findings, differential diagnosis, current interventions ordered, and available laboratory and radiographic findings. For novice APN students, having the data recorded and visible on a blackboard helps keep them on track as the scenario unfolds. If additional players are needed, such as a respiratory therapist, nursing assistant, or patient care secretary, a faculty member or another student may fill these roles. The students rotate through all three main positions, giving them exposure to three scenarios during one session. Some interaction between the team leader, the nurse, and the scribe may be permitted. Team building is an expectation of simulation, so interaction between the APN and bedside nurse and ancillary staff is encouraged. However, establishing guidelines is important so that the assisting staff members do not inform the team leader of the answers or direct the scenario.

Prior to the simulation, a time frame is identified for the scenario itself and for debriefing. A typical scenario runs for 15 to 20 minutes for advanced students, and 30 to 45 minutes for novice students. In the beginning, when working with novice students, the facilitator may take a "timeout" to encourage or facilitate certain behaviors. This approach is used in the first clinical course to help students develop their diagnostic reasoning skills. For example, following the completion of the patient history, the scenario may be paused and faculty may request that the team leader list several differential diagnoses. The scenario may be stopped again at the completion of the physical examination, to refine the differential list to the most likely diagnosis. Instructor involvement in the simulation room lessens and planned "timeouts" for teaching become more infrequent in the second semester; minimal to no interruptions are included in the final clinical course.

If a student is not meeting the expected outcomes for a scenario, the faculty member has several options. First, the faculty member can have the simulated patient ask a question, offer additional information, or develop additional signs and symptoms that might assist the student in his or her decision making. Second, the faculty member can provide information or observations via another scenario participant, such as a family member, telemetry technician, or respiratory therapist. Third, the faculty member may permit the consequences of the omission or error to occur and the patient's condition to deteriorate. These decisions may or may not be planned in advance of the simulation experience. Usually, permitting the patient to deteriorate or die is a consequence that is reserved for students in their final semester during their last one or two simulation experiences.

Although allowing simulator death can be a useful learning experience, it is prudent to determine at which point allowing simulated death is most beneficial to the learner. It is important to take into consideration the level of the learner and his or her comfort with simulation. In addition, the learner objectives should be considered when deciding whether death and the issues surrounding death are more important to review than the preplanned objectives. Implementing a phased approach to simulator death enables instructors to pair up learner objectives with the curriculum without impeding the learning process by disrupting novice learner confidence or students' acceptance of the simulated environment. Thus novice students are not subjected to simulated death until they gain a certain level of proficiency or when death is absolutely unavoidable.

OPTIMIZING THE SIMULATION ENVIRONMENT

Creating a full-immersion simulation facility requires paying considerable attention to detail so that the learners can become fully immersed in a simulated environment and suspend their disbelief. When the clinical environment and clinical details are recreated faithfully, the users of the simulation facility experience situational immersion and benefit further from the scenarios. Typically a full-immersion simulation center (see Figure 12-3) consists of three areas: the simulation suite, the control room, and the debriefing room. Other configurations may also be employed if necessary. Ideally the three areas will be adjacent to one another, with the shared walls having one-way mirrors mounted that allow the simulation suite to be viewed from either the control room or the debriefing room. These areas are used in conjunction to deliver the educational objectives of the desired clinical teaching scenario.

Figure 12-3   Typical Simulation Center Configuration

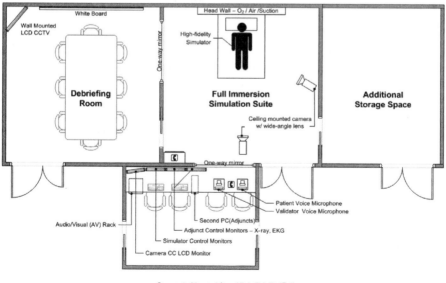

Suggested Layout for a High-Fidelity/Full
Immersion Simulation Suite

The Simulation Suite

The simulation suite houses the simulation mannequin(s), appropriate equipment, and medical supplies. It is usually equipped with video cameras, microphones, and a recording system so that the scenarios can be viewed during the debriefing or in real time by students and instructors, either on site or remotely.

The Control Room

The control room is the area where the simulation is manipulated. Personnel within this area modify simulator settings as appropriate and serve as the voice of the simulator. The sessions are recorded and viewed within this room. Subsequently, these recordings are used during the debriefing to highlight areas of interest and as evaluation tools so that students can watch and grade their performance. The control room contains the majority of the information systems infrastructure.

The Debriefing Room

The debriefing room typically contains a conference table, a television for video playback, and appropriate teaching aids, such as a whiteboard and reference materials. Its video display system is usually connected to the recording of the simulation suite so that additional learners may view the current simulation and benefit from the experience of the other students.

Not only does the feed play live via closed-circuit television, but the patient simulator's vitals are also displayed by the monitor, overlaid on top of the video feed so as to allow all students to witness the real-time physiological effects of interventions and scenario progression (see Figure 12-4). In addition, this area is equipped with a secondary display that shows the simulation adjuncts being displayed in the simulation suite (e.g., x-rays, lab values, EKGs). Another important aspect of conducting a simulation at the APN level is to have all learners, actors, and instructors wear appropriate clinical attire, whether that is hospital scrubs or professional dress. When a higher level of participation is required, the provider–simulator interaction is further strengthened; suspension of disbelief is also facilitated by recreating an environment with which the learner is familiar and comfortable.

Simulation Adjuncts

A simulation adjunct is any image, sound, video, or piece of equipment that, when viewed or used by the learner, tends to improve the realism of the

Figure 12-4 Video Display with Patient Vital Overlay

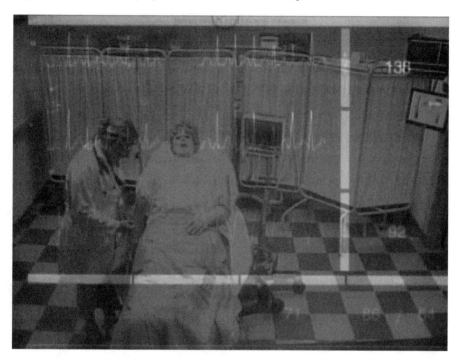

simulation experience. Visual adjuncts used in patient simulation include, but are not limited to, the following: patient laboratory data, x-rays, CT scans, EKGs (12 or 15 leads), and physical assessment photos. The purpose of including extra materials stems from the understanding that patient simulator is an exceptional, yet incomplete tool. It provides the basic framework to immerse students in a "simulated clinical experience." The adjuncts and attention to detail that surround the simulator elevate the educational delivery of content.

From an operations standpoint, it is important to be able to create an intuitive and useful catalog of the simulation adjuncts so that they can be accessed quickly and easily. This can be accomplished in a variety of ways, ranging from creating a database to manage all of the documents and images to using a computer operating system (Windows or Macintosh) and its folders to systematically manage the documents manually. Figure 12-5 displays a file-tree structure for organizing electronic files associated with delivering a complex full-immersion simulation.

Figure 12-5   File Tree Structure Used to Manage Simulation Files and Adjuncts

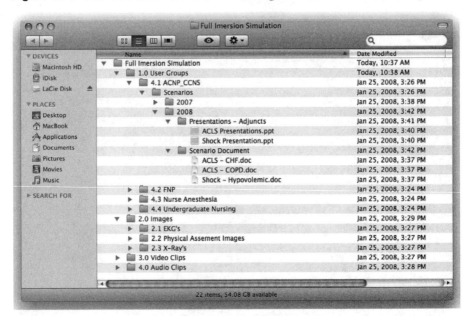

Using Standard Computer Presentation Hardware and Software to Improve a Simulation

One particularly useful adjunct is the use of a computer that is configured to output to four monitors—one primary monitor and three secondary monitors. This computer system is used in conjunction with the appropriate presentation software package (Apple's Keynote or Microsoft PowerPoint) and is controlled by the simulation personnel in the control room to display the appropriate simulation adjuncts during the simulation.

On the primary monitor, the presentation software package is configured to control the navigation of the presentation. The secondary monitors display content for the learners and facilitators (x-rays, EKGs, patient lab data; see Figure 12-6).

To achieve this display, the computer must be equipped with a specialized video card that is able to output graphics to two monitors. The output from the secondary video signal is split using a standard VGA splitter, which then feeds two individual monitors displaying identical content. Of the three monitors, one monitor is located in the control room and one in the simulation suite. Refer to Figure 12-6 for an illustration of a typical layout.

Figure 12-6   Simulation PC Adjunct Monitor Configuration

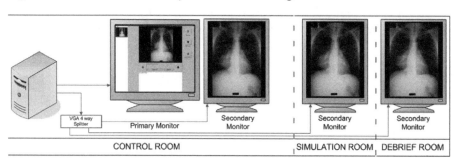

Hardware Configuration of a Simulation Center

The simulation facility is a highly specialized area that contains a large amount of audiovisual and computing technology equipment and infrastructure. It shares many of the same features of a television studio: It houses multiple repositionable cameras, microphones, video-scan converters, and hardware devices for video overlay, and it uses multiple methods for recording the generated media (i.e., the scenarios).

Many storage options exist when recording analog and digital video signals. In recent years, DVD/DVR systems have begun replacing traditional VHS recording systems for such applications, as they have better video quality, minimize the storage space needed, and are readily available. Because DVDs are relatively inexpensive, each student can be provided with a copy of his or her scenario for future review and/or self-evaluation and reflection. Furthermore, if the center uses digital video cameras, the generated media may be captured directly onto a hard drive or a server. This recording method provides the capability for instantaneous replay, the ability to easily edit the video footage for media generation and campaigns, and the capacity to stream the feed to any building via the Internet, thereby potentially increasing the number of learners. For example, a center that can accommodate only eight students at a time might potentially broadcast a simulation to a much larger audience in multiple lecture theaters.

Moreover, if the facility utilizes multiple types of equipment (i.e., analog cameras and a server for recording the footage), it can take advantage of hardware that converts analog video signals to digital signals in real time. Unfortunately, a reduction of video quality will inevitably occur when the analog signal is converted to its digital counterpart.

MAINTAINING A STATE-OF-THE-ART SIMULATION LAB

Moore's law (named after a one-time director of Intel) states that technology doubles its capacity every 24 months. Because of this rapid advancement, keeping abreast of technological changes is difficult and not always cost-effective for simulation facilities. For this reason, careful evaluation of all computer-based systems (e.g., databases, video equipment, computers) purchased and used by simulation facilities should be conducted so that the ability to expand and update the system is possible. Also, these systems inevitably need to be replaced, which means simulation centers should certainly consider strategies in light of the proposed technology replacement cycle.

Interprofessional Organizational Structure

The typical organizational structure of a high-fidelity simulation center is linear and places administrative and operational responsibilities on persons who are not typically trained in management (Jeffries, 2007). Many of these facilities employ traditionally trained, clinically proficient personnel—a registered nurse (RN), respiratory therapist (RT), physician (MD), or combination thereof—to manage and operate the facility. This model has been adopted because of many factors, such as fiscal constraints, lack of highly qualified nonclinical personnel in the industry, and the relative newness of high-fidelity (full immersion) simulation in health care. As such, clinical leaders who have identified the value and benefits of simulation are tasked with the administrative and operational components as well. Although this model is successful in practice, it assigns to individuals at least some responsibilities that are usually outside the realm of their education.

To overcome this problem, an interprofessional operational model has been developed. This model aligns the correct tasks with the appropriately trained individuals. For example, clinical personnel and faculty focus on the creation, delivery, and modification of the educational aspect of the simulation, whereas the administrative and technological staff handle the simulator operations and control, center management, and all associated maintenance. This differentiation of duties results in increased operational efficiency, as clinical experts are able to focus their energies and abilities solely on the education content, while operational team members stick to the operational logistics and management of technology. Furthermore, the wisdom of this model becomes readily evident when one considers the high level of complexity associated with APN high-fidelity simulation.

This model, as depicted in Figure 12-7, separates the clinical education components from the technological and operations components. The sizes of the circles in Figure 12-7 denote the direct impact each group has on the

Figure 12-7   Interprofessional Simulation Center Management Model

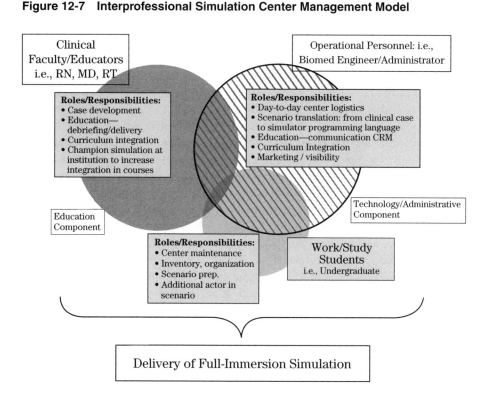

delivery of a simulation. Areas of overlap exist between the different groups, further strengthening the operation as each group relies on the others to aid in completion of their responsibilities. For example, the technical staff need basic functionality in clinical science and physiology, while the clinicians need basic functionality with the current technologies. In addition, a work-study student or volunteer may be employed to act as a center resource—organizing the scenario supplies and equipment, setting up the center, and acting in a scenario to further increase realism.

CHALLENGES IN ACUTE CARE ADVANCED PRACTICE SIMULATION

Despite the clear value of high-fidelity simulation, this technology should always be used as an adjunct to didactic preparation. Optimally, students should have some familiarity with the concepts and skills that are included in a given scenario prior to engaging in a clinical simulation. Even with prior introduction to the material being utilized, students and faculty may experience some degree of performance anxiety (Rauen, 2001). As discussed previously, providing an orientation to the simulation environment and demonstrating a typical scenario, either live or recorded, are helpful methods of allaying these fears.

Because simulation is an adjunct to classroom learning, additional time for simulation sessions must be afforded in the course or program curriculum. These experiences can be accommodated during normal class hours, special sessions, or individually scheduled simulation laboratory sessions. No matter which strategy is chosen, additional hours of faculty time are required to design and supervise sessions. Depending on the complexity of the simulation, several faculty members may be required to actualize the scenario. For example, one faculty member might be in the simulation room with the students working with the scenario, while another faculty member is in the control room providing the voice of the patient and delivering data that cannot be simulated. Still another faculty might be in the debriefing room with students, observing the enactment. In addition, optimal presentation of the scenario requires technical support from staff who know how to operate the patient simulator and other devices used to deliver data and create realism for the students.

Given today's faculty shortage, which is particularly acute in terms of APN faculty, few schools have adequate qualified personnel to staff an optimal simulation center. Moreover, many schools do not have enough funding or space to provide the type of facility discussed in this chapter. One solution to this problem is the formation of partnerships between schools of medicine and schools of nursing, or between nursing schools and hospitals, or between several nursing schools, to share facilities and staff. This strategy has been used successfully in North Carolina by Presbyterian School of Nursing at Queens University of Charlotte and Presbyterian Hospital (Queens University of Charlotte, 2007). Another strategy that can reduce the amount of faculty time needed to run the simulator is to utilize graduate and doctoral students to assist faculty members with simulation events. This approach has the added advantage of preparing a new generation of technologically savvy APN faculty for the future.

The biggest challenge for health care and for schools preparing future advanced practice providers, however, is the ongoing need to keep up with medical science, the latest evidence-based therapy, and all of the technology found in hospitals and practice settings. Even if faculties and schools of nursing are successful in staying abreast of all that is new, maintaining a simulation environment that truly reflects practice settings and situations will increasingly pose a challenge both intellectually and monetarily. Meeting this challenge is a must: The health of our nation depends on the quality of the providers of the future.

References

Benner, P., Hooper-Kyriakidis, P., & Stannard, D. (1999). *Clinical wisdom and interventions in critical care*. Philadelphia: W. B. Saunders.

Field, J., Hazinski, M. F., & Gilmore, D. (Eds.). (2006). *Handbook of emergency cardiovascular care for healthcare providers*. Dallas, TX: American Heart Association.

Hravnak, M., Tuite, P., & Baldisseri, M. (2005). Expanding acute care nurse practitioner and clinical nurse specialist education: Invasive procedure training and human simulation in critical care. *AACN Clinical Issues, 16*(1), 89–104.

Jefferies, P. (Ed.). (2007). *Simulation in nurse education: From conceptualization to evaluation*. New York: National League of Nursing.

Kleinpell-Nowell, R. (2001). Longitudinal survey of acute care nurse practitioner practice: Year 2. *AACN Clinical Issues, 12*, 447–452.

Lighthall, G., Barr, J., Howard, S., et al. (2003). Use of fully simulated intensive care unit environment for critical event management training for internal medicine residents. *Critical Care Medicine, 31*, 2437–2443.

Queens University of Charlotte. (2007). Queens and Presbyterian Hospital open house to unveil new patient simulation laboratory. Accessed January 31, 2008, from http://queens.edu/news_detail.asp?press_id=1997&section=nursing

Rauen, C. (2001). Using simulation to teach critical thinking skills: You can't just throw the book at them. *Critical Care Nursing Clinics of North America, 13*(1), 93–103.

Scherer, Y., Bruce, S., Graves, B., & Erdley, W. (2003). Acute care nurse practitioner education: Enhancing performance through the use of clinical simulation. *AACN Clinical Issues, 14*, 331–341.

CHAPTER 13

Regional Nursing Simulation Program

Susan Sportsman and Marcy S. Beck

In today's healthcare environment, which is characterized by both a nursing shortage and increasingly complex patient needs, many nurse educators are struggling to provide learning opportunities that reflect actual patient care in a safe and cost-effective way. Collaboration among individual nurse educators, nursing programs, healthcare organizations, and even state agencies can help educators address these challenges. This chapter describes how collaboration among a state agency, two nursing programs, and a regional hospital fostered the implementation of a Regional Simulation Center (RSC). The purpose of the RSC was to provide competency education and validation for both nursing students and hospital staff, using high-fidelity patient simulators. A description of the development of a specific scenario used in the RSC illustrates the effectiveness of the collaborative effort among partners of the RSC.

STATEWIDE COLLABORATION

The nursing education system in Texas has been the beneficiary of the settlement of the state's lawsuit against tobacco companies. Funds from this settlement were placed in the Permanent Fund for Higher Education: Nursing, Allied Health and Other Health-Related Programs. Under the direction of the Texas Higher Education Coordinating Board (THECB), the investment proceeds have been used to fund statewide grant projects to improve nursing education.

In 2004, THECB solicited proposals for projects to increase enrollment in initial RN-licensure programs, principally through creative and efficient use of existing and new faculty. The programs had to be easily and cost-effectively applied to other nursing programs and were expected to demonstrate partnerships with private and/or public entities (THECB, 2004).

REGIONAL COLLABORATION

In response to the statewide initiative to develop programs to increase admissions in Texas pre-licensure nursing programs, a university, a community college, and a regional hospital received a $1.27 million grant to collaboratively implement an RSC. The center was located in a 3410-square-feet, renovated nursing unit in the partnering hospital and was equipped with four adult and two child/infant high-fidelity patient simulators. Clinically strong, BSN-prepared lab mentors, working under the supervision of a MSN-prepared Director of the RSC, were made responsible for competency education and validation for associate degree and baccalaureate nursing students, as well as the hospital staff. The goals of the grant project were twofold: (1) to increase the number of students admitted to both the BSN and the ADN programs by reallocation of faculty workload, and (2) to improve the ability of students and hospital staff to practice safely, particularly related to clinical decision-making (Sportsman et al., in press).

The amount of time BSN and ADN students spend in the RSC varies, depending on the clinical objectives of specific courses. For example, during the first year of the grant, 100% of the BSN students' clinical experience in the health assessment course was handled by the lab mentors, rather than by faculty assigned to the course. Fifty percent of the clinical component of "fundamental" courses, which were traditionally taught in both school-specific laboratories, was instead supervised by center staff. Students in the BSN program spent 26.7% of their clinical time in the two required medical–surgical courses in the RSC, 8% in the maternal–child course, 13% in pediatrics, and 20%, in the final capstone course (Sportsman et al., in press).

Assigning students to the RSC for a component of their clinical experience allowed both ADN and BSN faculty to increase the total number of students assigned to them each semester, as at any given time a portion of the clinical group was scheduled for learning activities in the center, where they were supervised by the lab mentors. As a result, the number of potential students admitted to each program could be increased, without necessitating the difficult task of hiring additional faculty at the master's or doctoral level (Sportsman et al., in press). Faculty continued to maintain control of students' learning experiences in the RSC by writing learning objectives for specific scenarios and by working with the lab mentors to develop the scenarios.

As the implementation of the RSC progressed, the hospital nurse educators also began to use the center for competency validation. For example, hospital nurse educators and the RSC lab mentors developed and implemented sufficient scenarios to meet unit-specific goals for the clinical staff, along with the annual competency validation required by Joint Commission. This strategy allowed staff members to demonstrate their competency in a more realistic environment than the typical "table-top" skills fair previously offered. Such an outcome would not have been possible without collaboration between the lab mentors and the hospital nurse educators and without the availability of the RSC.

At the end of the three-year grant period, approximately 20,000 duplicated learner visits had been logged in the RSC. The partners assumed responsibility for the funding of the center, ensuring its continued operation without grant funds. The effectiveness of the collaboration transcended the grant period, assuring the ongoing availability of the RSC in the region.

USE OF COLLABORATION TO DEVELOP SPECIFIC SCENARIOS

The thread of collaboration as a strategy to meet the demands of current nursing education is not only evident in the operation of the RSC, but can also be seen in the development of specific scenarios used in the center. The discussion of the development of scenario-based simulation in the RSC will be illustrated here by a description of a specific scenario designed to teach diabetic management, using a hospital-approved protocol. This simulation scenario was designed to validate both student and hospital staff competence, demonstrating the importance of collaboration among the partners.

Selection of a Clinical Situation

The first step in developing a specific scenario is to identify a clinical situation, consistent with the content area to be addressed by learners (either nursing students or hospital staff). Clinical situations may be drawn from developers' professional experience; recommendations of accreditation or credentialing organizations; high-risk, low-volume or high-risk, high-volume situations; identified gaps in learner knowledge; or the introduction of new equipment, policies, or protocols. Because of the diversity of experience and perspectives, collaboration among the nurse educators and lab mentors is essential to developing a complex, yet realistic situation.

This collaboration, highlighting a variety of perspectives, is evident in the development of the diabetic management scenario. Initially, the hospital partner developed and implemented guidelines for the treatment and management of both hyperglycemia and hypoglycemia. After the initial implementation of the guidelines, two hospital chart audits demonstrated opportunities for improvement in implementation. As a result, hospital diabetes educators worked with the RSC lab mentors to develop a simulation scenario to reinforce the care principles necessary for effective utilization of the protocol by all nurses in the organization. Given that the initial education related to the protocol had been taught in a didactic forum without the opportunity to apply the protocol principles, the educators believed reinforcement using simulation would be an excellent teaching–learning strategy.

Even though this situation was designed with the specific purpose of improving implementation of the diabetic management protocol in mind, given the amount of resources required to develop scenarios, the developers hoped that the situation would have significant depth and breadth to be applicable in a variety of circumstances. Not only was the use of the protocol by hospital staff important for patient safety, but nursing students must also be competent in caring for diabetic patients. Therefore, this scenario was appropriate for both groups of learners being served by the RSC.

Scenario Design

Scenario Overview

Once the clinical focus of the scenario has been identified, the specifics of the scenario must be developed. In the development of the diabetic management scenario, the general information to be shared with the learners was outlined by the lab mentors. This information included (1) the current patient condition (assessment findings), (2) pertinent patient history, (3) medication or treatment orders, and (4) lab values, x-ray reports, and the results of diagnosis-specific examinations. It is important that the scenario include sufficient information to completely describe the situation, yet the data set provided must not be unrealistic or so large as to be distracting to the learner. Box 13-1 provides an example of the initial situation provided for the diabetic management scenario.

Learning Objectives

Learning objectives to direct the scenario must also be developed. In a review and synthesis of 109 research studies on the effectiveness of high-fidelity medical simulations, Issenberg and colleagues (2005) found that 6% of the articles cited the importance of having clearly stated goals with tangible outcomes measures to encourage learners to master the identified skills. These objectives must be behavioral in nature and include all outcomes that learners must successfully complete at the end of the scenario. The objectives should also be realistic given the time available for the simulation and the abilities of the learners. The objectives for the diabetic management scenario appear in Box 13-2.

Box 13-1   Diabetic Management Example—Initial Situation

Your patient is a 34-year-old female, who weighs 115 pounds and is 5 feet tall. She has been brought to the Emergency Department (ED) by her mother. Her mother states that her daughter had complaints of fatigue, cough, nausea, and vomiting for the past five days. The patient was diagnosed with diabetes mellitus, approximately 10 years ago. Since that time, her diabetes has been managed on insulin therapy TID and Lantus QD. Currently, she has been administering Novolog 5 units at meal times and Lantus 14 units in the evening. Five days ago, she began to cough, producing first clear, and then dark rust-colored sputum. She also states that she is experiencing overwhelming fatigue and intermittent bouts of nausea and vomiting. She has not been eating and omitted her evening insulin for the past four days because of "feeling so bad." She also did not take her insulin for the past 48 hours prior to arriving in the ED.

Baseline Assessment Findings

Body System Assessed	Patient Findings
Vital Signs	T: 100.8, HR 132 bpm, BP: 92/53, FSBG 900
Neurological/Sensory	Oriented but lethargic; speech clear but slow to respond to verbal stimulus
Cardiac	Apical pulse regular at rate of 132/min; radial and pedal pulse faint but palpable
Skin/Wound	Skin color pale, warm, and dry to touch; no bruising, skin tears, or wounds noted
Pulmonary	Rapid respiration at 32/min; forced inspiration and expirations; left lung clear to auscultation; course crackles heard in base of right lung. Pulse ox: 86%
Musculoskeletal	Weakened hand grasps bilaterally; otherwise, WNL
Gastrointestinal (GI)	Bowel sounds × 4 noted; states daily BMs
Genitourinary (GU)	Mother states "wet the bed last night;" incontinent of urine since brought to the ED last night.

Box 13-1   Diabetic Management Example—Initial Situation (continued)

Physician Orders: The ED physician takes the patient history, assesses the patient and writes initial orders as follows:

Date: Time: 1200 hours

Activity: Bedrest

Diet: NPO

VS: Q 30 minutes

O2 @ 2 L/min via NC

I& O: document hourly urinary outputs

IV of 0.9% NS; infuse 1 liter during first hour, and then decrease rate to 500 mL/hr.

Foley to bedside drainage

STAT CBC with diff; Survey 8; serum ketone level; U/sputum for gram stain and C& S

STAT ABG's

STAT ECG

STAT culture × 2 for T greater than 101.5°F

                                         Signed: J.B. Pierce, MD

Results from the diagnostic studies, which were performed STAT are below.

CBC and Differential Report

CBC	Result	Units	Expected Range
WBC count	14,000	k/ccm	4.8–10.8
Red blood cell count	4.7	m/cmm	4.2–5.4
Hemoglobin	15.2	Gms/dL	12.0–16.0
Hematocrit	48.6	%	16.0–37.0
MCV	83.4	Fl	80.0–94.0
MCH	29.8	Pg	27.0–31.0
MCHC	35.8	g/dl	33.0–37.0
Platelet count	347	k/cmm	150–400
Lymphs	5	%	20–50
Monocytes	5	%	2–9
Granulocytes	94	%	42–78

Box 13-1   Diabetic Management Example—Initial Situation *(continued)*

Survey 8 Report

Survey 8	Result	Units	Expected Range
Sodium	128	mEq/L	135–153
Potassium	6.7	mEq/L	3.5–5.3
Chloride	90	mEq/L	101–111
CO_2	4	mEq/L	22–30
Glucose	923	Mg/dL	70–110
BUN	43	Mg/dL	5–25
Creatinine	2.3	Mg/dL	0.5–1.5
Calcium	9.2	Mg/dL	8.0–10.4

Miscellaneous: Serum Ketones = 4+

Urinalysis Report

UA Chemstrip Screen	Result	Expected Range
Color	Colorless	Yellow
Clarity	Clear	Clear
Gravity	Less than 1.000	1.0005–1.030
pH	8	5–8
Leukocyte	Negative	Negative
Nitrite	Negative	Negative
Protein	Negative	Negative
Glucose	4+	Normal

Box 13-1   Diabetic Management Example—Initial Situation (continued)

UA Chemstrip Screen	Result	Expected Range
Ketone	4+	Negative
Urobilinogen	Normal	Normal
Bilirubin	Negative	Negative
Blood	Negative	Negative

Arterial Blood Gases (ABG) Report

ABGs	Patient Results	Units	Expected Range
pH	7.06		7.35–7.45
PaO2	112	mmHg	80–100
PaCO2	13	mmHg	35–45
HCO3 (Bicarbonate)	2.5	mEq/L	22–26

Chest X-Ray
Impression: Right lower lobe infiltrate

EKG
Impression: Sinus tachycardia with ventricular rate—132 bpm; otherwise no cardiac abnormalities.

Box 13-2   Diabetic Management Example—Learning Objectives

The objectives for the diabetic management scenario included the following:

i. Assess the patient and select the proper insulin dosage required.
ii. Describe the importance of coordinating the administration of insulin and feeding the patient.
iii. Differentiate among types of insulin used for the management of diabetes as indicated in the selected protocol.
iv. Interpret finger-stick blood glucose results and administer the correct insulin dosage per protocol.
v. Distinguish signs and symptoms of hypoglycemia and select the appropriate treatment per protocol.

Box 13-2   Diabetic Management Example—Learning Objectives *(continued)*

> vi. Distinguish signs and symptoms of hyperglycemia and select the appropriate treatment per protocol.
> vii. Select the proper treatment for special considerations demonstrated by the patient per protocol.

Staging the Scenario

Issenberg et al. (2005) found that 3% of the studies evaluating the effectiveness of simulation in medical education suggested that simulator validity was a factor in promoting successful learning. To this end, not only is it important to program the simulator to respond realistically to nursing interventions, but it is also important that the situations, including the responses of the simulators and the related equipment, be as realistic as possible. For example, for the diabetic management scenario, expired Glucose Calibration Verification Controls were available for learners to perform the finger-stick blood glucose (FSBG). Depending on which bottle was used, the FSBG value could be adjusted to meet the needs of the scenario.

Medical supplies and equipment typically used in actual patient situations should also be made available for learners' use. When the RSC was first opened, the lab mentors laid out the supplies and equipment needed to provide appropriate care. Learners commented that not only did they want a variety of types of supplies available to practice choosing the appropriate item, but they would also prefer to select the items from a supply cabinet as they would in an actual clinical setting (see Box 13-3).

Box 13-3   Diabetic Management Example—Equipment List

- Glucose gel
- Glucagon ampules
- $D_{50}W$ ampule
- Novolog insulin
- Insulin syringes
- Glucometer
- Glucose calibration solutions
- Lancets and glucometer strips
- Alcohol swaps
- Cotton balls
- Assorted food products that might be used in treatment: graham crackers, peanut butter, jello, orange juice, diet and regular sodas, plastic food for sandwiches, etc.
- Pulse oximeter

Preclinical Learning Activities

Particularly when nursing students are the identified learners, scenario developers may outline preclinical learning activities to prepare students to participate in the actual simulation. This preparation may include references related to drugs to be used in the scenario, signs and symptoms of the identified disease process and related pathophysiology, standards or guidelines for nursing management of the identified condition, potential complications, and potential ethical dilemmas. Similar to preparation for an actual clinical experience, the preclinical directions provide a structure for students to acquire the necessary background information, thereby allowing them to take maximum advantage of the learning opportunity of the scenario (see Box 13-4).

Box 13-4   Diabetic Management Example—Preclinical Preparation

The preclinical directions for the diabetic management scenario included written questions which nursing school learners were to answer, along with references, before coming to the RSC for the learning experience. The appropriate responses to each question are discussed with the students as a group, prior to their participating in the scenario.

1. **Based on the information in the scenario, should the nurse anticipate this patient to be classified as type 1 or type 2 diabetes? Provide the rationale for your responses.**

   Appropriate Answer:
   [Reference: Phipps (2006), pp. 1112–1115. Table 39-3, p. 1115; Venes (2005) has a table on p. 581.]

   This patient is classified as type 1: insulinopenic which depends on exogenous insulin on a regular basis for control/management; onset of DM was at an early age (= 30 y/o; thin individual).

2. **Differentiate between the clinical manifestations commonly seen in a patient with diabetes experiencing hypoglycemia versus hyperglycemia.**

   Appropriate Answer:
   [Reference: Phipps (2006), pp. 1111–1112 discusses s/s of hyperglycemia; pp. 1135-1136, Box 39-5: s/s of hypoglycemia.]

   Hyperglycemia:
   1. Three polys (polyuria, polydipsia, polyphagia)
   2. May experience nausea and vomiting
   3. Weight loss
   4. Headache
   5. Irritability

Box 13-4   Diabetic Management Example—Preclinical Preparation *(continued)*

6. Acetone odor on breath
7. Dyspnea
8. Orthostatic hypotension
9. Elevated blood glucose = 375 mg/dL inpatient

Hypoglycemia
1. Pallor, diaphoresis, feeling cold/piloerection
2. Tachycardia
3. Nervousness
4. Irritability, mental confusion
5. Weakness, trembling
6. Hunger
7. Headache, confusion
8. Diplopia
9. Irrational speech
10. Emotional lability
11. Convulsions
12. Coma
13. Extremely low blood glucose

3. **The patient in the scenario is probably experiencing hyperglycemia due to illness and changes in insulin management. Why?**

Appropriate Answer: Not feeling well, not eating, and not administering her insulin.

4. **Besides an insulin problem, what other physiologic issues might you expect the ED physician to assess/treat in this individual?**

Appropriate Answer: [Reference: Phipps (2006), pp. 1112–1114.]

This patient is experiencing hyperglycemia because of insulin deficiency. Besides hyperglycemia, the patient may experience osmotic diuresis, loss of H_2O and electrolytes, which could lead to ketonemia, ketonuria, dehydration, and hypovolemia leading to diabetic ketoacidosis (DKA), coma, and even death.

[Reference: Guthrie & Guthrie (2004), pp. 120–121.]
Insulin deficiency results in failure of nutrients to leave the blood and enter the cells.

- Elevated glucose in the blood; polyuria—excess urination
- Excess water loss: polydipsia—thirst
- Excess water loss carries electrolytes leading to hyponatremia
- Lack of glucose in cells causes starvation: polydipsia—hunger
- Cellular breakdown causes loss of potassium from cells to urine
- Fat breakdown will occur where they are converted to ketones by the liver leading to acidosis
- Most common causes of death in DKA: hypokalemia and cerebral edema

---

Box 13-4   Diabetic Management Example—Preclinical Preparation (continued)

5. **Complete the table below regarding Regular, Novolog, NPH, Novolin NPH, Novolin 70/30, Humalog Mix, and Lantus/Levenir.**

Type of Insulin	Onset (hr)	Peak (hr)	Duration (hr)	Appea-rance	Nursing Implications
Regular	30 minutes	2.5–3.5 hrs	6–8 hrs	Clear	Observe patient closely for s/s of hypoglycemia
Novolog (Aspart)	10 minutes	45 minutes–1.5 hrs.	3 hrs	Clear	Give when tray is in front of patient
NPH	1.5 hr	4–12 hrs.	24 hrs	Cloudy	Will need HS snack if dose is at supper
Novolin (NPH)	1.5 hr	4–12 hrs	24 hrs	Cloudy	Give 15–30 minutes before meal is served
Novolin 70/30	30 minutes Note: 70% NPH 30% Regular	1.5–16 hrs.	22 hrs	Cloudy	Give 15–30 minutes before meal is served. HS snack
Humalog Mix 75/25	10 minutes Note: 75% 25% Lispro (fast)	1–6.5 hrs.	22 hrs	Cloudy	Give when tray is in front of patient. HS snack
Lantus and Levemir (different meds but same information)	1 hr	None	24 hrs	Clear	Given once/day at the same time of day. Use pt preference. If no preference, administer at bedtime. Do not mix with any other insulin in syringe.

Additional information for preclinical questions: While visiting the triage ER nurse, the patient's mother stated that "her daughter had become difficult to awaken/arouse and keep focused, and was breathing fast and very deeply.... So I thought I should bring her to the hospital." Upon hearing this comment and seeing the general appearance of the patient, the triage nurse transported the patient directly to an ED treatment room.

Box 13-4   Diabetic Management Example—Preclinical Preparation *(continued)*

6. **While determining this patient history, what initial assessments would ED nurses perform?**

   Take vital signs, obtain FSBG, and perform head-to-toe physical assessment.

   Additional information: When asked about allergies, the patient's mother states that her daughter is allergic to penicillin.

7. **At this point, what does the nurse's assessment findings indicate may be happening in this patient?**

   Patient is experiencing signs of hyperglycemia because she is demonstrating signs and symptoms of a respiratory illness.

8. **This patient is experiencing a complication of diabetes mellitus due to insufficient insulin coverage during an acute illness. What are the common complications seen in diabetes, how are they classified, and what are the clinical manifestations of each?**

   Complications are classified as either acute or chronic. Acute complications include diabetic ketoacidosis (DKA) and hyperglycemic hyperosmolar nonketotic coma (HHNC), which is also known as hyperosmolar hyperglycemic state (HHS), when no coma is experienced. The clinical differences are addressed below.

Acute Complications

	DKA	**HHNC/HHS**
Onset	Gradual or sudden—less than 2 days	Gradual, usually greater than 5 days
Previous history of DM	85%	60%
Type of DM	Type 1	Type 2
Age of patient	Younger than 40 years	Older than 60 years
Mortality risk	1–15%	20–40%
Drug history	Exogenous insulin	Steroids; oral agents
Physical signs	Dehydration; Kussmaul's respirations; changes in mental status; fruity smelling breath; febrile	Dehydration; obtundation; hypothermia; no evidence of Kussmaul's respiration

Box 13-4   Diabetic Management Example—Preclinical Preparation *(continued)*

	DKA	HHNC/HHS
Glucose levels	Range is 250–1200 mg/dL	Range is 400–4000 mg/dL
Ketones	Present	Absent
Osmolarity	Mean is 320 mOm/L	Mean is 400 mOm/L
Arterial pH	Mean is 7.07	Mean is 7.26
HCO_2 (Bicarbonate)	Markedly low (less than 10 mEq/L)	Normal or greater than 10 mEq/L)
Anion gap	Less than 12 mEq/L	More than 12mEq/L

[Reference: Phipps (2006), p. 1118.]

Chronic Complications

Microvasular	Macrovascular
Diabetic retinopathy (blindness; retinal tears)	Dyslipidemia (elevated LDL; lower HDL contributes to atheroscleosis)
Diabetic nephropathy (renal disease)	Hypertension (contributes to renal dx; strokes; etc)
Neuropathies (Changes in nerve function, numbness)	Feet pathology (necrosis; gangrene; amputations)
Peripheral polyneuropathy	
Peripheral neuropathy	
Autonomic neuropathy	
Other (cranial nerve palsy; carpal tunnel)	

[Reference: Phipps (2006), pp. 1118–1123.]

Box 13-4 Diabetic Management Example—Preclinical Preparation *(continued)*

9. **How would the ED nurse prioritize nursing interventions for this patient to ensure that physician orders (found in the initial situation) are carried out in a timely fashion?**
   a. Start an IV access
   b. Draw the STAT venous specimens for labs
   c. Insert foley and collect sterile urine specimen

10. **Why would starting an intravenous access with a 22 gauge angio catheter be inappropriate for this patient?**

    A 22 gauge angio would not be large enough to care IV fluids at 500–1000 mL/hr rate. May also need to administer a volume expander. 22 gauge is appropriate for blood products but a larger gauge would be better for rapid infusion.

11. **What is the ED physician's rationale for ordering a STAT chest x-ray and sputum specimen?**

    Low grade fever, fast respiratory rate, diminished O_2 sat, forceful inspirations and expirations, coarse crackles auscultated in RLL, productive cough of rust-colored sputum for several days. A respiratory infiltrate could be the cause acute illness.

12. **Based on what you know about isotonic, hypertonic, and hypotonic intravenous solutions, why would the initial fluid choice for this patient be 0.9% saline?**

    [Reference: Phipps (2006), p. 1119.]
    Isotonic solutions (NL and RL) initially expanding vascular volume, remains in the vascular compartment, which is useful in hypovolemia. Be cautious the patient does not develop hypervolemia, too! Guidelines in Phipps (2006, p. 975) state, "Avoid hypotonic solutions (they are used to provide free H_2O and treat cellular dehydration) because they may cause cerebral edema."

13. **The abnormal values noted in the initial situation support the diagnosis of which complication of diabetes mellitus?**

    DKA due to high blood glucose (greater than 900), presence of serum and urine ketones (both are 4+); pH = 7.06; Bicarb = 2.5.

14. **Realizing the patient's probable diagnosis, because of the laboratory results, what emergency medical management and nursing management would the ED nurse anticipate?**

    [Reference: Guthrie & Guthrie (2004), pp. 121–122; Phipps (2006), p. 1119.]

    Medical Management

    • Maintain the airway if needed.
    • Establish fluid and electrolyte balance.
    • 0.9% NaCl initially for correction of dehydration.
    • KCL is added to fluids after patient starts producing urine. Monitor K+ by lab and electrocardiogram.
    • Reestablish carbohydrate metabolism (IV/lytes replacement and insulin infusion).

Box 13-4   Diabetic Management Example—Preclinical Preparation *(continued)*

- Insulin infusion 0.1–0.2 units/kg body weight/hour.
- Monitor FSBG hourly.
- Insulin adjusted to decrease glucose by 20–100 mg/dL/hr.
- Full recovery should take 24 hrs.
- When acidosis is relieved, IV fluids and insulin can be stopped and sub-q insulin started.
- When FSBG lowered to 300 mg/dL, feed patient and change IV fluids to D_5.45 saline to prevent hypoglycemia and cerebral edema.
- Use sliding scale or correction dose insulin as needed to maintain glucose level. (New terminology is "correction dose insulin." May continue to hear "sliding scale" in clinical areas.)
- If patient has never been on insulin: base starting insulin dose by patient weight.1–2 units/kg/day (children), 0.5–1.5 units/kg/day (adults).
- Administer first dose of sub-q 1–2 hours prior to discontinuing the insulin infusion.
- Na+ bicarb is only given if pH greater than 7.0.

Nursing Management
- Frequent monitoring of hydration.
- Frequent vital signs.
- Hourly urinary outputs.
- Performing and monitoring the EKG.
- Frequent FSBG monitoring.
- Serum ketones daily.
- Respiratory Assessment.
- Assess for mental status changes.

15. Which lab results support the diagnosis of an infectious process in this patient? Would you suspect the organism causing this infection to be bacterial or viral?

High WBC; high granulocytes and low lymphs show a "shift-to-left"; therefore, probably indicates a bacterial infection.

16. How would you interpret the patient's ABG results?

	Acidosis	**Alkalosis**
	pH ↓	pH ↑
Respiratory	$PaCO_2$ ↑	$PaCO_2$ ↓
Metabolic	HCO_3 ↓	HCO_3 ↑

↓ pH indicates acidosis; ↓ HCO_3 (bicarb) indicates metabolic; therefore, patient is in metabolic acidosis, which is consistent with DKA.

Box 13-4   Diabetic Management Example—Preclinical Preparation *(continued)*

---

17. **Why is the use of regular insulin as an intravenous push (IVP) bolus dose before the start of an infusion considered controversial in today's practice?**

    IV bolus of regular insulin has a half-life of 5 minutes and is considered of no value. (Remember, too, that a significant amount—20–50% of the insulin infusion will be lost because the tubing absorbs it.) Diabetes educators suggest that 50 ml of the insulin infusion be flushed through the tubing to saturate the tubing, before the infusion is started (Goldberg, et al., 2006).

18. **In current practice, are insulin infusions intended to be infused at a steady rate (ex: 15 units/hr × 9 hrs) or are they normally titrated based on a published protocol? Give the rationale for your answer.**

    Insulin drip rates are generally titrated based on hourly (or q2 hrs) FSBG results.

19. **Regarding the patient's insulin infusion: What dose would you expect the physician to order for the patient? The infusion bag contains regular insulin 100 units/100 ml of 0.9% NaCl. What should the infusion rate be?**

    Patient weighs 115# (52.3 kg.). Physician would order the infusion to start at 0.1–0.2 units/kg/hr (5.2–10.5 units/hr)

    Additional information: The patient is transferred to the ICU. The ICU nurse starts the insulin drip as ordered. The FSBGs and labs are repeated every two hours (odd hours) with the following patient trends noted during treatment:

Time	Glucose	pH	Na+	K+	CL	HCO_3	BUN/Creatinine
1315 hrs	923	7.06	128	6.7	90	2.5	43/2.3
1515 hrs	710	7.06	128	6.9	90	4	43/2.3
1715 hrs	492		132	6.8	101	6	41/1.7
1930 hrs	352	7.25	137	4.1	106	8	45/1.4
2200 hrs	303		139	4.7	114	15	27/1.2
0200 hrs	304		143	4.3	113	22	22/1.1
0400 hr	277	7.32	157	4.8	113	22	22/1.1

Box 13-4   Diabetic Management Example—Preclinical Preparation (continued)

20. How would you interpret this patient's response to treatment so far?

Until 1930 hrs, glucose is responding to insulin RS; pH and HCO_3 are moving toward normal values (metabolic acidosis improving slowly); Na+ is moving toward normal; K+ and CL levels are stable; creatinine is now within normal limits (WNL).

21. What clinical changes would you expect to assess in this patient as her DKA resolves?

Alert and oriented × 3; c/o hunger; ↑ BP; stabilized urinary output; lower FSBGs; negative ketones spilled.

Additional information: The patient has responded to medical management for her DKA. She is now transferred to the Medical/Surgical floor. Her glucose will be monitored and managed, using the Subcutaneous Hyperglycemia Protocol (see Appendix A) for the rest of her stay at the hospital. Her current weight is 120# (54.5 kg.).

22. Using the Subcutaneous Hyperglycemia Protocol, answer the following questions:

a. The goal of diabetes treatment is to maintain a preprandial glucose level at 70–110 mg/dL. What algorithm would the nurse expect to use for an increase in blood glucose for this patient? Why?

- Algorithm #1: Her weight is 115# = 52.3 kg.

b. The patient's FBSG at 0700 is 225 mg/dL. How much and when will the nurse administer her morning insulin?

- Novolog 5 units plus the additional 2 units = Novolog 7 units. Administer the Novolog when the patient's breakfast tray is present on her table. Lantus 14 units are administered at the same time every day. If she does not have a preference, administer at bedtime.

c. The patient's FSBG is 40 mg/dL. What should the nurse do?

- Retest the FSBG. Call lab for STAT blood glucose and treat patient with 30 grams of fast-acting carbohydrate. Notify physician. If next meal is more than one hour away, provide a protein and 15 gm carbohydrate snack in addition to above treatment.

d. The patient's FSBG is 60 mg/dL. What should the nurse do?

- Treat with 15 grams of fast-acting carbohydrate. Retest FSBG 15 minutes after treatment. If next meal is more than one hour away, provide a protein and 15 gm carbohydrate snack in addition to above treatment.

Box 13-4   Diabetic Management Example—Preclinical Preparation *(continued)*

e. **The patient's FSGB is 30 md/dL; she is unresponsive. What should the nurse do?**

   - IV access; 1/2 ampule of 50% dextrose IVP, observe patient for 10 minutes, if no response, repeat with the other 1/2 of the ampule. Repeat FSBG after meds given. No IV access; give 1 amp of Glucogon IV or SC. Patient may vomit, so use aspiration precautions. Repeat FSBG.

f. **Choose some food products that could be given to the patient that contains 15 gm of fast-acting carbohydrates.**

   - 1/2 cup fruit juice, 1.2 can nondiet soda, 1 tube glucose gel.

g. **Choose some diabetic snacks that could be given to the patient that contains 15 gm of carbohydrate plus protein.**

   - 1/2 meat sandwich (peanut butter, turkey, or roast beef), 1 container of yogurt, 2 packets peanut butter with 1 package graham crackers (one slice of bread = 14 gm CHO, 3 squares graham crackers = 14 gm CHO).

h. **If the patient is on a fluid restriction, and/or taking Precose or Glyset, what can you administer if they are hypoglycemic?**

   - One tube of glucose gel in buccal cavity and ask patient to swallow. Do not give patients on Precose or Glyset juice, cola, or sugar, because Precose and Glyset inhibit CHO digestion/breakdown, so need a "sugar" that is in the lowest state.

i. **What is the patient's ordered daily insulin for breakfast, lunch, dinner, and bedtime?**

   - Novolog 5 units at breakfast, lunch, and dinner. Lantus is 14 units. Do not mix these insulins. If the patient does not have a preference for Lantus, administer at bedtime.

j. **Using the Subcutaneous Hyperglycemia Protocol, when should the nurse notify the physician of the patient's condition?**

   - FSBG greater than 375 mg/dL.
   - FSBG less than 50 mg/dL after retest. Do not delay treatment with 30 gm of fast acting CHO before calling physician.
   - Patient is unresponsive and FSBG is greater than 70 mg/dL. Do not delay treatment before calling physician.

Action Prompts and Related Mannequin Changes

Issenberg et al. (2005) reported that 9% of the studies evaluated to determine the effectiveness of medical simulation found that a major advantage of simulation was the provision of an environment in which learners can make, detect, and correct errors without adverse consequences. In addition, 9% of the studies highlighted the importance of having reproducible, standardized educational experiences where learners are active participants, rather than passive bystanders. Action prompts and the related mannequin changes provide this type of environment.

Action prompts include three components: (1) an outline of the progression of the scenario, (2) questions the lab mentor may ask to prompt learner action and/or verbalization of clinical thinking, and (3) the actions or responses the learners should take during the scenario to successfully accomplish the objectives of the scenario. In this section, nurse educators provide notes or references to the lab mentors to ensure that the learners' actions are consistently performed correctly, using available evidence-based rationales. Specifically, the nurse educators collaborate with the lab mentors to outline the questions learners should be asked in an effort to stimulate their critical-thinking ability. The action prompts provide a mechanism by which the responsible nurse educators direct the learning experience and the evaluation of the learners even if they are not present during the competency validation.

As the learner responds to questions from the lab mentors related to the nursing care, the condition of the patient may change, either because of or in spite of the actions of the learner. This progression is perhaps the most effective portion of the simulation, because it provides the learner with an opportunity to respond to changes in the patient's condition in a safe environment.

Prior to the actual simulation, the scenario developers must define the specific physiological changes (positive or negative) that would occur in the patient in response to the learner's actions. A table that includes all body systems, as well as possible vocal comments, can be used as a framework for the developers to determine all necessary changes that might occur as the patient condition changes or time passes (see Box 13-5).

Debriefing

Issenberg et al. (2005) found that 47% of the 109 studies on the effectiveness of medical simulation identified feedback as the most important component of the teaching–learning process within simulation. This feedback, referred to as a debriefing, occurs immediately after the simulation experience and requires that the learners be led through a purposive discussion of the

**Box 13-5   Diabetic Management Example—Action Prompts
and Mannequin Changes**

The patient has been transferred to your medical/surgical unit after stabilization
in the intensive care unit. You are reporting for your shift at 0700. The breakfast
trays are expected to be delivered to the floor at 0800. At 0700, you go to the patient
bedside and complete your initial assessment. The patient did receive Lantus insulin
the previous evening.

Mannequin Settings

Body System Assessment	Patient Findings
Vital Signs	99-28–18, 124/78
Neurological/Sensory	PERRLA, oriented ×4, no reports of pain
Cardiac	RRR, pulses 2+. Capillary refill < 2 secs
Pulmonary	Bilateral crackles, pulse ox 97%
Musculoskeletal	Good strength and range of motion
Gastrointestinal (GI)	Active bowel sounds
Genitourinary (GU)	Amber urine
Skin/Wounds	Skin pink, warm, and dry; no lesions
Vocal Comment	"I'm fine."
Lab Results	FSBG: 162–170 mg/dL (use glucose calibration #D)

Expected Nursing Care:

- Obtain finger stick blood glucose (FSBG). (Note to Lab Mentor: Use the different
  glucose calibration solutions for the results the patient needs to obtain.)

Lab Mentor Discussion:

- Facilitate discussion of what FSBG indicate hypoglycemia in this patient.

Expected Nursing Care:

- Administer Novolog 7 U sub-q

Box 13-5   Diabetic Management Example—Action Prompts and Mannequin Changes *(continued)*

Situation Progression I

Patient becomes hypoglycemic either from not eating her breakfast or from not receiving the breakfast tray.

Expected Nursing Care:

- Obtain FSBG; Call lab for STAT blood glucose, treat with 30 gms of fast-acting CHO. Notify physician. Do not delay treatment for lab or physician notification.

Note to Lab Mentor: Have the various food products available for treatment. The student can select options to administer the 30 gm.

Lab Mentor Discussion

- Facilitate discussion related to the difference between treatment of a low glucose snack with either 15 or 30 CHO. Ask: Why would 30 gms be preferred in this situation?

Situation Progression II: The learner is expected to recheck the FSBG blood glucose 15 minutes after treatment. Results of the assessment include:

Body System Assessment	Patient Finding
Vital Signs	99-88-14, 120/60
Neurologic/Sensory	PERRLA, oriented ×4
Cardiac	RRR, Pulses 2+, capillary refill, < 2 secs
Pulmonary	Bilateral crackles, pulse ox 98%
Musculoskeletal	Good strength and range of motion
Gastrointestinal (GI)	Active bowel sounds
Gentourinary (GU)	Amber urine
Skin/Wound	Skin pink, warm, and dry
Vocal Comment	"I feel better."
Lab Results	FSBG: 83–139 mg/dL (use glucose calibration #C)

**Box 13-5   Diabetic Management Example—Action Prompts
and Mannequin Changes *(continued)***

Expected Nursing Care

- Obtain FSBG; provide a protein and 15 gm CHO snack. The learner is to pick the appropriate snack from the assorted foods for the patient, since she is 2 hours away from her next meal.

Situation Progression III: It is now 1630 and the dinner trays are expected at 1700. The learner enters the room to get the FSBG prior to dinner. The following are the results of the assessment:

Body System Assessment	Patient Finding
Vital Signs	99-90-14, 110/56
Neurologic/Sensory	PERRLA, oriented ×4, irritable
Cardiac	RRR, Pulses 2+, capillary refill, < 2 secs
Pulmonary	Bilateral crackles, pulse ox 96%
Musculoskeletal	Good strength and range of motion
Gastrointestinal (GI)	Active bowel sounds
Gentourinary (GU)	Amber urine
Skin/Wound	Skin pink, warm, and dry
Vocal Comment	"I feel quite nauseous."
Lab Results	FSBG: 324–540mg/dL (use glucose calibration #C)

Expected Nursing Care

- Obtain FSBG. The patient is hyperglycemic. Administer the appropriate amount of insulin per the protocol.

Lab Mentor Discussion

- Facilitate discussion on the findings for hyperglycemia in this patient.

**Box 13-5   Diabetic Management Example—Action Prompts
and Mannequin Changes *(continued)***

Situation Progression IV: It is 0800 the next day. You are caring for the same patient. Upon entering the room, the learner finds the patient unresponsive. Assessment findings are as follows:

Body System Assessment	Patient Finding
Vital Signs	99-112-14, 90/60
Neurologic/Sensory	PERRLA, unresponsive
Cardiac	RRR, Pulses 2+, capillary refill, < 2 secs
Pulmonary	Bilateral crackles, pulse ox 96%
Musculoskeletal	Weak
Gastrointestinal (GI)	Active bowel sounds
Gentourinary (GU)	Amber urine
Skin/Wound	Diaphoretic, pale
Vocal Comment	Unresponsive
Lab Results	FSBG: 25–41mg/dL (use glucose calibration #A)

Expected Nursing Care

- Obtain FSBG; Call lab for STAT blood glucose, Administer 1 ampule Glucagon IM or sub-q. Initiate aspiration precautions, notify physician, and do not delay treatment waiting for lab or physician.

Lab Mentor Discussion:

- Facilitate discussion the indications for treatment of an unresponsive hypoglycemic patient: D$_{50}$W vs. Glucagon. (The patient does not have an IV.)

Box 13-5   Diabetic Management Example—Action Prompts and Mannequin Changes *(continued)*

Situation Progression V: It is 15 minutes later. The learner checks the FSBG for response to treatment. Assessment findings are as follows:

Body System Assessment	Patient Finding
Vital Signs	99-80-14, 124/60
Neurologic/Sensory	PERRLA, orientated ×4
Cardiac	RRR, Pulses 2+, capillary refill < 2 secs
Pulmonary	Bilateral crackles, pulse ox 97%
Musculoskeletal	Good strength and range of motion
Gastrointestinal (GI)	Active bowel sounds
Gentourinary (GU)	Amber urine
Skin/Wound	Skin warm and dry
Vocal Comment	"I feel better."
Lab Diagnostic Results	FSBG: 83–139mg/dL (use glucose calibration #C)

Expected Nursing Care

• Obtain FSBG. Provide patient with breakfast.

learning experience, so that they can reflect upon it (Lasater, 2007). During the debriefing, students have an opportunity to express their feelings about both positive and negative experiences, which can help them to cope with their emotions and integrate the meaning of their learning experiences (Hertel & Millis, 2002). Lab mentors can also use this time to allow students to document care provided during the simulation. This exercise often stimulates further discussion regarding lessons learned or personal anecdotes. In addition, lab mentors may use the debriefing session to restate the learning objectives for the simulation, provide outlines from current research or clinical guidelines, or offer helpful visuals or other reinforcement activities.

ENSURING AN EFFECTIVE SIMULATION

Although the quality of research regarding the effectiveness of simulation as a learning strategy in clinical education is generally weak, most educators believe that simulation facilitates learning if certain conditions are in place (Issenberg et al., 2005). According to Issenberg and colleagues (2005), these conditions include provision of feedback, repetitive practice, curriculum integration, a range of difficulty levels, multiple learning strategies, clinical variation, controlled environment, defined outcomes, and simulator validity.

The development and implementation of the RSC suggests that collaboration should be added to the list of conditions for effective learning in simulation. The RSC became a reality thanks to collaboration among a state agency, a university, a community college, and a regional hospital. In addition, operation of the RSC, including development of specific scenarios and competency education validation for students, requires collaboration between the RSC lab mentors and the nurse educators who are ultimately responsible for the learning experience. In fact, this collaboration has been critical to the extent to which learners have had access to scenario-based stimulation. If the nurse educators (either hospital nurse educators or university/community college faculty) had been required to develop and implement the scenarios without the assistance of the lab mentors, there would have been far fewer learners served and scenarios developed, and the complexity of the scenario, as illustrated by the diabetic management scenario, would not have been as high. Certainly, collaboration was critical in the success of RSC.

References

Hertel, J. P., & Millis, B. J. (2002) *Using simulations to promote learning in higher education: An introduction.* Sterling, VA: Stylus.

Issenberg, S. B., McGaghie, W. C., Pertrusa, E. R., Gordon, D. L., & Scalese, R. J. (2005). Features and uses of high fidelity medical simulations that lead to effective learning: A BEME systematic review. *Medical Teacher, 27*(1), 10–28.

Lasater, K. (2007). High-fidelity simulation and the development of clinical judgment: Student experiences. *Journal of Nursing Education, 46*, 269–276.

Sportsman, S., Bradshaw, P., Bolton, C., et al. (In press). Regional simulation center partnership: A collaboration to improve staff and student competence. *Journal of Continuing Education in Nursing.*

Texas Higher Education Coordinating Board (THECB). (2004). *Nursing innovation grant program grant application.*

Hyperglycemia Protocol (Subcutaneous Insulin Orders)

1. **Discontinue all previous insulin orders.**

2. **Finger-stick blood glucose monitoring. Select one or more of the following options:**

   Before meals and bedtime (0300)

   ☐ Every 6 hours (0000–0600–1200–1800) if patient NPO

   ☐ _____ hours after meals

3. **Scheduled insulin dose (units):**

   Lantus _____ units subcutaneous at _____ (Please specify time to be given.)

   Do not mix Lantus with any other insulin in the same syringe.

4. **Correction dose algorithms for subcutaneous Novolog insulin:**

   For algorithm assignment, preferred criterion = total daily insulin dose (TDI), adding all scheduled components.

   Alternative criterion = body weight.

Insulin	Breakfast	Lunch	Dinner	Bedtime
Novolog				
Novolin NPH		xxxxxxxxxxxx		
Novolin 70/30		xxxxxxxxxxxx		xxxxxxxxxxxx
Humalog Mix 75/25		xxxxxxxxxxxx		xxxxxxxxxxxx

Algorithm 1 (TDI) < 28 units or wt < 56 kg	Algorithm 2 (TDI) 28–36 units or wt 56 to 73.9 kg	Algorithm 3 (TDI) 37–55 units or wt 74 to 111.9kg	Algorithm 4 (TDI) 56–90 units or wt 112 to 181.9 kg	Algorithm 5 (TDI) 91–144 units or wt > = 182 kg	Algorithm 6 (TDI) > 144 units	Algorithm 7
BG units	BG units	BG units	BG units	BG units	BG units	BG units
150–224 1	150–209 1	150–189 1	150–199 2	150–209 4	150–199 5	
225–299 2	210–269 2	190–229 2	200–249 4	210–269 8	200–249 10	
300–374 3	270–329 3	230–269 3	250–299 6	270–329 12	250–299 15	
375–449 4	330–389 4	270–309 4	300–349 8	330–389 16	300–349 20	
> = 450 5	> = 390 5	310–349 5	350–399 10	> = 390 20	> = 350 25	
		> = 350 6	> = 400 12			

Algorithm may be selected or revised according to clinical judgment and response to previous therapy.

Notify physician if BG > 400 mg/dL.

5. **Use URHCS hypoglycemia protocol if BG < 70 mg/dL or if patient is symptomatic.**

   i. If FSBG > 50 and < 69 mg/dL, treat with 15 g of fast-acting carbohydrate.

   ii. If FSBG < 50 mg/dL, retest FSBG, call lab for stat blood glucose, and then treat with 30 g of fast-acting carbohydrate. (Note: Do not delay treatment pending lab drawing.) Notify physician.

   iii. Retest FSBG 15 minutes after treatment. If FSBG < 70 mg/DL, repeat treatment based on result (as above).

   iv. If next meal is more than 1 hour away, provide a protein and a 15-g carbohydrate snack in addition to the above treatment to prevent recurrent hypoglycemia.

   v. If patient is unresponsive and BG < 70 mg/dL:

      1. Give 50% dextrose IV push, $\frac{1}{2}$ ampule. (Observe patient for 10 minutes, and if patient remains unresponsive, repeat $\frac{1}{2}$ ampule of 50% dextrose IV push. Repeat FSBG after medication is given.)

      2. If no IV access, give 1 ampule Glucagon IM or SC (may cause vomiting). Utilize aspiration precautions and turn patient on his or her side. For child < 20 kg, use 1/2 ampule (0.5 cc). Administer in gluteus, thigh, or deltoid.

   vi. Special considerations: When a patient is on fluid restrictions, use 1 tube of glucose gel in buccal cavity and ask patient to swallow.

   vii. If patient is using acarbase (Precose) or miglitol (Glyset), use 1 tube of glucose gel in buccal cavity. (Do not use juice, cola, or sugar.)

   viii. A patient with renal or liver compromise may experience reoccurring hypoglycemia even past treatment and will require continued observation for several hours.

      - If FSBG < 80 mg/dL, give insulin immediately after a meal is consumed.
      - Novolog and Humalog: Mix 75/25; needs to be given when the tray is in front of the patient.
      - Novolin 70/30 insulin should be given 15–30 minutes before a meal is served.

Signature: _____ Date: _____
Time: _____

CHAPTER 14

Interdisciplinary Simulation Center

Marilyn McGuire-Sessions and Paula Gubrud

The landmark Institute of Medicine (IOM) recommendations for health professionals' education discuss the importance of interdisciplinary education as a means to prepare learners to meet the IOM competencies (Greiner & Knebel, 2003). Specifically, the IOM's *Crossing the Quality Chasm* report (2001) describes a future healthcare environment in which practitioners function as effective team members and learn to "understand the advantage of high levels of cooperation, coordination and standardization to guarantee excellence, continuity and reliability" (p. 83). In addition, Greiner and Knebel (2003) suggest that effective interdisciplinary teams are composed of members from different professions with varied and specialized knowledge, skills, and approaches to addressing patient care problems. Effective teams integrate their observations, bodies of knowledge and expertise, and value the contribution each makes to the decision-making process. The process for shared decision making, which includes assuming accountability for the outcome of decisions, requires skills related to coordination and communication with the intent to optimize care for a patient or a group of patients.

Interdisciplinary simulations provide an opportunity for students to gain an understanding of the unique contribution each profession makes to addressing patient needs while developing the collaborative relationships required among members of those disciplines in the practice environment. Students rarely have exposure to what expert practice looks like as part of the curriculum, nor do they have the opportunity to dissect the reasoning patterns that expert practitioners use to make sound clinical judgments when interacting with the intraprofessional team. To overcome this shortfall of the nursing curriculum, Bransford, Brown, and Cocking (2000) have advocated for students' training in community-centered environments that include experts as mentors and teachers. Simulation and debriefing can be used to provide students with exposure to the actions, reasoning, and judgments that define expertise in interdisciplinary environments.

The Oregon Simulation Alliance (OSA), by design, is an interdisciplinary, simulation-focused organization that organizes regional interdisciplinary community-based simulation users through a statewide organization. The OSA was established in 2003 by the Governor's Healthcare Workforce Initiative, and has as its statewide mission "to ensure quality patient care for all Oregonians through the use of simulation technology and practice to help healthcare workers be more confident, competent, and compassionate in providing patient care." The OSA is both an advisory group and an oversight committee, combining the strength and expertise of key players in the state. The OSA's Governing Council includes representatives from the state's community colleges, public and private four-year colleges and universities, healthcare provider organizations, and simulation users. Since its inception, the Governing Council has been an interdisciplinary group whose members represent the nursing, emergency services, medicine, and respiratory therapy disciplines. One of OSA's stated mandates is the integration of simulation capacity into healthcare curricula so as to train and network simulation faculty, while recognizing the interdisciplinary nature of health care.

Defining the goals and characteristics of an interdisciplinary simulation center inevitably poses a challenge, however. As the development and use of high-fidelity clinical simulation environments have increased, the concept of an interdisciplinary simulation center has been implemented in a number of forms. The most common variation is the clinical simulation center that has, as its primary user group, one particular discipline (i.e., nursing or medicine). Members of other disciplines may also participate in clinical simulation in these settings, but their sessions are scheduled around the primary users' schedules. The variations found among interdisciplinary simulation centers can be linked to the beneficiaries of this clinical teaching modality, who can most readily be identified by determining who is participating in the clinical simulation experience. This chapter looks briefly at two types of simulation programs: (1) hospital-based, practitioner simulation programs and (2) academic settings where student practitioners provide clinical care in a simulated environment.

THE HOSPITAL-BASED INTERDISCIPLINARY SIMULATION CENTER: SIMULATION FOR PRACTITIONERS

Using high-fidelity clinical simulation in the hospital setting with the disciplines that practice there has been a way for hospitals to demonstrate their ability to develop and maintain proficiency in the five core areas of practice identified in the IOM's 2003 report, *Health Professions Education: A Bridge to Quality*—namely, delivering patient-centered care, working as part of interdisciplinary teams, practicing evidence-based medicine, focusing on quality improvement, and using information technology (Greiner & Knebel, 2003). Along with the five core areas identified by the IOM, the Joint Commission on Accreditation of Healthcare Organizations (JCAHO) supports enhanced safety and quality of health care by incorporating technology as a fundamental support component of the practice setting. Hospital-based clinical simulation experiences can be used to emphasize the interdisciplinary aspect of hospital care, which directly impacts patient outcomes.

Clinical simulation experiences can also occur "in situ," referring to the use of clinical simulation in a specific care environment. This type of simulation allows practitioners to use indigenous equipment, supplies, and access points in the exact area of care where clinical situations will occur. In situ simulation environments also create an opportunity for interdisciplinary simulation experiences, as employees representing various disciplines simply participate in simulation at the unit where they are assigned to work.

THE ACADEMIC-BASED INTERDISCIPLINARY SIMULATION CENTER: SIMULATION FOR STUDENTS

The nature of the high-fidelity clinical simulation environment for the pre-licensed, healthcare student has provided an additional level of clinical teaching and learning to healthcare education. In such a clinical environment, the student truly works at the patient's bedside and is required to make, in the moment of care, clinical judgments that might have previously been intercepted, to ensure patient safety, by the instructor or practitioner in the hospital or clinical setting. This type of teaching and learning has brought a new purposefulness to clinical education. The educator can identify for a particular day the type of patient, family, and interdisciplinary interactions that will be presented to the students, thereby enabling the educator to actually have students implement theory and evidence-based practice in close proximity to a clinical experience.

INTERDISCIPLINARY INFUSED HIGH-FIDELITY CLINICAL SIMULATION SCENARIOS

Use of high-fidelity simulation is applicable to all disciplines of health care and can be implemented to help learners develop new knowledge and skills, and acquire better understanding of the relationships and dynamics that support effective teamwork (Gaba, 2007). Recent landmark studies and comprehensive reports by Kohn, Corrigan, and Donaldson (2000) and the Institute of Medicine (2001) describe the importance of teamwork training as a means to improve patient outcomes. Learning experiences in simulation environments are increasingly being used to facilitate communication and collaboration between disciplines, a factor that is known to improve the effectiveness of care delivery, thereby positively influencing patient care outcomes (Jankouskas et al., 2007).

Key Objectives for an Interdisciplinary Infused High-Fidelity Clinical Simulation

As with any teaching/learning modality, identifying the learning outcomes is essential when an organization decides to adopt simulation as a training tool. When infusing the interdisciplinary nature of health care into a simulated clinical experience, identifying those care points where an interdisciplinary interaction would most likely take place heightens the fidelity of the care experience. Faculty members' expectations of students in the simulated care experience would then be the ability to deploy members of the interdisciplinary team appropriately and the demonstration of interdisciplinary communication skills. The use of a progressive simulation, known as an unfolding case scenario, can provide that mechanism. When this type of simulation is coupled with the illness trajectory framework (Corbin & Strauss, 1992), nursing care priorities that are linked with other disciplines along a care trajectory can be identified and demonstrated by students through this mechanism.

Guidelines for Interdisciplinary Scenario Development

Interdisciplinary simulation experiences should deliberately integrate one or more key concepts that describe effective interdisciplinary collaboration. The scenario template should provide prompts to assure that scenario authors develop learning objectives related to the knowledge, skills, and attitudes involved in interdisciplinary collaboration. Scenario templates can also be designed to emphasize the key concept of communication between providers. In addition, scenario templates should be designed to facilitate the development of an interdisciplinary care team by identifying designated roles for the various professionals who will be involved in the care. Finally, guidelines for debriefing should include discussion questions that assist learners to identify the characteristics of effective collaboration between disciplines.

The literature dealing with simulation design offers guidelines for designing interdisciplinary simulations. Recent articles indicate that learning objectives should be developed first as the foundation that drives the scenario storyline (Henneman & Cunningham, 2005; Jeffries, 2007; Salas, Wilson, Burke, & Priest, 2005). Salas and associates (2005), for example, noted that scenario design should begin by determining what knowledge and skills are held by the participants. When designing interdisciplinary scenarios, simulation developers are encouraged to assess the learners based on their skills and attitudes related to interdisciplinary communication. Next, faculty developers should identify learning outcomes that reflect the gap between what the participants know and can do and what they need to learn. Put simply, learning in high-fidelity simulation environments creates the opportunity for faculty to design learning experiences that fill in the gap between what students know and what they need to learn. The scenario storyline can then be developed to incorporate collaborative behavior and communication between various professionals.

Jeffries (2005, 2007), who was the lead investigator in a multisite study that addressed the implementation of simulation in nursing education, has proposed several guiding principles regarding scenario development. First, the scenario storyline should be constructed with the learning objectives in mind. As students progress in their knowledge and skills, the simulation scenarios should likewise become more complex and include a level of uncertainty that triggers the participants' need to make clinical judgments. The amount of relevant information given to the participants before the scenario should increase over time during the scenario enactment. The complexity of the scenario and the amount of relevant information provided before the simulation experience begins depend on the participants' experience and level of proficiency with a problem (Jeffries, 2007). Interdisciplinary simulations can be created to emphasize information that participants must communicate as the storyline unfolds.

Jeffries (2007) posited that patients in real life are not likely to exhibit all of the textbook signs and symptoms for a particular problem when the nurse first encounters a situation. For this reason, clinical information should be given to simulation participants over time, much in the same way that they are likely to encounter the information in reality. Thus scenarios should be designed so that participants are allowed to investigate questions freely while working in tandem with one another and to employ questions in any sequence. If participants become stuck and cease to gather additional information or to employ the clinical reasoning needed to make a judgment that would be enhanced by interdisciplinary approach, faculty members should provide a prompt that fits within the scenario storyline. Henneman and Cunningham (2005) also suggest that if students do not respond appropriately to the cues provided by the mannequin, faculty participants in the scenario may assume the role of a healthcare provider, such as the charge nurse or physician, in an effort to redirect students' thinking and action. Using experienced faculty members to provide discipline expertise through entrance into the scenario storyline creates new opportunities to recognize the expertise each discipline has to offer related to particular patient problems.

The use of prompts and cues represents an educational judgment made by faculty on behalf of the students' learning. Instructors sometimes demonstrate a tendency to redirect students when they are about to make a mistake, thereby enabling the learners to avoid the consequences of their action. However, seeing the consequences of one's mistakes can lead to a more powerful learning experience. Salas and associates (2005) advocate that teachers resist the temptation to rescue students from the untoward consequences of their errors. Jeffries (2005) suggests that prompts be considered when students are stuck or immobilized (meaning that they are unable to make any decision at all) and that students be allowed to make mistakes in simulation. During the simulation experience, interdisciplinary faculty should create an environment that promotes collaboration and communication and allow students to work through their differences and conflicts and resist the temptation to intervene prematurely. Ground rules for debriefing should also be established to ensure that any difficulties with communication and collaborative skills and attitudes are uncovered and discussed in an environment that is free of blame and accusations.

Henneman and Cunningham have created a framework for developing simulations (2005, p. 174), based on their experience with scenario development and implementation of high-fidelity simulation. In developing this model, they identified principles that should be included in scenario development, where those principles are derived from crisis resource management principles, which are themselves utilized to promote team collaboration in high-risk situations in anesthesia. Crisis resource management principles have been integrated into anesthesia training, including simulated learning experiences, for several years, with the intent of facilitating team functioning and improving patient safety (Gaba, Fish, & Howard, 1994). These principles suggest that scenarios be developed to assure that participants have an opportunity to be prepared for what they may encounter in practice, with a focus on the importance of team communication. Henneman and Cunningham (2005) designed their scenarios to assure that students received some information about the patient before beginning care by simulating a change-of-shift report from the outgoing nurse immediately before the simulation begins. This report provides a summary of the patient's condition and progress toward meeting goals toward recovery.

Interdisciplinary scenarios can be designed to emphasize the art of providing condition reports between disciplines. In addition, scenarios should ensure that students are encouraged to assign the appropriate tasks to the most qualified member of the team. This approach creates opportunities for students to gain an understanding of what each professional contributes in meeting the complex needs of patients in high-risk situations, chronic care environments, and end-of-life settings.

Using Theoretical Principles in Interdisciplinary Scenarios

Several recent articles in the nursing education literature have identified the notion of integrating the characteristics of "situated learning" into clinical education (Cope, Cuthbertson, & Stoddart, 2000; Taylor & Care, 1999; Wooley & Jarvis, 2007). Cope and associates posit that experts do not operate by following rules that are derived from knowledge and higher-order cognitive process, but rather use "complex situation understanding, a mature and practiced dexterity that comes from their breadth and depth of experience" (2000, p. 855). In situated learning, experts focus the learner's attention on the salient features of the situation in question. One of the defining characteristics of cognitive apprenticeship is that experts make their situational or tacit knowledge explicit as they coach the learner. Coaching incorporates modeling expert performance and includes providing feedback on the learner's performance.

The notions of *scaffolding* and *fading* are essential components to cognitive apprenticeships. In scaffolding, the mentor offers support to the learner; as the learner gains competence and confidence, the expert then withdraws (fades) the support (scaffolds). Cognitive apprenticeships also include strategies such as articulation, reflection, and exploration (Cope et al., 2000). As the learner gains confidence and competence, he or she is encouraged to articulate his or her understanding and reflect on his or her acquisition of expertise. Additionally, as the learner progresses and begins to demonstrate recognizable competence, he or she is encouraged by the mentor to explore multiple approaches to addressing problems in practice. Much of this process involves the opportunity to learn from established members of the professional community (Cope et al., 2000).

Simulation learning environments provide an ideal setting in which to implement the characteristics of cognitive apprenticeship and situated learning in intraprofessional environments. Teams of experienced faculty or practitioners can model effective collaborative behavior in simulated experiences. As students indicate they are beginning to develop a foundation related to their own discipline's knowledge, skills, and values, simulations that incorporate common and straightforward patient care problems and require the delivery of interdisciplinary care can be designed for students to participate in. As students gain expertise in their own discipline's knowledge, simulation scenarios may present more complex and ambiguous problems for the interdisciplinary team to solve. As students gain confidence in their own professional roles, scenarios that create opportunities for students to explore role cross-over versus the need for role clarity can then be introduced.

Another simulation activity that enhances the characteristics of situated learning involves interdisciplinary rounds on patients. Each patient's story can be designed to promote a greater understanding among the professions regarding what each practitioner knows and does in the actual care environment. The simulated rounds can include both faculty and student participants and can incorporate several patients with similar problems. This design enables students to develop pattern recognition related to the normal trajectory of a particular illness or health problem as well as a more in-depth understanding of the contribution each discipline makes relative to a particular kind of patient situation. The storyline of each case might, for example, emphasize solutions to patient care problems that help students appreciate the contribution each profession makes in today's complex healthcare environments. With this type of scenario, debriefing should emphasize the communication that both enhanced or created barriers toward achieving shared patient care goals. In addition, debriefing should be designed so that all participants become familiar with the unique knowledge and approach each discipline contributes toward providing holistic and comprehensive care.

The Interdisciplinary Simulation Scenario

Regardless of the simulation setting, the following scenario illustrates how the interdisciplinary nature of health care can be infused into a simulated clinical experience for the pre-licensure nursing student. In this high-fidelity, progressive clinical simulation scenario, the students care for the same patient over three points in the illness trajectory framework. At each point on that trajectory, students must address nursing and interdisciplinary implications for the clinical experience.

The first clinical encounter with the patient is when "Alice Nyman" is in the hospital for biopsy. The second clinical encounter occurs when the same patient is in active treatment. The last encounter is when, as part of the natural course of the disease, the patient is actively dying. Depending on the number of students experiencing clinical simulation on any given day, two to three students may actively care for this patient during each clinical encounter, while the remaining students actively observe the care their colleagues are providing. Students should be able to demonstrate the identified objectives for each clinical experience in approximately 20 minutes, leaving 30 minutes for each debriefing session. Because of the nature of the progressive clinical simulation experience, the students have an opportunity to "know" their patient in a way

Figure 14-1 Sample Scenario for an Interdisciplinary End-of-Life Situation

Scenario Title	Progressive Simulation: Oncologic Patient—Trajectory *(Infused with interdisciplinary care across the trajectory)*
Patient Name	Nyman, Alice
Medical Record #	**DOB:** **Age:**
Patient Type and Acuity	Oncology patient—disease trajectory—death and dying
Level	**Course:**
Author , w/email	
Keywords— Theory	Palliative, End-of-Life Care, Cancer Treatment and Symptom Management, Active Dying
Keywords—Skills	Therapeutic communication, medication administration, hydration, handling chemo waste, post-mortem care, interdisciplinary care
Patient Case History:	68-year-old female patient who is to undergo a bronchoscopy for biopsy of 2 cm pulmonary nodule found on her left upper lobe found on a follow-up chest x-ray last week. The patient is completely asymptomatic.
Medical History:	Patient is a 68-year-old female 45 months s/p r-upper lobectomy for resection stage IB–IIIA Non-small cell lung carcinoma (NSCLC). At that time she first presented with cough and hemoptysis leading to the diagnosis of a 4.5 cm r-upper lobe NSCLC. At that time there was no evidence of mediastinal involvement and she showed no evidence of metastatic disease. She had smoked a pack of cigarettes per day for 45 years but had stopped 2 years prior to her diagnosis.

Allergies:		PCN, ASA, Demerol	**Height:**	5′7″	**Weight:**	63 kg
Meds:						
VS:	**BP** 135/88	**HR** 90	**RR** 18	**T** 37.4	**SpO₂** 97	
Labs:						

Figure 14-1 Sample Scenario for an Interdisciplinary End-of-Life Situation *(con't)*

FIRST SEQUENCE

Physician Orders: Alice Nyman   **DOB:** 02/14/1938   **Allergies:** PCN, ASA, Demerol   (Dr. Rasmussen)

1. Admit to Same Day Surgery
2. DX—S/P NSCLC R-lung—r/o recurrent lung cancer L-lung
3. VS q 4 hrs
4. IV NS at 125 cc/hr
5. NPO
6. Morphine 0.5–4 mg IV q 2–4 hr prn pain
7. Phenergan 12.5–25 mg IV q 4–6 hrs prn nausea
8. Ativan 1 mg IV on call for OR
9. Notify Physician: SBP > 140 < 80, DBP > 90 < 50; HR > 120 < 50; RR > 22 < 8; T > 38.5; UOP < 30 cc/hr × 8 hours

Initial Computer Setup (first sequence)

VS:	BP	140/90	HR	92	RR	18	T	37.4	SpO$_2$	97
Lungs:	**Lt:** normal		**Rt:** normal			**Bowel sounds**			normal	
Heart:			**Rhythm:**							
Ectopy:			**Waiting:**							
Other:										

Report to start scenario:	Alice is a 68-year-old female who is to undergo a bronchoscopy for biopsy of a 2-cm pulmonary nodule found on her left upper lobe found on a follow-up chest x-ray last week. She is 45 months s/p r-upper lobectomy for resection of a 4.5 cm stage IB–IIIA NSCLC.
	She is very nervous that the cancer has spread. Knows that smoking was not a good habit and she quit 2 years ago. She's NPO. The surgeon has talked to her about the procedure. She has lorazepam 1mg IV on call to OR. She has not complained of any pain or other discomfort.
	Note: Student(s) need to start the IV, complete the pre-op check list, and get her prepared for surgery
	Interdisciplinary infused care: Surgeon, Anesthesia, Pathology, O.R. staff

Figure 14-1 Sample Scenario for an Interdisciplinary End-of-Life Situation *(con't)*

Alice Nyman First Sequence		
Priorities (in order)	**SN Interventions**	**Patient Responses**
Introduction, assessment	Introduce self Baseline VS Assess for discomfort	"I can't believe the cancer has spread." "I don't want to go through another surgery." "I should never have started smoking—don't ever smoke—you don't smoke, do you?"
Start IV and IVFs for surgery		
Pre-op check list	Go through pre-op check list, ask patient if there are any questions related to the surgery	"I don't have any questions." "The doctor explained it well." "I don't want to die of cancer."
Contact surgeon and/or anesthesia with consent questions/ clarifications	SN makes sure consent is signed properly and patient does not have questions before giving Ativan	
		"I am nervous. Can I have something to calm me down?"
	Open ended questions to help patient talk about why she is nervous Explain that there is an order for medication that will calm her before the surgery	
Interaction with the OR staff regarding transport and readiness of patient for surgery	OR calls to say they will come up to pick up patient	
Prepare to give Ativan Double check pre-op check list	Give Ativan IV Push with proper technique, 5 rights, etc.	"Will this help me calm down?" "I can't believe I have another surgery to go through." "I hope its not more cancer."

Figure 14-1 Sample Scenario for an Interdisciplinary End-of-Life Situation *(con't)*

Faculty Notes (theory, medications, etc.)
Debrief Priorities (facts, feelings, behaviors, priorities, noticing, interpreting, responding, evaluating, and reflecting—what went well, what would you do differently) 1. Communication with patient with prior history of cancer going in for procedure where more cancer may be found. 2. IV push administration—how did this go? 3. How to talk to patient who is blaming self due to smoking habit—techniques to be used. 4. Pre-op check list, consent form, and pre-op with Ativan. 5. Interdisciplinary care: how to accomplish all elements of care, communicate with the other disciplines involved in the care, and be available to a patient in distress.
Possible Increased Complexities for this Scenario:
1.
References:
1. Johnson, B. L. & Gross, J. (1998). *Handbook of oncology nursing* (3rd ed.). Sudbury, MA: Jones and Bartlett Publishers.
2. Fortenbaugh, C. C. & Rummel, M. A. (2007). *Case studies in oncology nursing.* Sudbury, MA: Jones and Bartlett Publishers.
Suggestions for Future Advanced Scenarios:

Figure 14-1 Sample Scenario for an Interdisciplinary End-of-Life Situation *(con't)*

Alice Nyman Second Sequence

68-year-old female patient who underwent a bronchoscopy 3 months ago for biopsy of 2-cm pulmonary nodule found on her upper left lobe found on a follow-up chest x-ray. The biopsy of the pulmonary nodule resulted in a diagnosis of small cell lung CA. A MRI of the brain which followed was negative which completed the staging of this different histological lung cancer from her initial diagnosis in 2003. She was admitted to the acute care floor to receive her second cycle of combination chemotherapy due to symptom management issues that occurred with her first round. She is also scheduled for a once-a-day radiotherapy (180 cGy per day) while she is in-patient.

Allergies:	PCN, ASA, Demerol		**Height:**	5'7"	**Weight:**	53 kg
Meds:						
VS:	**BP**	135/88	**HR**	90	**RR**	18	**T**	37.4	**SpO$_2$**	96
Labs:						

Second Sequence

Physician Orders: Alice Nyman **DOB:** 02/14/1938 **Allergies:** PCN, ASA, Demerol

1. Admit to ACU
2. DX: Symptom management related to chemotherapy for L-lung SCLC (3 yrs s/p R-upper lobe for NSCLC)
3. IVF—see chemotherapy protocol
4. Diet as tolerated
5. Up ad lib
6. EP (Etoposide and cisplatin) Protocol—combination chemotherapy regimen start after prophylactic antiemetic protocol
7. See antiemetic orders prior to starting chemotherapy
8. Compazine 2.5–5 mg IV q 4–6 hrs prn breakthrough nausea
9. Ativan 0.5–1 mg q 2–4 hrs prn breakthrough nausea
10. To start cranial radiation tomorrow q day till discharge
11. Social service consult
12. Notify HO: SBP > 140 < 80, DBP > 90 < 50; HR > 120 < 50; RR > 22 < 8; T > 38.5; UOP < 30 cc/hr × 8 hr

Figure 14-1 Sample Scenario for an Interdisciplinary End-of-Life Situation *(con't)*

Alice Nyman Second Sequence									
Initial Computer Setup									
VS:	**BP**	138/90	**HR**	94	**RR**	18	**T**	37.4	**SpO$_2$**	96
Lungs:	**Lt:** normal		**Rt:** normal		**Bowel sounds**	normal			
Heart:			**Rhythm:**						
Ectopy:			**Waiting:**						
Other:									
Report to start scenario:	*She has a central line in place. *There is 100 cc left in the bag of Cisplatin. When it is done infusing student(s) are to call the chemo nurse (Jane Smith) since she is qualified to handle the chemotherapeutic agents. *The scheduled antiemetic agents were given per protocol. *The saline lock is patent. *Continue with the protocol IV fluids when the cisplatin is done. *Alice has only had 100 cc of urine output since the cisplatin was started. ***Interdisciplinary infused care: Oncologist, Care Conference, certifications related to chemotherapy administration***								

Priorities (in order)	SN Interventions	Patient Responses
Focused Assessment, VS	Vital signs, IV fluid, CL, patient comfort (nausea pain) urine output	"I don't think the medicine they gave me is working." "I am feeling nauseous."
Administration of antiemetics	Follows five rights	
Reassessment r/t low urine output	Calls physician, follows protocol related to administration of Lasix IV, follows five rights	

Figure 14-1 Sample Scenario for an Interdisciplinary End-of-Life Situation *(con't)*

Priorities (in order)	SN Interventions	Patient Responses
Interdisciplinary: team communication—contact oncologist due to low u/o, contact social service physician regarding possibility of family conference related to patient wanting to stop treatment.		"I'm so sick, I just want to stop treatment but my daughter keeps wanting me to have all that can be done. I just want to feel better for as long as I have."
Accessing the nurse who is certified in chemotherapy to assist in the administration and completion of the chemo.		

Alice Nyman Second Sequence

Faculty Notes (theory, medications, etc.)

Debrief Priorities (facts, feelings, behaviors, priorities, noticing, interpreting, responding, evaluating, and reflecting—what went well, what would you do differently?)

1. Precautions with Cisplatin, (handling, nephrotoxicity, lifetime dose of; concern with low urinary output and need for infusing fluids at increased rate).

2. Qualifications of person able to handle chemotherapeutic agents—chemo certified nurse.

3. Antiemetic protocols for chemo and decisions for giving additional agents for breakthrough nausea and vomiting.

4. Discussion of Advance Directive.

5. Explore how to advocate for patient and family when differences in care occur, and to bring together the disciplines that are caring for patient/family.

Figure 14-1 Sample Scenario for an Interdisciplinary End-of-Life Situation *(con't)*

Possible Increased Complexities for this scenario:
References:
Suggestions for Future Advanced Scenarios:

Alice Nyman Third Sequence

Most recently this patient underwent a bronchoscopy for biopsy of 2-cm pulmonary nodule found on her left upper lobe found on a follow-up chest x-ray. The patient was completely asymptomatic. The bronchoscopy revealed SCLC in the l-upper lobe for which she received combination chemotherapy (EP protocol) and cranial radiation.

The patient completed 2 cycles of the chemo and received 2 weeks of cranial radiation before deciding to stop treatment a month ago. She was admitted to Hospice a week ago. Her family brought her in to the ED last night due to her agitation and difficulty breathing.

Allergies:	PCN, ASA, Demerol	**Height:**	5'7"	**Weight:**	49
Meds:					

VS:	**BP**	109/78	**HR**	110	**RR**	30	**T**	38.9	**SpO₂**	88
Labs:										

Figure 14-1 Sample Scenario for an Interdisciplinary End-of-Life Situation *(con't)*

Physician Orders: Alice Nyman **DOB:** 02/14/1938 **Allergies:** PCN, ASA, Demerol—DNR

1. Admit to ACU
2. DNR—see written order
3. DX: SCLC—Dyspnea—Comfort Measures Only
4. NPO
5. Morphine sulfate 2–6 mg IV push q 1–2 hrs prn titrate to comfort pain or dyspnea
6. Ativan .5–1 mg 1–2 hrs prn titrate to comfort agitation or dyspnea
7. O_2 at 4 L per NC

Initial Computer Setup

VS:	BP	106/76	HR	112	RR	28	T	38.9	SpO$_2$	87

Lungs:	**Lt:** Gurgling rhonchi	**Rt:** Gurgling rhonchi	**Bowel sounds**	hypoactive

Report to start scenario:	Patient here for comfort measures only. Her family brought her to the ED last night due to her agitation and difficulty breathing. She is on hospice. Family went home due to being up all night with patient. One hour ago patient received 2 mg of morphine sulfate and 1 mg of lorazepam IVP for moaning and restlessness. Seemed to make her comfortable. Some peripheral edema, coarse rhonchi bilaterally. Responding only with moans. Dr. Rasmussen would like to be called when patient expires. Daughter will be back after getting a change of clothes from home. Organ donations called and she is not a candidate. ***Interdisciplinary infused care: Hospice, Pastoral care, Organ donation.***

Priorities (in order)	SN Interventions	Patient Responses
Focused assessment	Assess for comfort, vital signs, edema, auscultate lungs	Starts to be agitated and have difficulty breathing RR up to 32 SpO$_2$ down to 83
Assess need for medication	"Would you like to have something more to make you more comfortable?"	Mostly unresponsive, moaning, RR 34 SpO$_2$ 80
Critical thinking on what to give patient (morphine, Ativan, or both)	Give morphine and Ativan via correct technique via IV push	SM RR HR and BP decrease Has less difficulty breathing

Figure 14-1 Sample Scenario for an Interdisciplinary End-of-Life Situation *(con't)*

Priorities (in order)	SN Interventions	Patient Responses
Interdisciplinary focus: Hospice contacted, organ donation contacted, pastoral care is contacted	Continued comfort measures	Patient vitals and SpO_2 decrease slowly to being deceased
	SN follows protocol for postmortem care	

Alice Nyman Third Sequence

Faculty Notes (theory, medications, etc.)

Debrief Priorities (facts, feelings, behaviors, priorities, noticing, interpreting, responding, evaluating, and reflecting—what went well, what would you do differently)

1. Care of dying patient.
2. Ethical "dilemma" on medication to give dying patient (morphine? Ativan? both?) making patient comfortable vs decreasing respirations "too much."
3. Postmortem care.
4. Interdisciplinary focus on the team caring for the dying patient and family—physically, emotionally, and spiritually.

Possible Increased Complexities for this Scenario:

References:

Suggestions for Future Advanced Scenarios:

that is not typical of a simulated experience as a result of the time spent both actively caring for and observing the care provided over the three key points in the disease trajectory. Prior to the students arriving for their day in clinical simulation, and due to the specific nature of this unfolding case, having faculty rounds prior to the care experience, if possible, can help faculty identify key objectives and roles that each faculty member will play during the simulated clinical day.

SUMMARY

The interdisciplinary nature of health care can be a complex and at times confusing concept to the pre-licensure nursing student. The current recommendations related to patient safety focus on interdisciplinary teamwork, including an emphasis on effective communication between disciplines. Researchers have found that pre-licensure students need opportunities to develop those collaborative skill sets that will prepare them for working in interdisciplinary practice environments. Unfortunately, nurse educators may not have a chance to provide consistent opportunities for students to practice this aspect of nursing, as such opportunities are often lacking in the hospital setting. The high-fidelity clinical environment, by contrast, can provide a clinical experience that focuses on interdisciplinary care and allows students to demonstrate the behaviors and communication skills that will prepare them for their future practice.

References

Bransford, J. D., Brown, A. L., & Cocking, R. R. (Eds.). (2000). *How people learn*. Washington, DC: National Academy Press.

Cope, P., Cuthbertson, P., & Stoddard, B. (2000). Situated learning in the practice placement. *Journal of Advanced Nursing, 31*(4), 850–856.

Gaba, D. M. (2007). The future of vision of simulation in healthcare. *Simulation in Healthcare, 2*(2), 126–135.

Gaba, D. M., Fish, K. J., & Howard, S. K. (1994). *Crisis management in anesthesiology*. New York: Churchill Livingston.

Greiner, A. C., & Knebel, E. (Eds.). (2003). *Health professions education*. Washington, DC: Institute of Medicine of the National Academies.

Henneman, E. A., & Cunningham, H. (2005). Using simulation to teach patient safety in an acute/critical care nursing course. *Nurse Educator, 30*, 172–177.

Institute of Medicine (IOM). (2001). *Crossing the quality chasm: A new health care system for the 21st century*. Washington DC: National Academy Press.

Jankouskas, T., Bush, M. C., Murray, B., et al., 2007). Crisis resource management: Evaluating outcomes of a multidisciplinary team. *Simulation in Healthcare, 2*(2), 96–97.

Jeffries, P. R. (2005). A framework for designing, implementing and evaluating simulations used as teaching strategies in nursing. *Nursing Education Perspectives, 25*, 96–103.

Jeffries, P. R. (Ed.). (2007). *Simulation in nursing education: From conceptualization to evaluation*. New York: National League for Nursing.

Kohn, L. T., Corrigan, M., & Donaldson, M. S. (Eds.). (2000). *To err is human: Building a safer health system*. Committee on Quality Health Care in America, Institute of Medicine. Washington, DC: National Academy Press.

Salas, E., Wilson, A., Burke, S. C., & Priest, H. A. (2005). Using simulation-based training to improve patient safety: What does it take? *Journal on Quality and Patient Safety, 31*, 363–371.

Taylor, K. L., & Care, W. D. (1999). Nursing education as cognitive apprenticeship. A framework for clinical education. *Nurse Educator, 24*(4), 31–36.

Wooley, N. N., & Jarvis, Y. (2007). Situated cognition and cognitive apprenticeship: A model for teaching and learning clinical skills in a technologically rich and authentic learning environment. *Nursing Education Today, 27*, 73–79.

CHAPTER 15

Planning and Creating a Scenario: The Institute of Technical Education Experience

Yvonne Lau, Suppiah Nagammal, and Tan Khoon Kiat

This chapter outlines the process that the authors undertook when planning and creating scenarios based on the nursing curriculum at the Institute of Technical Education (ITE) in Singapore (ITE, 2006). The ITE, a statutory board under the Singapore Ministry of Education, is a postsecondary institution that provides pre-employment training to individuals who leave secondary school and continuing education and training to working adults. Since its establishment in1992, ITE has become an internationally recognized institution as a result of its model of "Hands-on, Minds-on, Hearts-on" college education. By creating opportunities for school leavers and adult learners to acquire skills, knowledge, and the values of lifelong learning, we have nurtured and produced many graduates with the education and skills needed to face the challenges of the global workforce.

The nursing faculty in the college administer a full-time, two-year National ITE Certificate (Nitec) in nursing program that comprises two components: 40 weeks of institutional training and 36 weeks of supervised clinical practice at healthcare institutions. Our graduates are employed as Enrolled Nurses in various healthcare organizations and hospitals and have the opportunity to apply for progression to the Higher Nitec in Paramedic & Emergency Care course or the Diploma in Nursing course at other academic institutions.

IDENTIFYING DEVELOPERS

A core team of lecturers was selected by the administration of the school to lead the training of other faculty members in high-fidelity patient simulation training. The selection cycle utilized the following inclusion criteria:

1. The core team had to show interest in working with technology.
2. Faculty had to be working in the school for at least one year.
3. Faculty needed to understand the syllabi and the curriculum enough to adapt to and modify the learning needs of the students.

4. Faculty had to have hands-on experience in curriculum review.
5. Faculty had to have experience with clinical teaching with students in the hospitals.
6. Faculty had to provide students with purposeful and appropriate learning experiences and develop a conducive environment for learning,
7. Faculty had to be able to guide students to assess and apply information from various sources and enable them to learn independently.
8. Faculty had to provide opportunities for students to explore and cultivate enthusiasm for learning, team effectiveness, and communication skills.
9. Faculty had to inculcate in students an attitude of change and a spirit of innovation and entrepreneurship.

These guidelines were considered crucial, as the experience of the team would be called upon to fully integrate simulation training in the two-year Nitec in nursing program.

The chosen faculty had to undergo an intensive, five-day, train-the-trainer course offered by Medical Education Technologies Inc. (METI) to ensure that they would be able to use the high-fidelity patient simulators. The simulation process, however, took more than five days to master. Impromptu revisions and refresher courses helped the staff learn more about the capabilities of the high-fidelity patient simulators. To further enhance staff capability, selected staff members were given the opportunity to travel overseas to visit established schools in the United States that have been using high-fidelity patient simulation technology to enhance their teaching methodology; those staff members also attended a course at the Institute of Medical Simulation (located in Boston) to learn more about the teaching techniques that can be used with high-fidelity patient simulation.

IDENTIFYING LEARNERS

Before planning a scenario, nurse educators have to assess the learners who will participate in that scenario. Each organization may identify different learning outcomes for its learners. Thus, before scenario developers can identify the learners, they are required to address a multitude of learning outcomes across technical, methodological, and social skills; in addition, they must ensure that the goals and objectives of the simulation are specific, measurable, and achievable. Clearly, there is a direct connection between the performance task and the intended learning outcomes. For example, the learning outcome for a student enrolled nurse would not be of the same depth as the outcome expected of a registered nurse, as their job scopes vary dramatically. Learners come with different levels of expertise and experience; hence, it is important to identify who the learners are—the student nurse, the undergraduate nurse, the enrolled nurse, the registered nurse, the medical student, the doctor, and/or the member of a multidisciplinary team. Planning and creating an appropriate scenario must take into consideration both what the learners' competence level is and what the facilitator intends for them to learn.

IDENTIFYING LEARNING NEEDS

ITE conducts "industry sensing" to understand the training needs of the various sectors of Singapore's economy. This effort may include a literature search to identify the emerging trends, which then serve as industry inputs to ITE's Academic Advisory Committees, and feedback from roundtable discussions with industry representatives. As demand for healthcare services is clearly increasing, there is a perceived need to strengthen the training and education of healthcare professionals, and thus the need to innovate and revamp our current teaching methodologies. The goal is to ensure that the competency profile of every trained nurse consists of technical skills and knowledge, critical-thinking skills, reasoning ability, communication skills, and a service attitude.

While traditional classroom-based lessons can equip students with the technical competencies, they are inadequate in preparing nurses for the complexities of real work (Jeffries, 2005). Van Merrienboer, Clark, and Crook (2002) describe complex learning with multiple performance objectives as dealing with learning to coordinate and integrate a set of separate skills that constitute a real-life performance. A well-designed training program for complex learning (such as nursing skills) should ensure that all learners acquire the ability to use all the skills in a coordinated and integrated manner in real-life contexts (Merrienboer et al., 2002).

Exposure to a real work environment through clinical attachments is necessary for trainee nurses to experience the integrated practice of complex nursing skills. Unfortunately, the availability of such clinical placements is limited; even when they are available, the nature of the student's precise learning experience depends on the clinical situations encountered—which are largely unpredictable. Simulation training can compensate for this shortage of clinical placements to some extent. It can also help standardize the learning experience of students. When combined with a clinical scenario-based role-play strategy, simulation enables healthcare educators to teach clinical skills and critical-thinking skills in an integrated manner.

IDENTIFYING LEARNING OBJECTIVES

Before identifying learning objectives, it is best to review the educational taxonomies that define these objectives (see Box 15-1). At ITE, the objectives

Box 15-1   Educational Taxonomies

Cognitive

The cognitive domain involves knowledge and the development of intellectual skills. This includes the recall or recognition of specific facts, procedural patterns and concepts that develop intellectual abilities and skills. Objectives in this category address the following areas:

- Knowledge—shows recall of data
- Comprehension—shows understanding of the meaning
- Application—shows use of a concept in a process, new situation, or unprompted use of an abstraction
- Analysis—shows ability to distinguish between facts and inferences
- Synthesis—shows ability to put parts together to form a new whole, with emphasis on creating a new meaning
- Evaluation—shows ability to make judgments about the value of ideas or materials

Affective

This domain includes the manner in which we deal with things emotionally, such as feelings, values, appreciation, etc. The five categories include (Bloom et al., 1964):

- Receiving phenomena—shows awareness
- Responding to phenomena—active participation of learners
- Valuing—ability to show the worth or value a person attaches to a particular object
- Organization—ability to organize values into priorities
- Internalizing values—shows a value system that controls behavior

Psychomotor

The psychomotor domain includes physical movement, coordination, and use of the motor-skill areas. There are seven major categories (Simpson, 1972):

- Perception—shows the ability to use sensory cues to guide motor activity
- Set—shows readiness to act
- Guided response—displays early stages in learning a complex skill that includes imitation and trial and error
- Mechanism—displays intermediate stage in learning a complex skill
- Complex overt response—displays skillful performance of motor acts that involve complex movement patterns
- Adaptation—displays skills well-developed so that they can be modified
- Origination—able to create new movement patterns to fit a particular situation or specific problem

Box 15-2   Care of Patient on Blood Transfusion

1. Define blood transfusion.
2. State the purposes/indications of blood transfusion.
3. List the different types of blood and blood products used in blood transfusion.
4. Demonstrate the skills in caring for the patient who is on blood transfusion.
5. List the signs and symptoms of various types of transfusion reactions.
6. Outline the nursing actions to be taken when blood transfusion reactions occur.

Source: Copyright © 2006, ITE Nursing Curriculum, Version 3.

that we utilize when crafting our scenario are specific instructional objectives (SIOs). These SIOs indicate the intended learning aims of the module and task performance level. Thus, by incorporating the targeted skills set into the scenario, nursing teachers are able to visualize whether the nursing student has the ability to integrate his or her care of the patient in a holistic manner. Examples of SIOs for the care of a patient receiving a blood transfusion are found in Box 15-2.

The principles of writing objectives into our scenarios have been incorporated into the desired learning outcomes for each scenario. An example of the learning outcomes that students are expected to achieve upon completion of the scenario on Dengue fever are found in Figure 15-1.

SCENARIO CRAFTING

A well-written scenario addresses the intended learning outcomes for the learner. However, it is not enough to just look at task analysis; scenario developers must also focus on the delivery of care, the strategies for decision making used, the transfer of learning that occurs, and the overall integration of skills, including communication, that takes place during the enactment of the scenario. Opportunities for enhanced learning will be created if the delivery of the scenario is explicitly detailed by the nursing faculty.

To effectively engage the learner, the scenario must allow for the student's reflection on and self-evaluation of the analytical process used; this additional step ensures that learning is truly effective and meaningful. The clinical scenario-based role-play strategy and high-fidelity patient simulators at the ITE-METI Centre for Healthcare Simulation Training showcase elements of a real-world situation that have been recreated to enable trainee nurses to learn through real work practice in a nonthreatening, safe environment. The design

Course: *NITEC* In Nursing
Module: Clinical Practice 1.1
Topic: Comfort and Body Temperature

Figure 15-1   Example of a Scenario on Dengue Fever

Learning Plan and Lesson Outcomes

Scenario File Name: Vital signs—Dengue Fever

Lesson Plan:
CP 1.1 Lesson Plan: Vital signs—Dengue Fever

Learning Ooutcomes:
At the end of this lesson, leaners should be able to:

1. Apply principles and techniques of measuring, temperature, pulse, respiration, and blood pressure.
2. Document vital signs accurately.
3. Demonstrate skill in performing tepid sponging.
4. Demonstrate skill in measuring, reporting, and recording urine output.
5. Demonstrate skill in measuring, reporting, and recording vomitus.
6. Apply principles of safety precautions.

Lesson Duration: One and a half hours

Pre-Reading for Students:
Tabbner's Nursing Care—Theory and Practice
Nursing Studies Clinical Handbook.
http://en. wikipedia.org/wiki/Dengue_fever
http://www.who.int/mediacentre/factsheets/fs117/en/
http://www.hpb.gov.sg

Overview

Synopsis:

This simulated clinical experience involves 22-year-old Indian national construction worker, Mr. Sanjay Ramasamy. He is admitted via Accident & Emergency Department (A&E) for persistent fever without running nose or cough. His temperature has been 38 to 40 degrees Celsius for the past 2 days.

He also complains of severe headache and generalized myalgia. This morning he noted red dots appearing on his body. His appetite has been poor and he vomited a small amount of blood once just before arriving in A&E.

His platelets count indicates thrombocytopenia and serology test results are positive for Dengue. He has been admitted to a medicald ward for further management.

The learners are expected to perform vital signs measurements and initiate appropriate measures to promote comfort.

Figure 15-1 Example of a Scenario on Dengue Fever (*continued*)

Equipment and Set-Up

Patient Selected: Mr. Sanjay Ramasamy

Clinical Setting: Medical Ward 48

Patient History:

This simulated clinical experience involves 22-year-old Indian national construction worker, Mr. Sanjay Ramasamy. He is admitted via A&E for persistent fever without unning nose or cough. His temperature has been 38 to 40 degrees Celsius for the past 2 days.

He also complains of severe headache and generalized myalgia. This morning he noted red dots appearing on his body. His appetite has been poor and he vomited a small amount of blood once just before arriving in A&E.

His platelets count indicates thrombocytopenia and serology test results are positive for Dengue. He has been admitted to a medical ward for further management.

Staff Nurse passes over report to students (Refer to case-sheet/charts)

Role-play requires:
1. Two Year 1 nursing students.
2. Once staff nurse.

Medical Equipment and Supplies:

Sponging trolley
Parameter trolley
Measuring jug

Stationery:

Medical and nursing case notes
TPR and hourly parameter chart
I/O chart
IMR

Simulator Setup:

Ward setting
I/V drip in progress

Petechiae—bright red dots on body
Urine bag 3/4 full
Blood stained vomitus in a kidney dish
Signages: CRIB, FP, no toothbrushing, no I/M injection

Choose patient 'Sanjay Ramasamy' and then scenario 'Dengue Fever'.
Click on the state 'Baseline'.

Figure 15-1 Example of a Scenario on Dengue Fever (continued)

Scenario States

Pre-role play pointers: **Instructor Reference (to reiterate principles)**
1. Review normal range of temperature, pulse, respiration, and blood pressure.
2. Briefly discuss signs and symptoms of dengue fever and complications of dengue hemorrhagic fever.

Simulator States/Events	Simulation Zone		Staff Nurse/Doctor Action	Learning Points
	Students (Actions)	Patient Mr Sanjay Actions		
State: Baseline BP: 130/80 mmHg HR: 95/min RR: 24/min T: 40 degrees C	Introduce self to patient. Check identity. Proceed to take parameter. Measure and record parameter. Inform Staff Nurse of abnormal vital signs. Perform tepid sponge. Stop sponging when pt shivers. Ensure 3C.	Patient to shiver during tepid sponging.	Staff nurse to voice over T 40 degrees. Noted patient's temperature of 40 degrees C. Instruct to do tepid sponge and will inform Dr.	Apply principles and techniques of measuring temperature, pulse, respiration, temperature, blood pressure, and pain. Document vital signs accurately. Demonstrate skill in performing tepid sponging. Know when to stop tepid sponge.
Simulator shiver: Mechanism activated and deactivated when appropriate.	Reassures patient, props up and offers a kidney dish. Observe, measure, record, and report vomitus. Offer a mouth gargle. Educate patient on CRIB and the risk for bleeding.	Patient to complain of nausea. "Nurse, I feel like I want to vomit ......" Patient to vomit 50 ml of blood stained content. Patient to request to put cotside down to go to toilet to brush teeth. Patient to prompt for mouth gargle if not offered.	Staff nurse to instruct student to provide mouth gargle if not done.	Demonstrate skill in measuring, reporting, and recording vomitus. Identify and apply knowledge of dengue signs and symptoms. Apply principles of safety precautions.
State: After tepid sponge BP: 120/70 mmHg HR: 68/min RR: 18/min T: 38.1 degrees C	Note nature of urinary drainage 3/4 full. Drain, measure and record urine output. Repeat temperature taking 30 minutes later.			Demonstrate skills in emptying a urinary drainage bag. Measure and record urine output.
End of Scenario				

Source: Copyright © 2008, Institute of Technical Education.

of the scenarios and their enactment help to frame learning in the context of clinical practice and promote collaborative learning and teamwork.

At ITE, faculty-contributed case studies of various patient conditions that instructors have encountered during their clinical supervision of students in the hospitals were placed into a repository. These case studies were reviewed and sorted based on the competencies that could be assessed (i.e., single versus multiple competencies, level of thinking, and decision-making skills). Feedback and input from various faculty specialty experts were then obtained, enabling scenario developers to create an accurate sequence of events that became part of the final scenario.

Learning outcomes in simulation training depend as heavily on the design characteristics of simulation training as they do on teacher and student factors (Jeffries, 2005). In the ITE simulation pedagogy model, simulation sessions involve a group of 20 students. Some students are stationed in the simulation room, where they are actively involved in "hands-on" practice on the high-fidelity patient simulators, performing assessment and managing the patient's condition. The remaining students remain in the adjoining debriefing room, where they observe the proceedings through a glass partition and on a plasma television, which broadcasts a video recording of the simulation taking place. Communication in the simulation zone is picked up by microphones and channeled into the debriefing room so that the students can review the process. They are expected to remain "minds-on" as they learn through observing the experience, critique the actions (or inactions) of the role-players, and reflect on how care might be delivered more effectively.

After the scenario is complete, all role-players return to the debriefing room. As a group, all of the students then watch a video playback, share their feelings about the event, and discuss the reasoning that led to their decisions and actions. Their "hearts-on" sharing is an integral part of the learning process and elucidates their affective responses to the scenario. As other students take their turn in role-playing the next scenario, the scenarios can be repeated with a higher level of difficulty so as to maintain an element of challenge, yet provide opportunities for the students to consolidate their earlier learning.

ITE's mission for its simulation center is to assimilate clinical reality with high-fidelity patient simulators in the classroom. Simulation training is based on experiential learning, which typically includes a planning or briefing stage, an implementation or action stage, and a debriefing stage.

The briefing stage includes activities aimed at identifying objectives for the experience, providing students with a time frame, familiarizing students with the mannequins, providing guidelines for role players and observers, explaining how the simulation will be monitored, and describing how the role is related to the theoretical concepts.

The action stage begins when the student starts the actual simulation role-play. During simulation, the facilitator may help the student progress through the activity by providing information (cues) related to the problem or complication.

Finally, the debriefing stage involves giving feedback to the role players using the video footage, thereby helping students understand the motivation for and consequences of their actions, and reflect about their experiences with the high-fidelity patient simulator. Students who were assigned to be observers are invited to give feedback to their peers related to their communication, teamwork, decision making, and clinical skills.

The students' reflective learning activities provide the structure and scaffolding for learning from experience. The added value of this technology-based training approach derives from its ability to promote a kind of reflection that results in deep learning.

Debriefing after a simulation session is seen as a key element of training with a high-fidelity patient simulator. The debriefing period must allow the student adequate time to voice any fears or concerns that may have arisen from a well-facilitated simulation (Jones, 2002). Debriefing activity reinforces positive aspects of the experience and encourages reflection, which in turn allows the participant to link theory to practice, think critically, and discuss how to intervene in very complex situations (Jeffries, 2005).

STORYBOARDING

As part of the ITE curriculum, the individual case scenarios are translated into a meaningful framework populated with states and events. The various *states* in the scenario refer to the condition of the patient at different points of time, according to the story being told in this scenario. *Events* refer to the technical input of physiological data into the simulator—for example, changing a parameter value or creating an airway complication. *Actions* are things that happen during the scenario and identify what faculty members expect learners to do and what skills they must perform. An instructor reference—another feature included in a scenario—comprises a step-by-step guide as to how the facilitator should proceed with the scenario. Prompts, questions, and teaching points are all utilized as guides for directing the students to achieve the learning objectives of the session.

Once the storyboarding is in place, the scripted scenario, which at this point is complete with the states, events, and transitions, is entered into the simulator database of scenarios. The physiological parameters are calibrated to manifest the appropriate readings as the event unfolds. As an example, a complete storyboard of the scenario on blood transfusion appears in Figure 15-2.

Course: *NITEC* In Nursing
Module: Clinical Practice 2.1
Topic: Blood Transfusion and Reaction

Figure 15-2 Example of a Scenario on Blood Transfusion

Learning Plan and Lesson Outcomes

Scenario File Name: Blood Transfusion and Reaction

Lesson Plan:
CP 2.1 Lesson Plan—Blood Transfusion and Reaction

Learning Outcomes:
By the end of this simulation training session, participants will be able to:

1. Assist the Doctor in the insertion of the intravenous cannula.
2. Prime the intravenous line.
3. Calculate the intravenous infusion rate and regulate the intravenous flow rate.
4. Demonstrate the skills in caring for the patient who is on blood transfusion.
5. Recognize the signs and symptoms of blood transfusion reactions.
6. Outline the nursing actions to be taken when blood transfusion reactions occur.

Lesson Duration: One and a half hours

Pre-Reading for Students:
Tabbner's Nursing Care—Theory and Practice
Patient Care: A Skills Handbook
http://www.sgh.com.sg/ForDoctorsnHealthcareProfessionals/EducationandTraining/PostgraduateMedicalInstitute/SGHProceedings/Haematological+Emergencies.htm

Overview

Synopsis:
Mr Alvin Bong, is an obese 56-year-old male, NRIC No S666666H. He returned from OT 32 hours ago after laparotomy and partial gastrectomy for a perforated gastric ulcer and acute peritonitis. He is in the high-dependency unit with hourly parameters monitoring, NGT passive drainage, urinary catheter, and two abdominal drains. He is on Nil By Mouth and is on intravenous Dextrose/Saline 500mls 6 hourly. He complained of pain over his abdomen and his wound was a little bit soaked. Later he complained of breathlessness, tiredness, and giddiness. His Hb was found to be low and thus blood was ordered. However, after initiating the blood therapy, patient developed mild reaction to the blood.

The learners are expected to identify signs and symptoms of a anemia and render nursing care related to the condition.

There are five states in the simulator setup:

1. Baseline
2. Deterioration
3. Improvement
4. Blood transfusion reaction
5. Post IM Promethazine

Figure 15-2 Example of a Scenario on Blood Transfusion (*continued*)

Equipment and Set-Up

Patient Selected: Mr Alvin Bong

Clinical Setting: High-Dependency Unit

Patient History:

Mr Alvin Bong, is an obese 56-year-old male, NRIC No S6666666H. He returned from OT 32 hours ago after laparotomy and partial gastrectomy for a perforated gastric ulcer and acute peritonitis. He is in the high-dependency unit with hourly parameters monitoring, NGT passive drainage, urinary catheter, and two abdominal drains. He is on NPO and is on intravenous dextrose/saline 500 ml 6 hourly. He complained of pain over the abdomen.

At 1:30 pm, 2 ITE Year 2 nursing students have just returned from lunch break when Mr Bong pressed the call bell. A student nurse went to attend to him.

Medical Equipment and Supplies:

Patient monitor with chest leads, BP cuff, and pulse oximeter

Injection trolley

Sterile gloves

Gamgee and Micropore

Oxygen face mask

Intravenous drip set with filter

Intravenous solution D/Saline 500 ml

NGT with tubing for passive drainage

Urinary catheter with urine bag

2 abdominal drains

1 unit of packed cells

Blood collection insulation box

IM Promethazine

Specimen bag

Stationery:

Medical and nursing case notes

TPR and hourly parameter charts

OT checklist

IMR

Blood card

Patient ID wrist band

Blood transfusion reaction form

Simulator Setup:

Ward setting

Simulator in operating gown

Open patient 'Mr Alvin Bong' and then Scenario 'Blood Transfusion and Reaction.'

Click on the state 'Baseline.'

Figure 15-2 Example of a Scenario on Blood Transfusion (*continued*)

Scenario States

Simulation Zone				
		Debriefing Room		
Simulator States/Events	Students (Actions)	Patient Mr Alvin Bong (Actions)	Staff Nurse / Doctor (Actions)	Learning Points
Click State 'Baseline' BP: 100/60 mmHg RR: 21 bpm HR: 120 bpm Sat: 90%	Approach patient. Obtain pain score.	"Nurse, any abdomen is painful." (5–7 pain score)		Provide psychological support, and assess for pain score.
	Inspect patient's abdominal area and note operation site. Wound dressing is slightly soaked. Inform Staff nurse.		Staff nurse to instruct student to reinforce dressing.	
	Place gamgee over the dressing site and secure with micropore.			Identify and implement appropriate wound dressing technique.
Click State 'Deterioration' BP: 80/54 mmHg PR: 127 bpm RR: 23 bpm Sat: 88%	Reassure patient. Monitor vital signs. Inform staff of the vital signs and SpO$_2$.	"I'm feeling tired and rather giddy and very breathless."	Doctor to see patient and to order face mask 35% oxygen and prepare requisites for IV cannulation KIV for Blood and blood taking: FBC, PT/PTT, U/E Cr, and GXM.	Attend to patient's psychological needs. Be familiar with requisites and procedures.

Figure 15-2 Example of a Scenario on Blood Transfusion (continued)

Scenario States

Simulation Zone		Debriefing Room		
Simulator States/Events	Students (Actions)	Patient Mr Alvin Bong (Actions)	Staff Nurse / Doctor (Actions)	Learning Points
Instructor Reference: Administer 35% oxygen through the simulator software system when ventimask is correctly applied.	Administer oxygen therapy 35%.			Administer oxygen therapy correctly.
	Assist doctor in cannulation and collection of blood for FBC, U/E/CR, and GXM.		Doctor to take the blood and to insert cannula KIV for blood transfusion. Doctor to order N/Saline slow drip to keep line patent for blood.	Ability to send blood specimens with correct forms.
	Prime IV administration set with filter with N/Saline.			Prime intravenous line using the correct solution; N/Saline 0.9%.
Instructor Reference: 30 mins later, Lab notifies patient's Hb: 7.5 g/dl. Staff nurse informs doctor and students. Doctor orders 1 unit of packed cells to be transfused prior to operation. Staff nurse informs lab.				
Instructor Reference: 20 mins later, lab calls to inform that the unit of blood is ready for collection. Instructs H.A to collect blood.				
Click State 'Improvement' BP: 95/56 mmHg PR: 122 bpm RR: 20 bpm Sat: 91% Temp: 36.5	Monitor patient's vital signs		Staff nurse to order another reading of patient's vital signs prior to preparation of patient for blood transfusion (if student misses this step).	Monitor improvement in patient's vital signs after oxygen.

Figure 15-2 Example of a Scenario on Blood Transfusion (*continued*)

Scenario States

Simulation Zone			Debriefing Room		Learning Points
Simulator States/Events	Students (Actions)	Patient Mr Alvin Bong (Actions)	Staff Nurse / Doctor (Actions)		
	Prime new IV drip set with filter for blood transfusion.				Prime intravenous line using the correct solution; N/Saline 0.9%.
	Connect intravenous solution. Maintain a slow drip.				
Instructor Reference: 15 minutes later, H.A comes back to ward with unit of blood for transfusion.					
	Student will stay with patient and continue to monitor parameters accordingly. Regulate IV blood accordingly.		Staff nurse to connect the unit of packed cells after checked by doctor and herself.		Monitor the patient every 15 minutes first hr followed by every 30 min second hour and then hourly. Know that blood must to infused in 2–3 hours.
Instructor Reference: 15 minutes later, patient presses call bell.					
Click State "Blood transfusion reaction" BP: 140/70 mmHg PR: 90 bpm RR: 21 bpm Sat: 86% Temp: 38.6 Decreased breath sounds bilaterally without wheezing Mild Stridor (bilaterally)	Examine patient and stop blood transfusion immediately and report to staff nurse.	"I feel itchy all over my body, and I have all these rashes over my body."	Staff nurse to report patient's condition to doctor, and to instruct student to prime a new IV drip set with N/Saline (if learner did not do so).		Recognize the signs and symptoms of blood transfusion reaction and perform the appropriate nursing action.

Figure 15-2   Example of a Scenario on Blood Transfusion (continued)

Scenario States

	Simulation Zone		Debriefing Room		Learning Points
Simulator States/Events	Students (Actions)	Patient Mr Alvin Bong (Actions)	Staff Nurse / Doctor (Actions)		Learning Points
	Prime new I/V drip set with N/Saline solution. Remove I/V blood set and unit of blood, and connect new I/V line.		Doctor to examine patient. Staff nurse to instruct student to obtain a urine specimen from patient and continue to monitor the patient.		
	Assist doctor to obtain blood specimens for blood transfusion reaction. Instructs patient to pass urine for a urine specimen.		Dispatch the unit of blood with blood and urine specimens to the lab.		Familiar with the procedure for post-blood transfusion reaction.
Click State 'Post IM Promethazine' BP:102/60 mmHg PR: 80 bpm RR: 18 bpm Sat: 93% Temp: 38.1 Stridor resolved	Administer the medication.		Doctor to order medication IM Promethazine administered to stop the itch. Staff nurse to inform student to collect the medication and serve after checking with her.		Five rights checked before serving medication.
	Continue monitoring of patient's condition.				
End of scenario					

Source: Copyright © 2008, Institute of Technical Education.

Upon completion of the storyboarding, the scenario is programmed into the computer system of the high-fidelity patient simulator to test the feasibility of the pathophysiological changes that were made while scripting the scenario. The testing phase is intended to ensure that the students are given sufficient time to perform the skills required to manage the changes of the state that occur in the simulator and to provide for the overall care management of the patient.

CONCLUSION

As the scenarios are enacted during simulation sessions, nursing faculty may find it necessary to review and tweak the events based on the learning objectives. This review process may necessitate a return to the storyboard to make significant changes. The scenario may need to undergo many revisions to enable the learners to meet the stipulated learning outcomes successfully each time. Ultimately, scenarios are a tool to be utilized to meet the learning objectives. It takes skill, time, and patience to script challenging, clinically sound, realistic simulated clinical scenarios. A dedicated team, supported by technical and domain experts, is necessary for the successful implementation of the scenarios.

References

Institute of Technical Education (ITE). (2006). *ITE nursing curriculum, Version 3.* Singapore: Author.

Jeffries, P.R (2005). A framework for designing, implementing and evaluating simulations used as teaching strategies in nursing. *Nursing Education Perspectives, 26*(2), 96–103.

Jones, N. (2002). The facilitation of interactive simulation. Retrieved August 20, 2008, from www.patientsimulation.co.uk/4653/7006.html

Simpson, E. J. (1972). *The classification of educational objectives in the psychomotor domain.* Washington, DC: Gryphon House.

Van Merrienboer, J. J. G., Clark, R. E., & Crook, M. B. M. (2002). Blueprints for complex learning: The 4C/ID model. *Educational Technology, Research, & Development, 50*(2), 39–64.

CHAPTER 16

Simulation in the Hospital Setting

John M. O'Donnell and Beth Kuzminsky

There are approximately 300,000 nursing students enrolled in various educational institutions at any given time in the United States. While this group of learners has captured much of the initial interest of simulation nursing educators, the larger opportunity for changing practice and transforming patient care may actually be found in the professional nursing domain. The approximately 3 million professional nurses in the United States have entered the profession through a wide variety of educational pathways and possess what has been described as an "alphabet soup" of credentials. This heterogeneity of preparation, in concert with the increased practice complexity encountered by nurses, represents both a challenge and an opportunity. The national focus on patient safety and the need for more effective training designed to promote improvement in patient outcomes have also fueled interest in simulation educational methods for healthcare practitioners at all levels.

Professional nursing educators face challenges distinct from those faced by educators in traditional undergraduate and graduate settings. Nehring (2008) emphasizes the emerging trends in undergraduate education and points out that a paradigm shift is emerging, of which integration of simulation education serves as a core component. This paradigm shift is warranted based on the need for highly competent bedside providers combined with the public demand for safer health care.

Professional nursing educators face multiple challenges including, but not limited to, an aging nursing workforce, a national nursing shortage, and competing demands for finite resources. Often they face the task of managing orientation groups made up of personnel with varying educational backgrounds and experiences. These educators are charged with the dual roles of verifying competency among the existing workforce while making up for gaps in new graduate knowledge and ability. This point is emphasized in the work of Dorothy del Bueno (2005), who developed the screen-based Performance Based Diagnostic System (PBDS) for nurse competency evaluation. Del Bueno suggests that nursing faces a crisis as a result of inadequate preparation of new nurses. She further asserts that only 35% of new nursing graduates "regardless of educational preparation and credentials" are able to effectively meet entry level expectations for employment (del Bueno, 2005).

TARGETS FOR SCENARIO OR COURSE DEVELOPMENT FOR PROFESSIONAL NURSES

Given this spectrum of issues, it is important that professional nursing educators understand the driving forces behind, and other motivators for, adoption of innovative methods such as simulation. Professional nursing educators must provide a clear rationale when they propose the use of new educational approaches. Without this justification, it may prove difficult to obtain buy-in from bottom-line-conscious Chief Nursing Officers (CNOs). Factors that support infusion of simulation methods in professional nurse training can concurrently be integrated into scenario design and include the following elements:

- The Institute of Medicine (Kohn, Corrigan, & Donaldson, 1999), Institute for Healthcare Improvement (2007), and elements of the National Patient Safety Movement
- The National Quality Forum (2008) report on 28 Never Events
- Joint Commission sentinel events and their root-cause analysis (Joint Commission, 2008b)
- Joint Commission National Patient Safety Goals (Joint Commission, 2008a)
- Structured communication methods
- Institutionally derived incident reports with patient safety recommendations
- Provider safety
- Workplace violence
- Competency evaluation

In addition to the need for a review of relevant evidence within the literature supporting simulation initiatives, nursing educators need clear and easy-to-follow directions for the development of a simulation course. This chapter highlights a variety of tools, templates, and checklists that can shorten the development process for simulation educators who are teaching professional nurses. Specifically, the following elements of scenario development are discussed:

- The development of scenario objectives
- Scenario selection and design
- The "simulation bus" analogy

- Simulator selection
- Scenario development timelines
- Use of constructions in scenario development (e.g., the nursing process, critical thinking, and task analysis and checklist creation)
- The scenario QuickView Tool
- The Development Triangle Tool
- Alpha testing and instructor preparation
- Beta testing to evaluate scenario flow and final content validation
- Making sure that the scenario is ready to use in the final development phase

DEVELOPING SCENARIOS FOR USE WITHIN A PROFESSIONAL NURSING SIMULATION COURSE

Curriculum development for professional nursing simulation courses can be challenging and time-consuming for both curriculum developers and subject matter experts (SMEs). This situation may be attributed to the fact that historically, education for nurses has not centered on creation of a curriculum in which simulation serves as the predominant means of delivery. Lack of exposure and experience in this area can make curriculum development for simulation courses a daunting task for the novice simulation educator. Thus a need exists for the development of tools or templates designed to improve the experience for educators and SMEs during the simulation course development process.

Simulation scenarios are the core elements of simulation curricula. However, scenarios alone do not provide a complete learning experience; to flesh out the curriculum, additional supportive elements are usually included. These support elements act in concert with the scenario to provide a more complete learning experience for the participant. The exact constitution and deployment of these resources require careful selection and thoughtful execution.

Development of Scenario Objectives

Specific learning objectives lay the foundation for scenario development. An objective is a clear and unambiguous description of the educational expectations for the participant. When written in behavioral terms, it includes three main components: the expected participant behavior, the conditions for the performance, and the criteria for the performance. Most objectives refer to a particular educational taxonomy such as that developed by Bloom (cognitive domain), Krathwahl (affective), Gagne (learned capability), or Harrow (psychomotor), depending on the overall goal of scenario (Dietrich, 1980;

Duan, 2006; Harton, 2007; Housel, 2002). While selecting specific scenario topics, the development team should establish an overall scenario objective as well as specific participant objectives within each scenario. These objectives will, in turn, inform development of all supplemental materials.

Objectives are typically written in the active tense and are associated with a specific taxonomy. They define both the overall curricular target and the points of assessment necessary within each scenario.

Scenario Selection and Design

Development of professional nursing simulation courses typically follow one of two pathways: (1) a problem is identified from the top down because of a need to meet accreditation or regulatory requirements or through acquisition of risk management data or (2) clinical educators or clinicians identify a training need and turn to simulation as a surrogate for the actual clinical event. In either case, the simulation course is proposed. A logical process of scenario development must then be followed that will culminate in a successful course benefiting participants, the institution, and, most importantly, patients.

Scenario selection in the professional nursing domain can be driven by a variety of factors, including orientation requirements (either generic or targeted to a specialty area), annual mandatory training requirements [annual competencies, cardiopulmonary resuscitation, Advanced Cardiac Life Support (ACLS)], safety considerations [Joint Commission standards, national patient safety goals (NPSGs), failed communication issues, patient injury reports, near misses, sentinel events], risk management data (high-priority incident reports, institution-specific mortality and morbidity data), and other data sources (best evidence, closed claims data). Regulatory, safety, and competency targets also lend themselves to scenario selection and design.

After the focus of a new simulation scenario or course has been identified, important administrative and logistical decisions must be made. These points of contention include the length of the planned session, the number of participants per session, the number of sessions over time, the need for supplemental materials, the availability of simulators, the availability of props and the availability of technology (e.g., audiovisual, software, learning management systems). Most professional nursing simulation scenarios are authored by, or developed in conjunction with, experts on the subject area to be simulated. A development process can be initiated by individuals or by teams consisting of a leader or director plus a mix of subject matter experts (SMEs), content matter experts (CMEs), or a mixture of both. Although SMEs are recognized for having a wealth of knowledge and ability in a particular clinical area covered by the simulation, they may not be experienced in writing, teaching, or technology skills. To counter such shortcomings, a mix of didactic and clinical educational skills is required on the team, as well as skill in the areas of technology application, writing, coordination of complex processes, creativity, and data analysis. Most individuals do not possess this entire spectrum of skills, making the initial team selection process important to achieving success in scenario development. In forming a team, it is helpful to populate the group with a mix of qualities and skills and then capitalize on the team members' complementary strengths.

The phenomenon of "simulator purchased but still in the box" is all too common; it represents the realization, after the initial excitement of the purchase, that a curriculum is now required in which to use the simulation. To ensure that this fate does not befall your program, make sure that the appropriate team is in place and prepared to develop scenarios for the new tool.

The "Simulation Bus" Analogy

Because simulation is a new and novel educational method, many experienced nursing educators find themselves outside of their normal comfort zone when confronted with it. When approaching novice professional nursing simulation educators, curriculum consultants at the Winter Institute for Simulation, Education and Research (WISER) have used a "simulation course bus" analogy to introduce the primary roles and goals within a development team (see Figure 16-1).With this analogy, it is important to clearly convey the role of consultants in the development process as well as the roles of any team members involved in course development. The bus analogy initially emerged as a result of confusion about the services provided by our simulation institute. The misperception by the community of interest was that employees could be placed on a "bus to WISER," be driven to the center, disembark, receive the "magic" training, and return on the bus to their facility in a new and improved state. The bus analogy is a simple depiction of actual roles and goals that was constructed in response to these requests. This tool clearly identifies the roles and skill sets needed during development and implementation of a course.

The driver's seat in the bus analogy is occupied by the person charged with overall responsibility for course development (leader or course director). This is typically a unit-based or staff-development-office-based educator or leader who may also have subject matter expertise. Seat 1 is occupied by at least one individual with subject matter expertise who can provide input on the validity of simulation and instructional material content. Seat 2 is occupied (at least in spirit) by an administrative role. Without strong administrative support, it is difficult to develop and deploy a new educational method. Seats 3 through 6 represent the skill sets necessary for overall course development

Figure 16-1   The WISER Simulation Course "Bus" Analogy

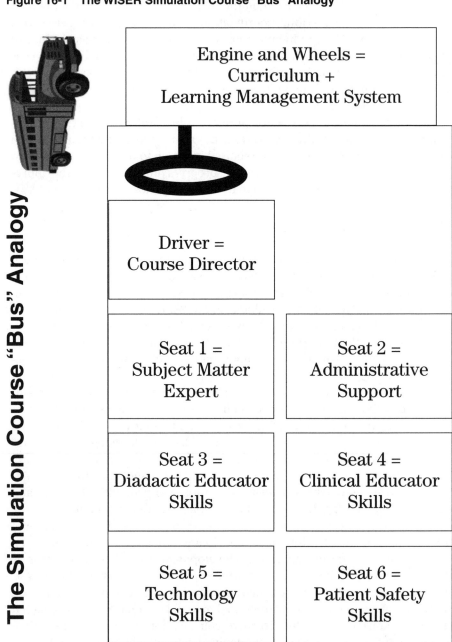

Source: Courtesy of Dr. Paul Phrampus,WISER.

and administration, which include didactic and clinical educator skills, technical skills, and experience in patient safety and human factors.

The engine of the bus is represented by the curriculum (scenarios and supplemental material) and a delivery method (learning management system). These materials often include up-front didactic content; reference materials; pre-, intra-, and post-course assessment tools; and defined simulation scenarios or skill activities. The learning management system is the part of the engine that allows for curricular delivery. It can be as simple as a course-specific binder or as sophisticated as an interactive, online learning environment.

The simulation center (WISER) or simulation consultants act in two capacities: dispatcher and mechanic. Direction is initially provided by the dispatcher role, which arises from mutual development of an overall scenario or course objective as well as specific participant objectives within the scenario. Once the bus is "in motion," the mechanic role involves consultation or intervention in the area of curricular development trajectory, assessment metrics, use of evidence, programming, logistics, fidelity, context, and selection of appropriate simulators, all of which allow the course bus to continue on its way to the intended destination.

Simulator Selection

Selecting the appropriate simulator for the learning objectives of the session is an important process. Lack of fit of the simulator to the task may result in degradation of the learning experience if the simulator interaction does not match up well with real-life experience. The degree to which simulator responses resemble real-life experience affects the ability of the participant to engage in the simulation process, suspend disbelief, and meet learning objectives. For example, most simulation mannequins are static and do not exhibit spontaneous movement or fluid joint motion. Therefore, use of a mannequin to simulate neurologic or musculoskeletal events is not yet an effective match of curriculum to simulator; even high-fidelity mannequins do not have realistic neuromuscular or neurologic findings (Alinier, Hunt, Gordon, & Harwood, 2006; Girzadas, Clay, Caris, Rzechula, & Harwood, 2007; Hravnak, Beach, & Tuite, 2007).

Scenario Development Timelines

It is important to provide individuals or teams involved in scenario or course development with a detailed timeline of activities, responsibilities, and completion targets. Many professional nurses who have taken on this role have *added* it as a responsibility, as their "real job" responsibilities may or may not include protected educational time.

Because no standard nomenclature has been established across the simulation industry as yet, it is important to agree on a "local" simulation nomenclature and to provide frequent summaries to the developers indicating milestones that have been achieved. For example, when describing center-specific nomenclature, the WISER "Expert Curriculum/Competent Facilitator" model is a good example. Development team members are typically unfamiliar with this concept. They are informed that the model consists of expert teams (SMEs and others) who are writing a curriculum for competent instructors to use during a scenario or course, which is the standard process for scenario and course development at the center (Dr. Paul Phrampus, personal communication, January 2007). This model also emphasizes the importance of using best evidence, practice standards, and standardized text sources in the development of scenarios and supplemental course materials.

Use of Constructs in Scenario Development

A variety of constructs can be used to assist simulation scenario development. A *construct* is a mental representation of a process (Merriam-Webster, 2008); it has also been termed an "operational concept." The value in using a construct lies in its ability to provide structure to the development, implementation, and evaluation processes. Three constructs will be discussed here: the nursing process, critical thinking, and task analysis.

Nursing Process

The nursing process is integrated within nursing education across the world. In the late 1950s and early 1960s, the work of nurses was described as a process and evolved from three steps to the current total of five or six discrete steps. These process steps were first outlined in the 1973 American Nurses Association (ANA) standards (Wilkinson, 2007). The nursing process is now routinely included in Nurse Practice Acts across the United States and is recognized internationally as describing the work done by a professional nurse (Wilkinson, 2007). The nursing process is taught in the U.S. nursing curriculum as well as in the curricula of many other countries, including the United Kingdom and Canada (Wilkinson, 2007). The nursing process embedded as a construct in scenario development was first reported by O'Donnell in 2003 (O'Donnell & Hoffman, 2003).

The steps in the nursing process typically include assessment, diagnosis, planning, implementation or intervention, and evaluation (summarized in the mnemonic ADPIE). With the advent of evidence-based practice, outcome identification has often been identified as a sixth step (ANA, 2004). The ADPIE structure was used to individualize simulation programming in the Laerdal SimMan operating system in a manner that would resonate with nurses, regardless of the type of educational program in which they were participating (Burns, Hoffman, & O'Donnell, 2005). Burns et al. (2005) described the use of the integrated ADPIE process combined with communication assessment (ADPIE-C) in teaching first-year undergraduate students (Burns et al, 2005). McCausland integrated the nursing process within a simulation course to create objectives for developing a heart failure simulation and in evaluation of student performance (McCausland, Curran, & Cataldi, 2004).

A significant benefit of using the nursing process as a model for scenario development is its broad acceptance as a description of nursing practice around the world.

Critical Thinking

Critical thinking is defined as a "thought process" that improves with ongoing professional nursing expertise. Improvement in critical-thinking ability is presumed to correlate with the progression of a nurse from novice through expert practice (Benner, 1982; Paul, 1993). The ability to analyze and process data and then make appropriate decisions within a specific context is an example of critical thinking. While difficult to objectively measure, critical thinking is valued by both clinicians and educators as a core attribute in expert decision making (Paul, 1993; Turner, 2005).

Because simulation education is by nature experiential, it offers an opportunity to evaluate context-specific decision making under controlled conditions. With thoughtful design, simulation scenarios can be created that present the student with realistic patient problems requiring accurate and appropriate decision making. One challenge in scenario development is to design situations that allow critical-thinking pathways to be evaluated in summative fashion.

One approach that can be used to measure progression through critical-thinking processes is the checklist. Checklists can help to evaluate participant decision making within a scenario through verification of task completion as well as in the order of task completion. Clay et al. (2007) describe the use of best practice checklists developed through simulation, which were then used in the clinical setting by critical care residents. Evaluator scores of resident performance were positively correlated with more frequent use of the checklists. Eaves and Flagg (2001) describe the use of performance checklists to maintain military ICU nurse competence in the face of decreasing clinical admissions. Gawande (2007) points out the historic resistance to use of checklists in health care but documents their remarkable effectiveness in improving care processes and enhancing patient safety.

Task Analysis and Checklist Creation

Development of accurate checklists representing best patient care practices is certainly challenging. One approach from the discipline of ergonomics that shows promise in facilitating this effort is systematic task analysis (Annett, Duncan, Stammers, & Gray, 1971; Shepherd, 1998; Stanton & Stanton, 2006). Accurate task analysis can help to evaluate the performance of individuals and processes in both simulated and real-world settings. In two studies of professional nurses, this approach was used to describe intravenous (IV) insertion and patient transfer. A 10-point best practices protocol was developed for each of these skills. This protocol was then used to evaluate IV insertion and patient transfer scenarios. In both studies, the 10-step process was used as a checklist within the scenarios to evaluate performance and provide rapid participant feedback (O'Donnell, Bradle, & Goode, 2007; O'Donnell, Goode, Odonohoe, & Choe, 2007).

SCENARIO QUICKVIEW TOOL

The Scenario QuickView Tool (see Table 16-1) supports scenario development, use, and programming (e.g., of Laerdal SimMan and SimBaby) by capturing all aspects of the simulation on a single reference page. This one-page document identifies the main scenario components and allows the instructor to rapidly prepare for the session. In addition, the tool provides a means for organizing each simulation scenario to ensure that all components are accounted for prior to starting the session. The intent is to provide a detailed, "scenario at a glance" means for organizing each component in a simulation scenario. SMEs, working in conjunction with curriculum developers, then populate this tool with the following details: scenario learning objective, specific behavioral objectives during the scenario, simulator requirements, setting/situation, patient description, event progression, key debriefing points, simulator vocal responses, and a column listing props and equipment that can be used as a checklist.

THE DEVELOPMENT TRIANGLE TOOL

The Development Triangle Tool facilitates progress mapping for the development team. This tool provides step-by-step direction on different phases of the scenario or course development process (see Figure 16-2). The development triangle displays development progression in a pictorial fashion, where each element is mapped to the framework of the course. The degree of progress in scenario development is tracked, so that all team members can

Table 16-1 Use of the *Scenario QuickView Tool* for Hemolytic Blood Transfusion Reaction Scenario. This one page snapshot represents all main scenario components allowing the instructor to rapidly prepare for the session. The props column can be used as a checklist function in environmental preparation.

Simulator	Patient Description and Event Progression	Specific Behavioral Objectives	Specific Debriefing Points	Vocal Responses	Physiologic Changes	Props Needed
		Trainee will follow the ADPIE (Assess, Diagnose, Plan, Implement/Intervene, Evaluate) steps to manage the scenario				
SimMan	**PACU Report:** Mr. Smith—57-year-old, 75 kg patient transferring to medical-surgical unit s/p hemi-colectomy. Oriented—sleeps between arousals. Operative course uncomplicated—duration 2.5 hours with use of general anesthesia. EBL = 650 ml. IV fluid replacement = 3400 ml.	**A: Assessment** Standard assessment for new surgical patient admission to medical-surgical unit **D: Diagnosis of Problem** Hemolytic Blood Transfusion Reaction **P: Plan of Care** 1. Standard post-op patient assessment	• Standard assessment post-op patient • Potential for complications from surgical procedures • Laboratory values • H & H critical values • Unexpected response to therapies	"My surgery site hurts." "My belly is upset." Post transfusion reaction:	Initial vital signs: Temp: 36.8°C HR: 116 bpm RR: 18 BP: 108/54 SpO$_2$ 94% @ 21, nasal cannula 3 mins. post start of blood transfusion: Temp: 38.1°C HR: 130 bpm RR: 24,	• 1 unit of blood with patient name and ID number • Patient ID • Allergy band • Jackson-Pratt drain • Bloody abdominal dressing • 4×4's • Surgical staples in a midline abdominal wound

351

Table 16-1 Use of the *Scenario QuickView Tool* for Hemolytic Blood Transfusion Reaction Scenario. This one page snapshot represents all main scenario components allowing the instructor to rapidly prepare for the session. The props column can be used as a checklist function in environmental preparation. *(continued)*

Simulator	Patient Description and Event Progression	Specific Behavioral Objectives	Specific Debriefing Points	Vocal Responses	Physiologic Changes	Props Needed
	IV fluids NSS @ 100 ml/hr. O_2 at 2L nasal cannula. PCA Morphine infusing at rate 1mg/hr. **Physical Exam:** Midline abdominal dressing moderately saturated-serous-sanguinous drainage. Incision intact with staples. Jackson-Pratt drain present with 75 ml of sanguinous fluid.	2. Labs review 3. Review physician orders 4. Administer blood 5. Standard assessment for patient receiving blood transfusion 6. ID patient reaction to blood product 7. Stabilize patient condition 8. SBAR communication to MD	• Standard assessment for blood transfusion candidates • Classic signs of hemolytic blood transfusion reaction • Interventions for patient experiencing hemolytic blood transfusion reaction	"I feel like I'm shaking." "I feel really hot."	BP: 88/50 SpO_2 92% @ 2 liters nasal cannula. Vital signs progressively deteriorate until blood transfusion is discontinued.	• NSS IV and drainage system • IV pump • Blood tubing/supplies for venipuncture/ blood collection tubes • Monitors and BP cuff • Pulse oximeter • Nasal cannula/ O_2 source • Stethoscope

Table 16-1 Use of the *Scenario QuickView Tool* for Hemolytic Blood Transfusion Reaction Scenario. This one page snapshot represents all main scenario components allowing the instructor to rapidly prepare for the session. The props column can be used as a checklist function in environmental preparation. *(continued)*

Simulator	Patient Description and Event Progression	Specific Behavioral Objectives	Specific Debriefing Points	Vocal Responses	Physiologic Changes	Props Needed
	PMHx: COPD, osteoarthritis, smoking × 30 pack-years, CAD, HTN. Allergy History: PCN, Ancef, Protamine. Past Surgical History: right knee arthoscopy 1979, CABG × 4 2005, EGD 2007 **Meds:** 1 baby aspirin qd, Plavix, Carafate qd, PRN Albuterol, Nitroglycerin SL	9. Provide reassurance to patient **I: Implement/ Intervene** 1. Standard post-op assessment 2. Standard blood administration steps 3. ID patient reaction to blood product 4. D/C blood transfusion	• Use of SBAR communication model • Provide patient/family centered care			• Thermometer • Medications labeled as: Tylenol suppository 325 mg • Benadryl 25 mg IV • Vancomycin 1 gm IV infusion • Morphine PCA syringe and tubing • PCA machine or pump

Table 16-1 Use of the *Scenario QuickView Tool* for Hemolytic Blood Transfusion Reaction Scenario. This one page snapshot represents all main scenario components allowing the instructor to rapidly prepare for the session. The props column can be used as a checklist function in environmental preparation. *(continued)*

Simulator	Patient Description and Event Progression	Specific Behavioral Objectives	Specific Debriefing Points	Vocal Responses	Physiologic Changes	Props Needed
	Baseline VS on admission: Temp: 36.8°C, HR: 116, RR: 18, BP: 108/54, SpO$_2$ 94% @ 2 liters nasal cannula. Pain = 4/10 **Labs and tests:** hemoglobin 9.2 gm/dl and hematocrit 27.6% Repeat values pending. Electrolytes: Na+ 145, K+-3.5, CL− 102, HCO3-20	5. Anticipate orders: Benadryl 25 mg IV, 325 mg Tylenol PR 6. Return blood to blood bank 7. Vital signs per institutional policy 8. SBAR communication to patient/family **E: Evaluate and Reassess** • Ongoing vital signs assessment				• Foley catheter and collection bag • Urine in foley bag (reddish brown tinge).

354

Table 16-1 Use of the *Scenario QuickView Tool* for Hemolytic Blood Transfusion Reaction Scenario. **This one page snapshot represents all main scenario components allowing the instructor to rapidly prepare for the session. The props column can be used as a checklist function in environmental preparation.** *(continued)*

Simulator	Patient Description and Event Progression	Specific Behavioral Objectives	Specific Debriefing Points	Vocal Responses	Physiologic Changes	Props Needed
	5 min post PACU transfer: Repeat H&H levels reviewed = hemoglobin 7.9 gm/dl and hematocrit 23.7%. Post-operative orders assessed, participant identifies need/reads physician order aloud for blood transfusion.	• Ongoing use of SBAR communication to patient , family, and physician • Emotional support to patient				

References:
1. Despotis, G. J., Zhang, L., & Lublin, D.M. (2007). Transfusion risks and transfusion-related pro-inflammatory responses, *Hematology/Oncology Clinics of North America, 21*(1), 147–161.
2. Guise, J. M., & lowe, N.K. (2006). Do you speak SBAR? *JOGNN - Journal of Obstetric, Gynecologic, & Neonatal Nursing, 35*(3), 313–314.
3. Sheppard, C. A., Logdberg, L. E., Zimring, J. C., & Hillyer, C. D. (2007). Transfusion-related acute lung injury. *Hematology/Oncology Clinics of North America, 21*(1), 163–176.
4. Spiess, B. D. (2007). Red cell transfusions and guidelines: a work in progress. *Hematology/Oncology Clinics of North America, 21*(1), 185–200.
Source: Courtesy of Dr. Paul Phrampus, WISER.

Figure 16-2   The WISER Development Triangle Tool. This tool provides progress mapping for the development team. This tool provides a pictorial representation of the scenario development process.

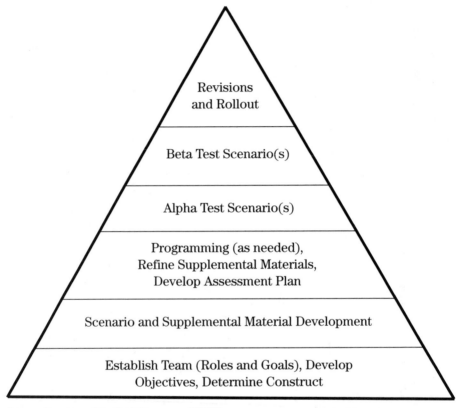

Source: Courtesy of Dr. Paul Phrampus, WISER.

readily see which tasks have been accomplished and which remain to be completed. Appendix A includes a sample scenario on hemolytic blood transfusion reaction that illustrates the development triangle.

ALPHA TESTING AND INSTRUCTOR PREPARATION

As the apex of the triangle is approached, the planning process culminates in alpha testing—that is, the first run of the scenario utilizing all supplemental materials. All didactic, simulation, and assessment elements must be tested during the alpha phase, and any feedback must be analyzed for ongoing scenario or course improvements. Typically participants who are asked to engage in the alpha-testing process are part of the development team or are experienced in the subject matter area.

Developing and adhering to a standardized evaluation process during the alpha-testing phase offers developers an opportunity to assess the need for revisions of the scenario, supports a "train the trainers" mission, and validates that the original course objectives have remained the focus. In addition to assuring the match of the original objectives to the scenario or course that was built, the SMEs who participate in the alpha-testing phase are asked to provide other feedback. These individuals are cooperatively engaged as partners in assuring that the course being evaluated and revised is valid according to current practice and is appropriate for the stated target audience. Further, they are asked to analyze and measure all course elements in light of nationally recognized protocols or best-evidence practice standards. All of this feedback is then considered by the course authors in making revisions to the scenario, but is not included in overall course participant data collection.

Many roles may need to be filled during development and running of a simulation session. The primary roles, for example, will vary from course to course and from simulation center to simulation center. Typical roles include a director (who runs the simulator and controls room events) and an instructor who interacts with participants in the room. Other roles can be added as needed depending on the scenario complexity and instructor and student availability.

Once scenarios have undergone alpha testing, those individuals who will be assigned as instructors within the final course require readiness training. Common instructor preparatory steps include the following measures:

- Take a tour of the facility/environment
- Attend a simulation course (as an observer and then as a participant)
- Complete a "Technology 101" session (audiovisual equipment, simulator hardware and software)
- Participate in a "meet the simulator session" (review of features)
- Review instructor behavioral expectations (safe learning, seriousness, professionalism, respect)
- Complete practice debriefing exercises (with expert oversight)

It is often useful for instructors to be placed in the participant role (in alpha, beta, or "live" courses) so that they can experience the scenarios from that perspective. In many professional nursing courses, instructors perform a "walk-through" of all scenarios prior to running them with participants. This offers the opportunity to practice both director and in-room instructor roles. Novice instructors are often assigned to work with more experienced instructors until they become more comfortable with the simulation process.

BETA TESTING: SCENARIO FLOW AND FINAL CONTENT VALIDATION

Beta testing is conducted after the alpha testing has been completed. The goals of the beta-testing phase are to finalize scenario flow, garner participant feedback (while explaining that the scenario is in beta—that is, a trial phase), and identify any problematic areas. Participant feedback is essential in assessing the practicality and value of the scenario and for determining whether the scenario makes sense. The beta testing can be conducted either with instructors or with a group of participants. It is often helpful to let the participants know that the course is in the beta-testing phase and to actively enlist their support in the testing process. Again, all didactic elements, scenarios, and assessments are evaluated, and the data are then analyzed for inclusion in a continuous quality improvement feedback loop.

FINAL DEVELOPMENT PHASE: IS THE SCENARIO READY FOR USE?

After the alpha and beta course evaluation data and feedback have been analyzed, final scenario revisions can be rapidly completed. Planning for fit of scenarios within an overall simulation course involves assessment of logistical and scheduling elements within a particular simulation environment as well as final verification that all components are complete and available to both participants and instructors. Regardless of the learning management system employed or the method used to deploy the simulation curricular elements, completion of key course components should be tracked. The WISER Professional Nursing Simulation Scenario Readiness Checklist (see Table 16-2) is an example of a tool designed to assist simulation scenario or course authors in their development work.

CONCLUSION

Many myths surround the process of developing scenarios and programs in simulation education. The most common misperceptions include the notions that simulation curricular material development is simple, easy, cheap (inexpensive), and efficient, and that "any educator" can jump into simulation work without any preparation and training.

Table 16-2 WISER Professional Nursing Scenario Checklist

Prior to Scenario Session

☐ Complete overall scenario and specific participant objectives
☐ Determine construct, algorithm, or best practice to be used in scenario development, use, and evaluation
☐ Verify completion of pre-scenario supplemental materials (QuickViews, quiz, survey, assessments, PowerPoint, pdfs, documents, debriefing guides)
☐ Load materials into learning management platform/create instructor manual
☐ Identify trainees and instructors
☐ Assign instructor roles and goals
☐ Verification of instructor training and readiness
☐ Identify, prepare, and package props according to simulation scenario
☐ A-V and technology checks (software and hardware including microphones, headsets, video, web)
☐ Verify completion of course preparation for both instructors and participants
☐ Describe participant behavior expectations (dress code, professionalism, etc.)
☐ Demonstrate simulator functionality to participants—conduct orientation
☐ Conduct instructor "huddle" to review specific scenario goals and describe session flow

During Scenario Session

☐ Have trainee read stem
☐ Initiate simulation with a clearly established start point
☐ Create an accurate record of the simulation (video, log file, checklist, etc.)
☐ Conduct simulation according to pre-established course flow
☐ Complete scenario after achieving clearly established endpoint

Post-Scenario Session

☐ Conduct debriefing and provide immediate feedback to participants
☐ Verify completion of post-scenario supplemental materials (quiz, survey, assessments, follow-up didactic materials)
☐ Verify that all recommendations for edits and adjustments are completed
☐ Reset simulation environment for following scenario

Source: Courtesy of Dr. Paul Phrampus, WISER.

To date, professional nursing simulation has not received the attention that undergraduate and graduate simulation has enjoyed due to a variety of factors—specifically, the sheer number of professional nurses, the competing demands for resources within healthcare institutions, and the overall shortage of nurses. These forces pull educators in many different directions. Nevertheless, several forces are also driving the use of simulation in professional nursing. The public is demanding safer health care and is no longer tolerant of conditions that permit near misses, sentinel events, or deaths due to inadequate provider preparation to occur. Further, the Joint Commission, which has more than 15,000 member facilities, is now requiring demonstration of competency-based training and establishing more rigorous standards of practice, education, and care (Joint Commission, 2008b). Professional nursing has a responsibility to acknowledge and accommodate advances in training and education that might potentially lead to safer care. In raising the bar for education and training, simulation promises to be a core element in improving and standardizing the process for provider training, competency validation, and other aspects of advanced education.

When working with novice educators to set up a simulation program, it is important to clearly establish expectations (including roles and goals) at the preliminary meeting. The value of the project for both the institution and the educator must be clearly conveyed. During the ensuing scenario development, use of tracking tools such as the Development Triangle may assist in documenting team successes and help to fuel excitement and motivation among the team members.

It is equally important to convey the timeline and the amount of effort required for scenario development. Adopting a philosophy of "under-promise and over-deliver" creates an environment supportive of success. Future developments in professional nursing simulation will be driven by demonstration of the utility and value of this approach for professional nurses. The simulation community has begun to recognize the need for developing a curriculum for the primary providers at the "point of care." The philosophy of the "right care for the right patient at the right time, every time" is congruent with the use of a training technology that allows providers to rise to this level of care delivery.

References

Alinier, G., Hunt, B., Gordon, R., & Harwood, C. (2006). Effectiveness of intermediate-fidelity simulation training technology in undergraduate nursing education. *Journal of Advanced Nursing*, *54*, 359–369.

American Nurses Association. (2004). *Nursing: Scope and standards of practice* (3rd ed.). Washington, DC: Author.

Annett, J. (1971). Acquisition of skill. *British Medical Bulletin*, *27*(3), 266–271.

Benner, P. (1982). From novice to expert: The Dreyfus Model of Skill Acquisition. *American Journal of Nursing, 82*, 402–407.

Burns, H., Hoffman, R., & O'Donnell, J. M. (2005, May). *Enhancing nursing knowledge acquisition through an innovative curricular approach using high fidelity human simulation.* Paper presented at the 23rd Quadrennial International Council of Nurses (ICN) Congress, Taipei, Taiwan.

Clay, A. S., Que, L., Petrusa, E. R., Sebastian, M., & Govert, J. (2007). Debriefing in the intensive care unit: A feedback tool to facilitate bedside teaching. *Critical Care Medicine, 35*, 738–754.

del Bueno, D. (2005). A crisis in critical thinking. *Nursing Education Perspectives, 26*, 278–282.

Dietrich, M. C. (1980). The affective domain in medical technology education. *American Journal of Medical Technology, 46*, 576–580.

Duan, Y. (2006). Selecting and applying taxonomies for learning outcomes: A nursing example. *International Journal of Nursing Education Scholarship, 3*, Article 10.

Eaves, R. H., & Flagg, A. J. (2001). The U.S. Air Force pilot simulated medical unit: A teaching strategy with multiple applications. *Journal of Nursing Education, 40*, 110–115.

Gawande, A. (2007). The checklist: If something so simple can transform intensive care, what else can it do? *New Yorker, 83*(39), 86–101.

Girzadas, D. V., Jr., Clay, L., Caris, J., Rzechula, K., & Harwood, R. (2007). High fidelity simulation can discriminate between novice and experienced residents when assessing competency in patient care. *Medical Teacher, 29*, 472–476.

Harton, B. B. (2007). Clinical staff development: planning and teaching for desired outcomes. *Journal for Nurses in Staff Development, 23*, 260–268; quiz 269–270.

Housel, N. (2002). *The effect of clinical instructor credentialing on the clinical performance outcomes of physical therapist students.* Doctoral dissertation, University of Central Florida, pp. 1–256.

Hravnak, M., Beach, M., & Tuite, P. (2007). Simulator technology as a tool for education in cardiac care. *Journal of Cardiovascular Nursing, 22*(1), 16–24.

Institute for Healthcare Improvement. (2007). *Reaping the harvest: A review of the 5 Million Lives Campaign's first year and a preview of what's to come.* Cambridge, MA. Retrieved July 7, 2008, from http://www.ihi.org/ihi

Joint Commission. (2008a). 2009 national patient safety goals. Retrieved July 7, 2008, from http://www.jcaho.org

Joint Commission. (2008b). Sentinel event: Reporting of medical/health care errors. Retrieved July 7, 2008, from http://www.jcaho.org

Kohn, L. T., Corrigan, J. M., & Donaldson, M. S. (1999). *To err is human: Building a safer health system.* Washington, DC: National Academy Press.

McCausland, L. L., Curran, C. C., & Cataldi, P. (2004). Use of a human simulator for undergraduate nurse education. *International Journal of Nursing Education Scholarship, 1*(1), 1–17.

Merriam-Webster (Ed.). (2008). International unabridged on-line dictionary. Springfield, MA. Retrieved July 20, 2008, from http://unabridged.merriam-webster.com

Nehring, W. M. (2008). U.S. boards of nursing and the use of high-fidelity patient simulators in nursing education. *Journal of Professional Nursing, 24*, 109–117.

National Quality Forum. (2008). Serious reportable events in healthcare: 2005–2006 update. Retrieved July 3, 2008, from http://www.qualityforum.org

O'Donnell, J., Bradle, J., & Goode, J. (2007). Development of a simulation and Internet based pilot intervention to evaluate adherence to a patient transfer protocol in the real world environment. *Simulation in Healthcare: The Journal of the Society for Simulation in Healthcare, 1*(1), 62.

O'Donnell, J., Goode, J. A., Odonohoe, O., & Choe, M. (2007). The impact of intravenous catheter insertion training modalities on clinical intravenous catheter insertion performance in graduate nursing students. *Simulation in Healthcare: The Journal of the Society for Simulation in Healthcare, 1*(1), 114.

O'Donnell, J. M., & Hoffman, R. (2003). *Enhancing professional competence through high fidelity human simulation.* Paper presented at the University of Pittsburgh Innovations in Education Teaching Excellence Fair, Pittsburgh, PA, January 2004.

Paul, R. W. (Ed.). (1993). *Critical thinking.* Santa Rosa, CA: Foundation for Critical Thinking.

Shepherd, A. (1998). HTA as a framework for task analysis. *Ergonomics, 41,* 1537–1552.

Stanton, N. A., & Stanton, N. A. (2006). Hierarchical task analysis: Developments, applications, and extensions. *Applied Ergonomics, 37*(1), 55–79.

Turner, P. (2005). Critical thinking in nursing education and practice as defined in the literature. *Nursing Education Perspectives, 26,* 272–277.

Wilkinson, J. M. (2007). *Nursing process and critical thinking* (4th ed.). Upper Saddle River, NJ: Pearson/Prentice Hall.

Simulation Scenario: Hemolytic Blood Transfusion Reaction in The Acute Care Hospital Setting

STUDENT LEVEL: ENTRY LEVEL PROFESSIONAL NURSE (ORIENTATION) TO EXPERIENCED RN (COMPETENCY)

OBJECTIVES

Following completion of this simulation session participants will:

1. Demonstrate the process for post-operative admission and evaluation of a patient on the medical–surgical unit.
2. Differentiate between type and cross and type and screen with respect to blood administration.
3. Identify the most common ABO blood groupings and surface antigens.
4. Follow the correct protocol for initiating a blood transfusion.
5. List the classic signs of a blood transfusion reaction.
6. Demonstrate an understanding of the most common causes for a blood transfusion reaction.
7. Demonstrate the ability to effectively communicate an emerging transfusion reaction using the SBAR communication process.
8. Explain the pathophysiology of transfusion-related immune suppression and transfusion-related lung injury.

Scenario Outline or Stem

Mr. Smith is a 57-year-old, 75 kg patient admitted to a medical–surgical unit s/p hemi-colectomy. He is oriented but sleeps between arousals. He has a midline abdominal dressing which is moderately saturated with a serous-sanguinous drainage. The incision is intact with staples in place. A Jackson-Pratt drain is in place and contains approximately 75 ml of sanguinous liquid. Past medical history is significant for chronic obstructive pulmonary disease, osteoarthritis, smoking 1 pack per day for 30 years, coronary artery disease, and hypertension. Allergy history includes penicillin, Ancef, and Protamine. Past surgical history includes right knee arthroscopy in 1979, coronary artery bypass grafting × 4 in 2005 and esophagoscopy last year. Meds include

1 baby aspirin every day, Plavix, Carafate, and as-needed Albuterol and Nitroglycerin. The operative course was uncomplicated with operative duration of 2 $\frac{1}{2}$ hours under general anesthesia. Blood loss was 650 ml and perioperative intravenous fluid replacement totaled 3400 ml of crystalloid solution. He has an intravenous of NSS running at 100 ml/hr in his right forearm. He has oxygen 2 liters by nasal cannula. A morphine patient controlled analgesia (PCA) pump is in place with a baseline infusion rate of 1 mg/hr. He received a total of 12 mg of morphine in the recovery room. He has a Foley catheter in place which contains 30 ml of amber, concentrated-appearing urine. Labs were obtained in the recovery room: hemoglobin of 9.2 gm/dl and hematocrit of 27.6%. Repeat values are pending. Electrolytes include Na+ 145, K+ − 3.5, Cl− 102, HCO3− 20. Admission vitals include heart rate: 116, blood pressure: 108/54. RR: 18, oxygen saturation: 94% on 2 liters nasal cannula. Temp: 36.8 degrees Celsius. Pain rating is 4/10.

Post-Operative Orders

- Intravenous of normal saline solution at 100 ml/hr
- Portable anterior to posterior chest x-ray
- Labs: Repeat hemoglobin and hematocrit (H/H), platelets, and international normalized ratio (INR)
- Patient controlled analgesia (PCA) orders: morphine PCA 1 mg/hr infusion. 1 mg morphine dose, 5 mg in 30 minutes, 5 minute lockout
- Vancomycin 1 g intravenous every 12 hours (last dose 4 hours ago)
- Transfuse with 1 unit of packed red blood cells if repeat H/H less than 8.5/25.5

Instructor Notes/Scenario Flow

Patient will complain of ongoing but moderate abdominal pain. Abdomen will be tender to palpation with absent bowel sounds. Heart rate will gradually increase before transfusion to 120 bpm. Respiratory rate increases to 20 bpm. After the participant completes their admission evaluation of the patient, the repeat hemoglobin and hematocrit values will be offered: 7.9 and 23.7. When blood is called for, participant will be informed that the type and cross has expired and a repeat sample must be sent. Participant must call an urgent report using the situation, background, assessment, recommendation (SBAR) structure to the physician to report status and will hang the unit of blood as ordered following facility protocol. After the transfusion is started, the patient will complain of chills/rigors and become febrile to 38.1 Celsius. Heart rate will increase to 130 bpm. Respiratory rate will increase to 24. Oxygen saturation and blood pressure will fall to 92% and 88/50 respectively. Vital signs will continue to deteriorate until transfusion is halted. Participants will be expected to make a follow-up call notifying physician of situation and requesting that physician come to evaluate the patient STAT and requesting interim orders. Improvement in patient condition will be seen with cessation of the blood, administration of oxygen at 4 liters nasal cannula, administration of Benadryl 25 mg intravenous and 325 mg Tylenol per rectum. Blood must be packaged appropriately and returned to blood bank for analysis.

Reading for the Participants

1. Despotis, G. J., Zhang, L., & Lublin, D. M. (2007). Transfusion risks and transfusion-related pro-inflammatory responses. *Hematology/Oncology Clinics of North America, 21*(1), 147–161.
2. Guise, J. M., & Lowe, N. K. (2006). Do you speak SBAR? *JOGNN - Journal of Obstetric, Gynecologic, & Neonatal Nursing, 35*(3), 313–314.
3. Sheppard, C. A., Logdberg, L. E., Zimring, J. C., & Hillyer, C. D. (2007). Transfusion-related acute lung injury. *Hematology/Oncology Clinics of North America, 21*(1), 163–176.
4. Spiess, B. D. (2007). Red cell transfusions and guidelines: a work in progress. *Hematology/Oncology Clinics of North America, 21*(1), 185–200.

Study Questions

1. What are the appropriate steps to take in the admission of a patient to a medical–surgical unit?
2. What are the differences between a type and cross and a type and screen assay?
3. How soon will you be able to give a unit of blood after a type and cross has been sent in your facility?
4. What are the most common blood types?
5. What do we mean by the term universal donor blood type?
6. When would you give uncrossed (no cross match) blood to a patient?
7. What signs and symptoms would indicate that a patient is a candidate for blood transfusion?
8. What hemoglobin and hematocrit values are normal and at what value would you call the physician STAT?

9. What are the steps for administering a unit of blood (in the correct order)?
10. What are three classic signs of a hemolytic blood transfusion reaction?
11. List and prioritize your top three immediate interventions if you suspect a hemolytic blood transfusion reaction is occurring.
12. What are the three most common reasons for a patient to have a hemolytic blood transfusion reaction?
13. How would you prepare a STAT report of hemolytic blood transfusion reaction using the Situation, Background, Assessment, Recommendation (SBAR) communication model?
14. What is the pathophysiology of transfusion related immune suppression?
15. What is the pathophysiology of transfusion related lung injury?
16. Describe the Situation, Background, Assessment, Recommendation (SBAR) communication model?
17. Why is structured communication important to patient safety?

Equipment, Supplies, and Props

- 1 unit of blood with patient name and identification number
- Patient identification band
- Allergy band
- Jackson-Pratt drain
- Abdominal dressing with bleeding
- 4×4's
- Surgical staples in a midline abdominal wound
- NSS intravenous and drainage system
- Intravenous pump
- Blood tubing/supplies for venipuncture/blood collection tubes
- Monitors and blood pressure cuff
- Pulse oximeter
- Nasal cannula and oxygen source
- Stethoscope
- Thermometer
- Sample medications labeled as: Tylenol suppository, intravenous or intramuscular Benadryl, Vancomycin intravenous drip, morphine for patient controlled analgesia
- Patient controlled analgesia machine or pump
- Foley catheter and collection bag

Programming Construct within SimMan Software System: ADPIE

- Assessment **upon arrival to medical–surgical unit:**
  - Standardized admission steps for admitting new patient to medical–surgical unit
  - Reviewed initial lab values of hemoglobin 9.2 gm/dl and a hematocrit of 27.6%
  - Vital signs taken
  - Pain assessment complete—4/10

- Assessment **5 minutes post-medical–surgical unit arrival:**
  - Identified abdominal dressing—moderately saturated
  - Pulse rate of 120; respiratory rate of 20
  - Bowel sounds assessed but absent
  - Pain assessment—tender abdomen
  - Repeat hemoglobin and hematocrit levels reviewed = 7.9 gm/dl and 23.7%
  - Post-operative order assessment—identifies need and reads physician order aloud for blood transfusion
  - Pre-blood transfusion assessment complete: intravenous site—correct catheter gauge in place/patent site; blood transfusion equipment; correct patient/correct blood type/expiration date—all assessed with verification of another RN

- Assessment **5 minutes post-administration of blood transfusion:**
  - Vital signs taken: 38.1 Celsius, heart rate 130, respiratory rate of 24, BP 88/50
  - Chills identified

- Diagnosis:
  - Blood transfusion reaction
  - Allergic reaction
  - Patient decompensation or deterioration

- Plan:
  - Stabilize patient condition
  - Urgent communication to physician using structured (SBAR) model
  - Provide reassurance to patient

- Interventions:
  - Discontinues blood transfusion
  - Initiates oxygen therapy
  - Administration of Benadryl 25 mg intravenous or intramuscular and 325 mg Tylenol per rectum
  - Blood packaged appropriately and returned to blood bank
  - Have situation and literacy-appropriate conversation in reassuring the patient

- Evaluation:
  - Ongoing vital signs monitoring
  - Review of systems appropriate to a medical–surgical unit
  - Follow-up patient interviews
  - Ongoing pain evaluation
  - SBAR to physician/patient/family in updating condition

Category/Topics Covered in the Scenario for the NCLEX-RN Blueprint

- Nursing Process: Integrated throughout the NCLEX-RN Blueprint
- Communication: Integrated throughout the NCLEX-RN Blueprint
- Reassurance: Element of Caring, which is integrated throughout the NCLEX-RN Blueprint
- Safe and Effective Care Environment
  - Establishing Priorities
  - Informed Consent
  - Collaboration with Interdisciplinary Team
  - Performance Improvement (Quality Improvement)
  - Consultation
  - Resource Management
  - Error Prevention
  - Standard/Transmission-Based/Other Precautions

- Physiological Integrity
  - Adverse Effects/Contraindications
  - Parenteral/Intravenous Therapies
  - Blood and Blood Products
  - Pharmacological Agents/Actions
  - Dosage Calculation
  - Pharmacological Pain Management
  - Expected Effects/Outcomes
  - Medication Administration
  - Laboratory Values
  - Potential for Complications from Surgical Procedures and Health Alterations
  - Vital Signs
  - Pathophysiology
  - Hemodynamics
  - Unexpected Response to Therapies

CHAPTER 17

Facilitated Debriefing

Judy Johnson-Russell and Catherine Bailey

"I didn't think he would respond by going into anaphylaxis."

"I should have studied on allergic reactions to antibiotics more."

"We didn't work as a team."

"Why did his respirations slow down when we gave the IV morphine too fast?"

These insightful comments were made by students in a facilitated debriefing. It is common to hear and read that debriefing is one of the most important aspects of simulation learning experience (Henneman, Cunningham, Roche, & Cumin, 2007). Although debriefing comes at the end of a simulated clinical experience, it is during this time when the learners begin to process the events of the simulation, and the real learning occurs. Although it may be conducted in a variety of ways, using a variety of techniques, a poor debriefing not only fails to assist students in the learning process, but may actually cause them psychological harm (Rall, Manser, & Howard, 2000). For these reasons, it is imperative that faculty seriously think about the goals and techniques they will use in a debriefing session and conduct it in a safe and productive manner.

Debriefing follows simulation whether a faculty member facilitates it or not. Students inevitably talk with peers about the simulation or reflect on the events themselves. With this kind of informal debriefing, however, the lessons learned may be incorrect and students' thoughts and verbalizations may be disorganized. The facilitated debriefing, by comparison, assists students to review specific objectives of the simulation, enhances learning through expression of feelings and thoughts, and fosters critical thinking and problem solving in a nonjudgmental and organized manner.

This chapter begins with a discussion of the historical origins of debriefing. This section is followed by a discussion of the importance of debriefing and an exploration of the process of debriefing. It concludes by summarizing best practices related to debriefing.

HISTORICAL ORIGINS OF DEBRIEFING

Debriefing, as a formal mechanism, began in the military. Following missions or during exercises, soldiers reconvened to analyze what had occurred and to develop new strategies for future missions. In more recent times, hostages and prisoners of war have been debriefed to learn more about their experience (Walker, 1990). Polit and Beck (2008) have recommended that debriefing should follow data collection if deception was used to explain the purpose of a research study or if participation in a study was stressful. Debriefing is also reported in the literature as it applies to the educational setting (Revell, 2008). After an experiential activity, the participants are brought together to discuss and process the activity. The debriefing session assists the participants in reflecting on their activity with the hope that they will be able to process the activity effectively. Today debriefing is also a recognized part of the simulation experience (Kardong-Edgren, Starkweather, & Ward, 2008).

IMPORTANCE OF DEBRIEFING

The students involved in simulation are usually adult learners. As learners with life experiences preparing for a profession, students expect to utilize what they already know and to be challenged with realistic situations that will allow them to add to their knowledge base so they may provide better care for patients. They typically benefit from learning experiences, like simulation, where they can apply what they know and are challenged by events presented during the scenario.

During a simulation, students participate with hands-on interventions in an often fast-paced simulated clinical experience. During the scenario there is rarely time to reflect on the events, to conceptualize, or to reconstruct one's cognitive frameworks (Waldner & Olson, 2007). Facilitated debriefing provides the time and the impetus for reflecting on what the students were feeling, what they were thinking, what they did, what occurred as a result, and how they can apply this new information to their care. Participating in the simulation provides the hands-on learning, but the facilitated debriefing is where the cognitive processes that lead to long-term learning and application occur. It is also where students discover the meaning of the events, the relationship between their interventions and the outcomes, and potential applications for future patient care.

Best Practices

There remain many questions about the most effective way to facilitate a debriefing (Fanning & Gaba, 2007). The literature seems consistent in agreeing that some elements are clearly important. Best practices include a quiet atmosphere away from the simulator bed where learners can sit, contemplate, and share the recent events. The ability to watch significant parts of the simulation on video playback is also helpful for self-assessment and understanding what *actually* occurred, as opposed to what the learners *thought* happened (Fanning & Gaba, 2007). It is important that learners feel that the debriefing environment is a safe place to discuss their thoughts and feelings about mistakes without criticism or ridicule from faculty or peers and to express fears that their performance, or lack of it, will affect the rest of their careers. Debriefing must be felt to be a time of shared learning and discovery, rather than a time of evaluation. Therefore ensuring safety and encouragement during the process is a major issue.

Goals of Effective Debriefing

A number of models and goals for debriefing have been reported in the literature (Dieckmann, Reddersen, Zieger, & Rall, 2008; Fritzsche, Leonard, Boscia, & Anderson, 2004; Haskvitz & Koop, 2004; Jefferies, 2005; Lederman, 1991; Mort & Donahue, 2004; Petranek, 1994; Thatcher & Robinson, 1985). Most focus on describing and analyzing the events that occurred, and assisting the student to transfer the learned information to their practice. The more commonly identified goals of debriefing are to recognize and release emotions, to reinforce simulation objectives, to enhance critical-thinking and problem-solving skills, to foster reflective learning, and to link events in the simulation to the real world. Each goal will be discussed in detail here.

Recognizing and Releasing Emotions

Participating in simulation produces a wide variety of emotions, which are commonly viewed as consisting of a post-simulation energy, excitement, or perhaps anxiety experienced immediately following the simulation. Thus it is important to allow the learners to express these feelings prior to beginning the more cognitive discussions. Assisting the learners to decompress, to remove themselves from the role they played in the simulation (Stafford, 2005), and to express their feelings and thoughts is, therefore, necessary at the beginning of the debriefing. Their comments (i.e., some related to the actual events of the simulation and others that pertain to their own actions) may be addressed again later as students begin to describe and analyze the simulated clinical experience (SCE).

Reinforcing Simulation Objectives

A major goal of debriefing is to reinforce the objectives of the SCE to ensure that the intended learning occurred. In well-written scenarios, the objectives are clearly spelled out. Usually these points are given to the learners ahead of time. Faculty may also remind the learners of the objectives at the beginning of the session or as they discuss events that occurred as a result of the defined objectives. Questions can be asked that will encourage the learners to think about and discuss how they met specific objectives. Asking them to focus on a particular objective will enhance their learning related to it.

Clarifying Information

As the learners discuss the SCE, questions usually arise about events that occurred during the experience. Learners can then share their perceptions of these events and answer one another's questions. Faculty members function as facilitators during the debriefing, just as they do during the simulation. Therefore, to allow the learners to discover the answers to their own questions, references and resources should be available in the debriefing room, just as they are in the simulation suite.

Questions posed by the faculty should lead to students' own discovery of the answers, rather than faculty's explicit provision of the answers. For beginning students, it may be more appropriate to provide more information and prompts to assist them in this discovery process. Learners may also have missed some of the events of the scenario while performing their personal role (such as preparing to give a medication) and, therefore, remain unaware of the whole picture (Peters & Vissers, 2004). Clarifying those missing links may be necessary for the learner to understand the whole experience. Learners tend to remain focused on the description of events and may need encouragement to analyze the cause of the events. A deeper understanding and an increase in knowledge will occur when they move beyond the description phase into analysis and application.

It is often difficult to determine the appropriate approach when learners have settled on incorrect information. Providing them with alternative actions or content information may be necessary when they are unable or unwilling to identify appropriate behaviors and actions. Thus learners may need to be directed to look up the answers using the resources in the room.

Enhancing Critical Thinking and Problem Solving

One of the major differences between clinical teaching and simulation is that simulation provides time to stop and allow the learners to consider the meanings of findings, to think critically about the situation, and to consider alternative actions. Afterward, debriefing sessions are an excellent means to identify what the learners were thinking when they performed specific tasks. Recognizing the motivations behind their actions allows the learners to rethink the situation, to analyze it and their own actions, and to develop alternative interventions. This self-evaluation or reflection encourages active participation, which is necessary for learning to occur. It may also bring out emotions and the students' own understanding of the parts they played in the outcomes of the simulation.

If a student was assigned the role of documenter during the simulation and a portable whiteboard or flipchart was used to record new data, using that information during debriefing can aid the learners in examining specific details. For example, they might take a closer look at the lab data that were received during the simulation and correlate these results with physical findings and the healthcare provider's orders. This analysis might then lead them to determine another meaning to the event and result in students' prioritizing and planning care differently for the next time.

A review of the videotape that isolates a specific event could also lead the learners into a discussion of the causes for an unexpected outcome. As they analyze and problem-solve the causes, they may also decide on a different plan of care and alternative interventions.

During the debriefing, all learners should be encouraged to express their own perspective on the various events. Because each learner has a unique frame of reference and background, students' perceptions are important to the discussion. By sharing this information, they learn from and about one another. They can then discuss and arrive at conclusions that may entail different or perhaps more effective interventions.

Fostering Reflective Learning

Reflective thinking is thought by some to be at the heart of clinical judgment. The amount and quality of the learner's reflective thinking are directly related to improved patient care outcomes (Pesut & Herman, 1999). As a matter of fact, learners who question what they could do differently in the future tend to be better practitioners. The reflective thought process, as encouraged during debriefing, might focus not only on the pathophysiology of the condition, the interventions applied, and the outcomes of those interventions, but also on students' performance as both individuals and team members.

Facilitative questions about students' individual performance and their work as a part of the team are important to ask if the information is not volunteered. When learners mention their own deficiencies, asking how those shortcomings could be resolved is helpful for the students and encourages them to take responsibility for correcting their stated limitations.

Questions about how students communicated and how they provided or sought assistance from other team members can provoke additional reflective thinking opportunities. As responding to patients' and family members' questions is often difficult for new learners, the act of role-playing more effective communication during the debriefing may be beneficial. Encouraging the person who played a family role in the simulation to describe his or her reactions and feelings to the learners' responses—or lack thereof—may also be helpful.

Linking Events to the Real World

Adult learners need to know that the information they are being provided and are expected to learn has true relevance in the real world. They want to be able to add new information to the knowledge and experience they already have and to apply it to the endeavors in which they are currently engaged. If significant information does not seem relevant, then the faculty can ask appropriate questions, such as "Could this ever happen to a patient with ventricular tachycardia?", that will allow the learners to make connections to the clinical area and to similar patients.

Faculty sometimes forget that learners cannot envision the many applications to patient situations that a simulation has presented. Spending time in discussing how the lessons learned in the SCE can be generalized to patient care and patients with a variety of conditions/problems is, therefore, extremely important. Extending their new knowledge into broader concepts may assist the learners in applying it to their everyday practice. For instance, the new experience of seeing the results of a kinked chest tube may lead to a discussion of assessing for obstructions in tubes in other types of patients. When working with less experienced learners, it may be appropriate for the faculty to give accounts of similar patients or events from their own practice.

Faculty may also need to acknowledge the unreality of the simulator and the circumstances surrounding the SCE to enable the learners to suspend their disbelief and move to generalization. Of particular concern to some learners is the artificial nature of the mannequin (Henneman & Cunningham, 2005).

Considerations in Debriefing

Location

Although it may be appropriate to debrief students at the bedside when a specific procedure, piece of equipment, or other skill needs to be correctly demonstrated, effective debriefings are more likely to occur when the learners are seated away from the distraction of the simulator and the environment. A demonstration at the bedside, if necessary, may be followed by a sitdown discussion in another area. Concentration and communications are enhanced if the learners and faculty are positioned in a circle with video playback and other resources available. When a circle configuration is used, the faculty member becomes a peer and a facilitator rather than an evaluator or instructor. The setting should be both quiet and private. Most learners will not feel like sharing if, for example, they are in one corner of a lab within hearing distance of other students.

Resources that should be available in the debriefing room include hospital procedures/guidelines, standards of practice, drug books, PDAs, textbooks, and the documentation of the events during the simulated clinical experience as recorded on a whiteboard, smartboard, flipchart, or patient's chart. Any of these materials may be referenced or revisited at opportune times during the debriefing.

Time

Debriefing should occur as soon as possible after the simulation so that information and the feelings associated with it will not be lost. Although debriefing is recognized as very important to simulation, often faculty do not schedule enough time for students to fully process information. The amount of time allotted for this exercise should be commensurate with the objectives, level of the learners, number of learners, and complexity of the SCE. Learners at the beginning of their programs may need longer debriefings to understand and accomplish the objectives of the SCE, whereas those students who are nearing completion of their programs may need longer to process the complex patients and their care. Simulated clinical experiences that deal with death and dying or other emotional issues will also require additional time for debriefing.

It will take much less time to debrief five students than to debrief ten students, or an entire class of student observers. No less than 30 minutes should be scheduled for the debriefings, and often one hour is preferable. Some educators suggest that the debriefing should be two to four times as long as the simulation. While that allocation of time is realistic for a short SCE, it may not be for simulations lasting for more than an hour. Contingency plans should always be made for debriefings that go longer than planned. If topics are being addressed that students are actively engaged in discussing, then it may be advantageous to allow the debriefing to continue past the original time scheduled. If more than one SCE is run during the day with the same learners, the debriefing should occur after each SCE.

Faculty in the Debriefing

It is always preferable to have the faculty members who were present in the simulation lead the debriefing. Otherwise, the specifics of the simulation or concrete events cannot be addressed and the individual needs of the students may remain unmet. The presence of two faculty members during simulation and debriefings always adds to the richness of the experience. Their observations and perceptions of the events may be different and can contribute significantly to the discussions. If more than one facilitator participates in the debriefing, they will need to come to some agreement prior to the simulation on the amount of time they will spend on various parts of the debriefing, the major content to cover, questions to ask, the methods they will use, and their individual roles in the process. If these issues are not decided prior to the debriefing, then students may become confused by the lack of continuity.

Learners in the Debriefing

All of the learners who participated directly in the simulation should be debriefed together (i.e., primary roles and participant observer roles). Some SCEs provide minimal expected behaviors for each state. Students may be given these expectations and observe for them during the simulation. During the debriefing, they can then report on behaviors that they observed or that were omitted. This peer feedback, if given appropriately, can be very beneficial to the primary participants.

If additional classroom learners have observed the simulation, then they may be debriefed separately or with those who were providing care, or if time permits, a combination of both. Techniques such as debriefing the groups independently and then bringing them together for a dialog about their observations, if carefully supervised, can provide valuable insights for a large number of learners.

If the primary participants are debriefed only with the larger viewing audience, then they may fear criticism and hesitate to express their true feelings and thoughts in front of the larger group. It is also imperative for instructors to ensure the safety of the primary participants, as the audience may tend to be critical of their performance. At the same time, feedback from the audience may be beneficial for the primary participants, if it is given in a helpful manner. Rules of conduct may be discussed prior to the debriefing and role-playing employed to demonstrate how to offer constructive criticism to peers.

Observation forms given to the audience prior to the simulation may direct their attention to specifics of the SCE, which can later be discussed in the debriefing. These forms tend to be more general and contain space for learners to make notes about requested observations. The forms may also contain questions about observers' own level of knowledge and the preparation that would be needed prior to their caring for a similar patient.

Larger viewing groups are sometimes divided into smaller groups and given specific questions to answer related to their observations or the content of the scenario. After a period of discussion, a spokesperson for each group can report on the questions they answered to the larger group.

Types of Debriefing

The most common form of debriefing, and the one thought to be most effective, is the verbal debriefing following immediately after the simulation. A written debriefing sometime follows the verbal debriefing. The written debriefing, where learners answer specific questions, is thought to be especially beneficial for learners for whom English is a second language. The added time to process thoughts and express them in a written form enhances learning for many. Questions such as "List five things you learned during the simulation" also assist the learner in evaluating the experience. The written debriefing often assists learners in answering questions on a more personal basis. Petranek (2000) developed a worksheet that specifically addressed key concepts of the simulation; students then wrote about their learning in relation to these concepts. Further learning occurred when the faculty members returned the students' papers with additional comments.

In another form of verbal debriefing, learners are given specific topics or events to report on following the simulation. They may or may not be told about these issues prior to the SCE, but the report is to include observations from the SCE just viewed.

Flight crews and medical teams have used the plus/delta method in their debriefing sessions. With this approach, various behaviors that occurred during simulation are listed in two columns. The plus column identifies those behaviors that were done well; the delta (the Greek word for change) column lists behaviors or actions participants would like to improve on and identifies how they would change them (Fanning & Gaba, 2007).

Written debriefing is popular with some faculty. Again, specific questions that address the SCE objectives may be given to the students to answer. Although the answers are sometimes turned in to faculty, who then respond to them, other instructors prefer to have the questions answered on an Internet-based bulletin (discussion) board. With the latter approach, other learners can view all the answers and provide additional comments.

Journaling is another form of written debriefing. This activity tends to promote more intense self-assessment and may show learning over time. Review of students' journals also provides a more private or personal exchange with the faculty.

Faculty Role in Debriefing

The role of the faculty member in debriefing is as a facilitator or catalyst who asks questions, stimulates thinking, and leads learners to a deeper, more thorough analysis. How much involvement the facilitator has during the debriefing depends on the initiative taken by the learners. Adult learners like to be responsible for their own learning and may independently discuss the key elements of the simulation. However, some groups may show little initiative and, therefore, may need more faculty involvement. A word of caution is in order in such cases: Faculty all too often revert to being lecturers in debriefing.

Assisting the learners to become actively involved in their own learning is crucial to their understanding and retention of new information. If appropriate resources are available, learners may also answer questions by accessing the resources rather than simply being given the answer by the facilitator. In addition to answering unresolved questions, assuming such an active role assists students in learning how to use resources appropriately when they are working in the clinical area.

The general rule for faculty is not to facilitate more than absolutely necessary and to allow the learners the opportunity to lead the discussions as long it is relevant and meeting the objectives. Providing learners with a thorough "introduction" to debriefing (see the discussion of the process of verbal debriefing later in this chapter) will also assist in their understanding of the expectations for them to be active participants in the discussions.

EFFECTIVE DEBRIEFING TECHNIQUES

Faculty members use a wide variety of techniques to facilitate successful verbal debriefings. Most of these methods are designed to stimulate group interactions, individual reflection, and maximize learning. Among the most important techniques are asking open-ended questions that stimulate thought and frank discussions. Posing thoughtful questions in the beginning of the session can help learners identify their feelings and the reasons for them. For example, the instructor might ask, "Jenny, I noticed you frowning when Mrs. P. asked you about her husband's nasogastric tube. What you were thinking and feeling at that time?"

Questions assist students in looking at what happened to the patient, how it happened, why it happened, and what they did that influenced the outcomes. For example, the instructor might ask the following questions: "What does the group think caused Mr. W. to vomit?" "When you inserted the nasogastric tube, what did you expect to happen?" "How did you prioritize your care after that happened?"

Appropriate questions can also inspire learners to look at their own behavior and the way they functioned within the team setting. To this end, the faculty member might say, "Sam, how was the information about the patient's bleeding communicated among team members?" Finally, open-ended questions can be used to help the learners evaluate the overall experience and its relationship to the real world—for example, "When could you see this type of situation occurring in the hospital?"

Facilitators must always be aware of their tone of voice, nonverbal behavior, and words if they are to foster effective learning. "Tell us more about what you were thinking when the patient's wife kept telling you that he had pain?" expressed in an interested tone will encourage the learners to reflect, whereas "What were you thinking when you refused to give the patient pain medication?" in a critical tone will more than likely cause the learner to become defensive and stifle learning. Keeping communication nonjudgmental is important if learners are to feel safe and continue to share their thoughts (Kuiper, Heinrich, Matthias, Graham, & Bell-Kotwall, 2008).

Asking too many questions and asking them directly of specific students can lead the learners to respond only to the instructor rather than stimulate a discussion among all of the participants in SCE. Addressing questions to the group as a whole and allowing several individuals to give their perspectives are helpful techniques in this regard. Encouraging students to respond to one another's comments may also be necessary: "Betty, did you see things the same or differently than Sally?" This type of prompting is especially important with learners who tend to be quiet.

Another important technique, especially after asking a question, is to provide time for learners to think and absorb before answering. Too often faculty answer their own questions without giving the learners adequate time to develop their answers. The respect and use of silence encourages learners to do the same for one another (Steinwachs, 1992).

Rephrasing, reflecting, rewording, echoing, and repeating part of what has just been said are other techniques that focus learners on specifics and encourage them to further explain their points. Learner: "We didn't answer his questions!" Facilitator: "You don't think you communicated with the patient adequately?"

Learners frequently experience uncomfortable feelings during simulation. Assisting them to recognize, confront, and deal with these feelings in debriefing will provide them with strategies and confidence for recognizing and acting on these same feelings in the clinical area (Henneman & Cunningham, 2005).

Maintaining a trusting relationship while identifying a learner's knowledge base, assumptions, and feelings may be difficult for instructors, particularly in a situation where the learners' actions are in question. Rudolph, Simon, Dufresne, and Raemer (2006) suggest that facilitators adopt a "stance of curiosity" where the learner's mistakes become puzzles rather than serious errors. They further recommend that facilitators utilize this curiosity or inquiry in conjunction with advocacy; advocacy includes the facilitator's statement of his or her objective observations and subjective judgments related to the mistakes.

Praise and pointing out behaviors that the group or individual did well are always important in the debriefing. Learners are particularly pleased if the facilitator publicly acknowledges improvements in their performance. This is especially true if the group or an individual discussed a problem in an earlier SCE and was able to change this performance in the current simulation.

Expressions of acceptance and empathy are also important, as learners may struggle to relate their feelings and limitations. They may need to be reassured that this simulation was carried out for learning purposes and that mistakes are a part of the learning process. Sometimes sharing similar mistakes made by someone in a different setting both broadens students' understanding of its possible occurrence and decreases their feelings of failure.

Constructive criticism from peers is always powerful; however, learners may not be adept at providing it. Thus it may be necessary for facilitators to lead a discussion with some role-playing on giving constructive criticism to others during the debriefing session. Taking the situation out of the simulation debriefing and talking about giving constructive criticism to a team member in the hospital, and then role-playing the exchange, may also provide the necessary practice that will help students engage in an appropriate dialog during debriefing.

Another way to deal with learners criticizing each other is for the facilitator to say something like this: "Everyone has times when they become overwhelmed. As the primary care nurse, how could you have assisted your team member?" Alternatively, the facilitator could say to the student being criticized, "Who on your team could have assisted you?" These responses are aimed at fostering empathy and teamwork as well as support.

Often one or two learners will tend to dominate the debriefing session. As adult learners, these participants typically try to focus the discussion on topics they feel they need to understand. These issues, however, may be somewhat different from those of concern to the facilitators. If the dominant students are leading the session in productive ways and all the learners are interested in their discussion topics, then there is no need to intervene. However, if they are preventing others from talking, it may be necessary to remind those students that it is important to encourage and listen to the thoughts of others on their team. Sometimes it is possible to engage them in eliciting comments from their peers. If these students continue to dominate the discussion in a nonproductive way, it may be important to make an appointment with them after the debriefing, so that they may continue their discussion.

Techniques to Be Avoided

There are several techniques that prevent learners from sharing information and increase their anxiety rather than stimulate discussions. These include the facilitator becoming an instructor and teaching content, asking closed questions, answering questions before the learners have a chance to process their answers, using judgmental and critical or belittling statements, and focusing entirely on errors (Rall, Manser & Howard, 2000).

THE PROCESS OF VERBAL DEBRIEFING

This final section of the chapter presents a synthesis of the process of debriefing. A verbal debriefing consists of four parts: the introduction, sharing of personal reactions, discussion of events, and the wrap-up. Although the first three components are sometimes discussed simultaneously, all should be covered at some point in the debriefing.

Introduction

The introduction sets the stage for students to share their thoughts, feelings, and analysis of the SCE. The faculty must clearly communicate their expectations that all learners will participate in the reflective process. They must reassure the learners that this is a safe place to discuss their thoughts and actions and that mistakes are a part of the process. Learners need to know that the debriefing is not being graded and they are not being evaluated. They must feel confidant that the purpose of the debriefing is to enhance their learning and that the faculty's questions are intended to stimulate thinking. Faculty must also remind the learners that their role is one of a facilitator, rather than an instructor or evaluator at this point in the simulation—that they, too, are learning about the learners and discovering how they may be of further assistance to them.

It is imperative that the learners know that the discussion of their behavior and limitations will not be shared with other learners or faculty members. To assure that this expectation is met by all parties, they may be asked to sign a confidentiality statement. Often this confidentiality statement tries to protect the integrity of the SCE by stating that the learner will not discuss the simulation, so that all learners may experience it equally. The establishment of clearly stated expectations and the development of trust are essential to the facilitate debriefing.

Sharing of Personal Reactions

In the immediate post-simulation period, the sharing of personal reactions decreases the excitement, anxiety, and tension that built up during the SCE. Once students have described what happened to them and talked about their feelings, it is often possible to assist them in analyzing their comments further. Facilitator questions might then focus the discussion on the relationship of their feelings to the events. For example, these questions might relate to individual functioning, to team functioning, to communication with team members, to communication with the patient and family members, or to patient events and outcomes. Assisting students to delve deeper into the events that led to their reactions provides valuable learning for all. Their responses may also provide a nice segue into the discussion of events.

Discussion of Events

While personal reactions focus on the learner, the discussion of events focuses on the patient, his or her condition, and the interventions employed by SCE participants. Questions about how familiar students were with the patient's condition, treatments, and complications prior to the SCE could be asked during this part of the debriefing. Asking them to give specific examples of when not knowing this information might have jeopardized the patient's safety is the type of thought-provoking inquiry that is appropriate at this time. Additional questions might include "How well did you anticipate potential patient problems or complications?" and "How well did you institute a plan to manage them?" "What might you have done differently?" is a question that may be applicable in many different contexts.

Adult learners know what they want to learn. Given this fact, it is important to let them take the lead in the debriefing discussions as much as possible. Students will want to discuss the experiences and knowledge they already have and determine how the new information they obtained from SCE fits into their existing frame of reference. Toward the end of the discussion of events, the facilitator should take the discussion to a broader level of thought beyond the just-completed SCE. Generalization of students' new knowledge and experiences is discussed in light of other patients and situations as part of this effort. In this way, the learners transfer their learning to other situations and to the real world.

Videotaping in Debriefing

While some study findings have suggested that oral debriefing without video technology is just as valuable as debriefing with video (Savoldelli, Naik,

Park, Joo, Chow, & Hamstra, 2006), other researchers suggest that reviewing portions of the videotaped SCE may enhance the learners' perception of what actually transpired and how they contributed to it. Learners, however, must be made aware that they are being videotaped and give their written consent to this recording. They must be told exactly who will view the tape and when it will be destroyed. Generally, the video record is viewed only by the learners and faculty directly involved in the SCE during the debriefing session and then destroyed immediately afterward. Erasing the tape in front of the learners provides additional peace of mind for the participants. If the video is to be saved or used for another purpose, the learners must know and agree to that usage.

Viewing portions of the videotape and collaboratively critiquing the learners' performance during debriefing is especially beneficial when errors of omission, procedural problems, missed cues, or poor decision making occurred during the simulation. Reflecting on the problems presented, discussing alternative plans for care and interventions, and correcting procedural errors are all thought to be more effective following the actual viewing of the problems. It is not unusual for learners to believe that they have followed a procedure correctly during the SCE, only to realize that they omitted a step while watching the video. Having learners record the time between a patient's request—medication for pain, for instance—and the actual satisfaction of that request is also an eye-opening experience for many students. Time passes more quickly when they are involved in the SCE. For the facilitator, a counter or other way to tag significant events is important so that time will not be lost during the debriefing sessions attempting to find the part of the tape the facilitator wishes the learners to view.

Wrap-up

The wrap-up summarizes the important information learners discussed during the debriefing. It generally includes highlights of the simulation or things they did well, in addition to areas they say they need to improve. While a faculty member most often gives this summary, the learners themselves could also present it. The wrap-up may also mention elements of the objectives, the things the students learned, and the most important points of the SCE. Thanking the students for their participation in the SCE and the debriefing is an excellent way to end the session on a positive note.

Evaluation forms that allow the learners to evaluate the total experience should be provided. Their responses should be anonymous, yet allow the learners to adequately evaluate the quality of the total learning experience.

SUMMARY

Debriefing is recognized as a vital part of the simulation experience. Although it is carried out in a variety of ways with different models and techniques, debriefing is where the learners process the objectives of the SCE, learn about themselves, link new knowledge with previous knowledge, and generalize new knowledge to the real world. If these goals are to be realized, then it is imperative that the facilitator be knowledgeable about the process and carefully plan for the debriefing.

References

Dieckmann, P., Reddersen, S., Zieger, J., & Rall, M. (2008). Video-assisted debriefing in simulation-based training of crisis resource management. In R. R. Kyle & W. B. Murray (Eds.), *Clinical simulations: Operations, engineering, and management* (pp. 667–676). Boston: Elsevier.

Fanning, R. M., & Gaba, D. M. (2007). The role of debriefing in simulation-based learning. *Simulation in Healthcare, 2*, 115–125.

Fritzsche, D. J., Leonard, N. H., Boscia, M. W., & Anderson, P. H. (2004). Simulation debriefing procedures. *Developments in Business Simulation and Experiential Learning, 31*, 33–338.

Haskvitz, L. M., & Koop, E. C. (2004). Students struggling in clinical? A new role for the patient simulator. *Journal of Nursing Education, 43*, 181–184.

Henneman, E. A., & Cunningham, H. (2005). Using clinical simulation to teach patient safety in an acute/critical care nursing course. *Nurse Educator, 30*, 172–177.

Henneman, E. A., Cunningham, H., Roche, J. P., & Cumin, M. E. (2007). Human patient simulation: Teaching students to provide safe care. *Nurse Educator, 32*, 212–216.

Jefferies, P. R (2005). A framework for designing, implementing, and evaluating simulations used as teaching strategies in nursing. *Nursing Education Perspectives, 26*(2), 96–103.

Kardong-Edgren, S., Starkweather, A., & Ward, L. (2008). The integration of simulation into a Clinical Foundations of Nursing course: Student and faculty perspectives. *International Journal of Nursing Education Scholarship, 5*(1), 1–16. Retrieved September 20, 2008, from http://www.bepress.com/ijnes/vol5/iss1/art26

Kuiper, R. A., Heinrich, C., Matthias, A., Graham, M. J., & Bell-Kotwall, L. (2008). Debriefing with the OPT model of clinical reasoning during high fidelity patient simulation. *International Journal of Nursing Education Scholarship*. Retrieved September 1, 2008, from http://www.bepress.com/ijnes/vol5/iss1/art17

Lederman, L. C. (1991). Differences that make a difference: Intercultural communication, simulation and the debriefing process in diverse interaction. Workshop conducted at the Annual Conference of International Simulation and Gaming Association, Kyoto, Japan.

Mort, T. C., & Donahue S. P. (2004). Debriefing: The basics. In W. F. Dunn (Ed.), *Simulators in critical care and beyond* (pp. 76–83). Des Plaines, IL: Society of Critical Care Medicine.

Pesut, D. J., & Herman, J. (1999). *Clinical reasoning: The art and science of critical and creative thinking*. Albany, NY: Delmar.

Peters, V. A., & Vissers, G. A. N. (2004). A simple classification model for debriefing simulation games. *Simulation & Gaming, 35*(1), 70–84.

Petranek, C. F. (1994). Maturation in experiential learning: Principles of simulation and gaming. *Simulation & Gaming, 25*, 513–522.

Petranek, C. F. (2000). Written debriefing: The next vital step in learning with simulations. *Simulation & Gaming, 31*(1), 108–118.

Polit, D., & Beck, C. (2008). Nursing research: Generating and assessing evidence for nursing practice. Philadelphia: Lippincott Williams & Wilkins.

Rall, M., Manser, T., & Howard, S. K. (2000). Key elements of debriefing for simulator training. *European Journal of Anaesthesiology, 17*, 515–526.

Revell, K. (2008). "Leadership cannot be taught": Teaching leadership to MPA students. *Journal of Public Affairs Education, 14*(1), 91–110.

Rudolph, J. W., Simon, R., Dufresne, R., & Raemer, D. B. (2006). There's no such thing as "nonjudgmental" debriefing: A theory and method for debriefing with good judgment. *Simulation in Healthcare: The Journal of the Society for Medical Simulation, 1*(1), 49–55.

Savoldelli, G. L., Naik, V. N., Park, J., Joo, H. S., Chow, R., & Hamstra, S. J. (2006). Value of debriefing during simulated crisis management: Oral versus video-assisted oral feedback. *Anesthesiology, 105*, 279–285.

Stafford, F. (2005). The significance of de-roling and debriefing in training medical students using simulation to train medical students. *Medical Education, 39*, 1083–1085.

Steinwachs, B. (1992). How to facilitate a debriefing. *Simulation and Gaming, 23*, 186–195.

Thatcher, D. C., & Robinson, M. J. (1987). *An introduction to games and simulation in education.* Hants: Solent Simulations.

Waldner, M. H., & Olson, J. K. (2007). Taking the patient to the classroom: Applying theoretical frameworks to simulation in nursing education. *International Journal of Nursing Education Scholarship, 4*(1), 1–14.

Walker, G. (1990). Crisis care in critical incident debriefing. *Death Studies, 14*, 121–133.

CHAPTER 18

A Curriculum for the Pre-licensure Nursing Program

Thomas J. Doyle and Kim Leighton

Simulation has been utilized by healthcare educators for decades to supplement the clinical experiences of pre-licensure nursing students (Bond, Kostenbader, & McCarthy, 2001); however, it is only within the last decade that computer-driven patient simulators have allowed for repetitive practice and immediate feedback without risk to patients. The use of high-fidelity patient simulation has not yet become a standard part of the curricula in most U.S. healthcare education programs. When Nehring and Lashley (2004) surveyed nursing schools identified as owning patient simulators, they found that no formal simulation curriculum was in use at the respondent schools. In fact, more than 75% of these schools had used a simulator in less than 10% of their total curricula (Nehring & Lashley, 2004).

In the short time since that survey, Medical Education Technologies, Inc. (METI) has designed a curriculum of simulated clinical experiences (SCEs) for undergraduate nursing programs, providing opportunities for nursing educators to quickly and easily integrate simulation throughout their curriculums. Integration of patient simulation throughout the nursing curriculum is consistent with trends in nursing education nationwide (Peteani, 2004), as it provides opportunities for students to experience patient care situations that they might not otherwise encounter in the traditional clinical environment.

This chapter outlines the challenges facing nursing education today, describes the importance of patient simulation to pattern recognition and enhanced learning, defines the benefits achieved by use of patient simulation, describes the creation of an undergraduate nursing curriculum for simulation, and provides examples of how simulation is integrated into a nursing curriculum.

CHALLENGES FACING NURSING EDUCATION

Nursing education faces many challenges today, including a shortage of nursing faculty and clinical sites, medically complex patients, scientific and technological advancements, differing expectations of today's students than in the past, and the expressed concern that nursing graduates are not prepared for the realities of practice.

The current and projected nursing shortage has been well documented. Despite the nursing shortage, an estimated 147,000 qualified nursing school applicants were turned away in 2005, an increase of 18% over the number who were not admitted in such programs in 2004 (National League for Nursing [NLN], 2005). To overcome this problem, many nursing schools have attempted to increase enrollments, but have found that a shortage of faculty impedes those efforts. In a 2002 American Association of Colleges of Nursing (AACN) survey, 41.7% of responding schools reported that a lack of qualified faculty was the main reason for not accepting all qualified applicants (Berlin, Stennett, & Bednash, 2003). The nursing faculty deficit has become critical, as current faculty members' ages increase and the pool of replacement faculty decreases (AACN, 2005). Other reasons for the inability to accommodate all applicants in suitable nursing programs are a lack of appropriate clinical placement sites and a dearth of classroom space (AACN, 2006).

Nursing schools struggle to find adequate clinical placements for nursing students (Rhodes & Curran, 2005). Often, the patients available for students to care for are too medically complex for the novice nursing student. Hospitalized patients are more acutely and critically ill than in the past, creating situations in which nursing students lack the knowledge to safely care for those patients and may, in fact, be prohibited from providing any care for the patient (Feingold, Calaluce, & Kallen, 2004).

In the recent past, scientific and technological advances have helped to increase longevity of life. As a result, the medical profession has been presented with more severely ill patients, patients who have experienced more chronic illnesses, and patients who require technologically complex care; despite their greater acuity, however, the average length of a hospital stay decreased from 7.6 days to 5.8 days between 1980 and 2000 (Institute of Medicine [IOM], 2004). This decreased length of stay requires nurses to provide more complex care in shorter periods of time. As a result, the nursing educator often assigns a student to care for a particular patient, only to return the next day and find that the patient has been discharged. In addition, students must provide care in a compacted period of time and often do not see the outcomes of their decisions and care provided.

Student learning expectations are also different than they were in the past. According to Prensky (2001), the educational system was not designed to teach today's students, who grew up immersed in technology. Meanwhile, the majority of nursing educators have adopted technology to various degrees over the past decade. As a result, multitasking students who desire random access, immediate gratification, and frequent rewards often struggle in classrooms taught by educators who teach how they were taught—usually in a step-by-step lecture format culminating with formal testing.

The many challenges facing nursing education are clearly daunting. Moreover, employers of nursing graduates express concern over their inability to manage the expectations and competencies required in the new graduate role (Morton & Rauen, 2004). The presence of newly graduated nurses with little or no exposure to the types of illness, disease, or complications that a patient experiences further compounds the risk for preventable adverse effects. Although nursing schools have been charged with preparing graduates qualified for entry-level practice, it has not been uncommon for those graduates to find themselves in situations they were unprepared to handle.

Baigis and Caines (2000) conducted a study using focus groups consisting of new graduates (practicing less than one year), managers, preceptors, and clinical educators. They identified a large gap between new graduates' expectations and the reality of their job. New-graduate participants verbalized concerns about escalating responsibility too soon after being employed and not having enough time to provide patients with holistic care. Managers and preceptors of newly employed nurses reported that the new graduates exhibited difficulties with time management, prioritization, delegation, multitasking, and organizational skills. Employers believed that the graduates were inadequately prepared in school for their role and responsibilities.

Information gathered by Casey, Fink, Krugman, and Propst (2004) further emphasizes the concerns voiced by nurses. Those authors studied stresses and challenges experienced by 270 new-graduate nurses in several large hospitals in one Midwestern city. Participants reported that lack of confidence in skill performance and deficits in critical thinking and clinical knowledge were their greatest stressors and challenges. They further reported that it took approximately 12 months of employment for them to become comfortable and confident in caring for their patients.

PATTERN RECOGNITION AND LEARNING

It is critical to provide a variety of clinical experiences for students so they will develop pattern recognition. In other words, learners are expected to improve their ability to quickly and accurately identify changes indicating deteriorating conditions through repeated exposure to the situation or surrounding circumstances (Gladwell, 2005). The Dreyfus and Dreyfus Model of Skill

Acquisition (1980), as adapted for use with nursing by Benner (1984), supports learning on a continuum progressing through novice, advanced beginner, competent, proficient, and expert stages. One of the hallmark findings of that work is that as someone becomes more competent, he or she moves from reliance on abstract principles to use of concrete experiences. Those with higher levels of competence identify problems more quickly, based on subtler cues (Larew, Lessans, Spunt, Foster, & Covington, 2006). The challenge to nursing educators always has been to provide enough experiences for the students to draw from, increase their exposure, and subsequently have a favorable impact on preventable adverse event reductions.

Undergraduate nursing schools have been unable to provide repetition of experiences in the apprenticeship model currently used. Furthermore, too often nursing students have been exposed to limited experiences with unusual or critical cases. Dunn (2004) has stated:

> Even within clinical training programs, learners must both understand and be able to execute physiologically sound practices within chaotic clinical environments any time of the day or night. Learners must acquire the necessary skills to deftly integrate the cognitive and manual skills required to create order from chaos in the context of complicated resuscitations, potentially anxiety-provoking environments of potentially great disorder, and immense disease complexity. (p. 15)

Unfortunately, it is often at those critical learning points when students are excluded from managing the patient because of the potential for increased patient risk (Gordon, Wilkerson, Shaffer, & Armstrong, 2001).

Healthcare consumers have stressed that nursing students should be provided education and technical training that enable competency (Pew Health Professions Commission, 1998). To ensure that this goal is met, nursing educators are challenged to reconsider their teaching methods.

The use of SCEs may bridge the gap between theory and practice. Supplementing traditional clinical experiences with risk-free SCEs increases the student's exposure to a variety of clinical situations. It is through repeated exposure to a situation that learning occurs (Benner, 1994; Bastable, 2003). Clark and Mayer (2003) agree that repetition of experiences is vital for learners to increase proficiency and suggest that learning experiences should be designed that offer many opportunities to practice, while recognizing that tasks of a more critical nature require more practice. "We must recognize that trainees at all levels learn by doing, not by listening and observing... . Knowledge comes from repeating the experience" (Fanaroff, 1999, p. 329).

SIMULATION AS A TEACHING STRATEGY TO ADDRESS THESE CHALLENGES

It is well documented that traditional approaches to teaching and learning no longer work with today's students. Instead, nursing educators must find new and innovative approaches to the acquisition of knowledge and facilitation of learning for nursing students. Human patient simulation is one such strategy to address the multiple issues that nursing education faces. Patient simulation allows educators to teach multiple objectives at once, brings learning alive in a multidimensional environment, and increases the confidence of the learner, which leads to competence (Alinier, Hunt, & Gordon, 2004).

Since high-fidelity patient simulations were initially introduced in nursing programs, faculty have struggled with adopting and integrating this pedagogy. The primary reason for this difficulty was the need to create the various simulations or scenarios needed to use the patient simulators. Given the demands on nursing faculty, unless they were allotted time for this activity as part of their workload assignments, scenario development just did not happen. As a consequence, often the simulators sat unused or were turned on simply for patient assessment. The real potential of using the simulators was, for the most part, unrealized.

As an education company, METI figured out early on that a turnkey solution was needed for nursing education. The Program for Nursing Curriculum Integration (PNCI)—METI's solution to this dilemma—was born in 2000 but would not become reality for several more years.

THE PROGRAM FOR NURSING CURRICULUM INTEGRATION

The PNCI is a commercial answer to the challenge of providing educators with the tools necessary to make the transition to patient simulation easier. This turnkey solution assists faculty with this transition and increases their efficiency as they embark on the use of this technology to facilitate learning and assess competency. One of the primary benefits of the PNCI is that it focuses on nursing educational concepts and competencies; no adjustments to the curriculum are required because it is already based on the same foundation. This standardized platform minimizes the impact on the existing curriculum while decreasing faculty resistance to adopting patient simulation, as PNCI requires minimal incremental work on their part.

Development of the PNCI

Development of the PNCI began with the identification of a primary partner who would make the vision a reality. METI found this partner in Texas Woman's

University–Dallas, a customer since 2003. Under the leadership of a Patient Simulation Task Force, the faculty had already begun to identify how and where various forms of simulation could be used in the undergraduate curriculum. Once an agreement was reached, the task force met with METI leadership on a monthly basis to finalize the outline describing where patient simulation could be used in the undergraduate curriculum. After nearly 14 months of work, in consultation with the existing standards and criteria from the National League for Nursing Accreditation Commission and the American Association of Colleges of Nursing's (2008) *Essentials of Baccalaureate Education for Professional Nursing Practice*, the initial plan was finalized. In concert with the development of the plan was the identification and creation of the initial simulated clinical experiences (SCEs), more commonly known as "scenarios."

The foundation of the PNCI is the Integration Roadmap, which is organized based on the concepts taught in undergraduate nursing across four semesters. In each semester, a specific SCE is identified by title that may be used to facilitate the indicated concept(s). If a specific SCE is not identified, it is then indicated that the concept will be integrated into other simulations during the same semester. For instance, the Patient Simulation Task Force determined that a SCE focused on the analysis of abnormal vital signs—a key concept in the second semester of study—in and of itself would not be educationally sound. In contrast, a SCE designed around postoperative nursing care including abnormal vital signs, such as tachycardia and hypotension, was identified as a better fit to bring learning alive for the students. Ultimately, the potential to do 100 SCEs in the undergraduate curriculum was identified. All areas of practice have also been identified and included in the design of various SCEs.

In the first semester, student nurses are introduced to the practice of professional nursing. The clinical nursing curriculum begins in this first semester and includes those courses that serve as the foundation for practice. For example, nursing assessment encompasses health assessment with patients of all ages, influences of culture, health promotion, and the nursing process. The second clinical course in this semester is a fundamentals course, which emphasizes a variety of nursing skills, pharmacology, and communication with patients, families and co-workers, and teaching–learning strategies for health promotion and maintenance.

The second semester focuses on the unique role and contributions of nursing to collaborative management of both adult and pediatric patients with acute health problems. In addition to understanding a variety of acute medical conditions, emphasis is placed on the development of clinical judgment, including the recognition of significant assessment and laboratory data, which adds to students' clinical nursing skill base. Learners are also introduced to families during childbearing and the collaborative management of events surrounding the birth of a child.

In the third semester, the focus switches from patients of all ages with acute problems to those with more chronic health problems. Emphasis is placed on knowledge of chronic health problems seen in various age groups. Assessment, clinical judgments, and nursing interventions not only stress health promotion and health maintenance, but also include more restoration and rehabilitation activities of patients in both inpatient and outpatient settings. In addition, learners are introduced to the nurse's role in the community working with diverse groups, addressing common problems found in urban and rural areas, and preparing for and responding to terrorism.

In the last semester, learners are challenged by caring for individual patients or groups of patients in acute care and critical care settings. Emphasis is on critical thinking, leadership skills, professionalism and accountability, recognizing and responding to crisis situations, becoming proficient performing nursing skills, and collaborative management of healthcare problems of all kinds.

Included in the design of all SCEs across the four semesters are patients from different cultures and with various health beliefs. Additionally, the learner must deal with psychosocial problems and manage issues related to personal and patient safety.

The Integration Roadmap is intended to provide faculty guidance on how patient simulation may be utilized in any nursing program. By intentional design, it provides an example of how and where patient simulation may be utilized to facilitate learning while still providing for faculty flexibility. The Integration Roadmap is meant to serve as a reference for faculty as they integrate simulation into their curriculum. It gives guidance for planning, implementation, and evaluation of student learning through the use of patient simulation.

Simulated Clinical Experiences

As indicated previously, the Integration Roadmap identifies 100 SCEs. The SCE is a process tool that enables faculty members to execute a learning strategy in such a way as to address multiple objectives. Each process tool provides instructors with an extensive overview and outline of the learning exercise and requires minimal faculty development time for use. All SCEs are presented in a standard format, which includes the following components:

- Software scenario file name
- Indication of which preconfigured patient should be applied for the simulation
- An overview of the SCE that provides a synopsis of the simulation, including the targeted audience and other key points

- Learning objectives, including the cognitive taxonomy addressed
- NCLEX-RN test plan categories addressed
- Clinical location in which the simulation occurs
- Suggested equipment, supplies, and simulator setup
- Monitoring required or desired
- Additional faculty notes to assist in the execution of the SCE
- Background patient history and information
- Healthcare provider's orders
- Scenario that identifies each state or "chapter" in the clinical story, the patient events (both simulator-enabled findings and other pertinent data), minimal behaviors expected of the learner, and faculty prompts and questions to facilitate learning either during the simulation or in a subsequent debriefing session
- Questions for the learners to prepare for the SCE
- Evidence-based references

These tools are provided as an electronic document, so that faculty may easily customize them. In addition to the complete version intended for faculty usage, an abridged version for learners includes the learning objectives, patient history and background information, questions for preparation, and references. All of the SCEs are evidence-based or evidence-informed, with the relevant reference citations being provided in both the instructor and student versions. Best practice standards have also been included to address regional variations in practice. The references are updated every two years and the SCEs modified to reflect changes in evidence-based practice.

Each of the SCEs has been designed so that it may be used for either learning or assessment purposes. Because minimal expected behaviors are identified for each state of the scenario, faculty can easily evaluate learners' performance. The PNCI also includes a group of supplemental tools—for example, the SBAR Communication Guide, a debriefing guide, and evaluation forms—designed to assist faculty members in integrating patient simulation into their curriculum.

SIMULATION ACROSS THE CURRICULUM

To date, little has been written about integration of simulation throughout an undergraduate nursing curriculum. The literature does, however, provide a few examples of how simulation is used in various programs, generally involving one course or part of a curriculum: simulation in the preclinical portion of a nurse anesthesia program to establish a uniform base of experiences (Lupien, 1998); a three-year curriculum designed to teach core competencies to emergency medicine residents (McLaughlin, Doezema, & Sklar, 2002); one year of an undergraduate medical program (Kozmenko, Yang, Chauvin, DeCarlo, & Hilton, 2005); undergraduate obstetric curriculum (Robertson, 2006); and a modular curriculum administered during an internal medicine clerkship (McMahon, Monaghan, Falchuk, Gordon, & Alexander, 2005).

Despite the expressed desire of nursing students to participate in more SCEs throughout their educational program, nursing educators have been slow to integrate simulation throughout their curricula. The availability of curricula such as the PNCI makes the process of integration easier. This turnkey program provides the nursing educator with multiple preprogrammed, evidence-based or -informed SCEs from which to choose. These scenarios are available for all levels of nursing students and encompass a variety of patient settings in which nursing care is provided. In short, the PNCI reduces faculty preparation time by eliminating the need for scenario development.

Learning processes in the SCE assist educators to identify curriculum gaps and areas of weakness. For example, Billings and Halstead (1998) observed that patient simulation assisted nursing students to apply content learned in the classroom to the clinical patient setting. Gaps in student learning become apparent when students perform poorly in the simulation setting and are unable to apply theoretical knowledge (Hunt, 2004). Chopra et al. (1994) also determined that patterns of error by participants learning with simulation were similar to patterns of error in the clinical environment. The true value of simulation lies in its ability to offer experiences throughout the educational process that provide students with opportunities for repetition, pattern recognition, and faster decision making.

Choosing Simulated Clinical Experiences

There are numerous opportunities to integrate simulation into the nursing curriculum. Courses with a clinical component are the most common starting point in many nursing programs; however, options also exist for nonclinical courses. Determining which SCEs to use often presents quite a challenge for the nursing educator.

To make effective decisions with regard to this technology, the nursing educator should closely examine his or her objectives for using patient simulation in his or her course, as this consideration will help determine which SCE to choose. Many nursing educators offer nursing students a SCE prior to the traditional clinical experiences in an effort to prepare students for that experience and to reduce their anxiety about providing clinical care. For this purpose, choosing an experience that closely resembles the type of patient that will be cared for in the clinical setting is important. Nursing educators also have the unique opportunity to offer low-volume, high-risk simulated patients that students do not often encounter in their clinical work, such as patients with amniotic fluid emboli or anaphylactic reaction to a blood transfusion. Other types of patients with complicated conditions can also be replicated in the simulation lab, such as those with diabetic ketoacidosis or acute respiratory distress syndrome.

When choosing SCEs, it is helpful for faculty members who teach theory courses to examine areas of poor performance on examinations by conducting an item analysis. That poor performance may indicate that students do not fully understand the material. If any such gaps in the curriculum are identified, nursing faculty can facilitate learning in the simulation laboratory to close them. An analysis of NCLEX-RN results will provide insight into nursing student areas of weakness as well. Furthermore, the SCE provides opportunities to improve communication and teamwork among nursing students.

Simulation in Courses with a Clinical Component

As the nurse educator begins to integrate simulation into a course, he or she will undoubtedly be concerned about where the additional time for preparing and completing simulations will come from. Because it is rarely possible to increase the amount of time available for a given course, it is vitally important that the nursing educator closely examine current methods of course delivery in the classroom, in the skills laboratory, and at clinical sites. Nursing students who are prepared for the SCE will have already learned about risk factors, assessment, medications, diagnostic studies, other interventions, complications, and patient education related to the patient condition being studied. Therefore, by holding nursing students accountable for that learning, the nursing educator does not need to spend classroom time lecturing on these same topics. Rather, this time can be spent enhancing the nursing student's understanding of the material through SCEs.

Many colleges begin to integrate simulation early in the undergraduate nursing program, while students are learning assessment techniques and fundamentals. Opportunities to learn abnormal vital signs, lung and heart sounds, or pulse characteristics are often limited when assessing peers. By contrast, use of a patient simulator allows students to learn about abnormal assessment findings, but within the context of a patient scenario. For example, learning about abnormal lung sounds, such as wheezing, takes on new meaning when the student is confronted with a patient with asthma. The student must ask subjective questions, interpret the answers, and perform an accurate assessment. By doing so, the student learns the meaning of the wheezing instead of simply what it sounds like.

Similarly, learning how to insert urinary catheters and perform dressing changes typically consist of following a checklist procedure. In the simulation laboratory, however, students can build on that knowledge. For example, when a urinary catheter is inserted and no urine returns, the student must use his or her problem-solving skills. Is the patient dehydrated? Did the patient just return from surgery where he or she lost a large amount of blood? Is the patient in renal failure? Or is there just a kink in the tubing? This type of simulated experience moves the learner beyond application of knowledge to the analysis level. In many nursing programs, skills and fundamental laboratories are built around rotating stations where students participate in various activities; in this case, the simulation laboratory becomes another such station.

Simulated clinical experiences can also be offered in the classroom by bringing a portable simulator to the room. Nursing students can participate by being chosen or volunteering to take on nursing roles in the management of the simulated patient. The remaining students can observe the interaction, offering suggestions or insight into the patient's care. For example, when learning about acute renal failure, medical–surgical nursing students might participate in a SCE to provide care for a pediatric patient with acute glomerulonephritis. Following the simulation, the instructor debriefs the group, including a discussion of the differences between adult and pediatric renal failure, distinguishing characteristics of acute and chronic renal failure, and concerns about the ability of the mother (a role played by the faculty member) to care for the child.

Nursing programs with nonportable simulators may consider investing in two-way interactive video, an option that allows a small number of students to care for a patient in the simulation laboratory while the remainder of the class group watches from the classroom. The observing students can offer suggestions or observe for specific interventions. For example, two students who are learning about death, dying, and bereavement might care for a patient at the end of life. The remainder of the class can observe via two-way interactive video, allowing them to see and hear what occurs in the simulation laboratory. While observing, they can take note of the physical care delivered to the patient as well as psychosocial aspects of the care provided.

Small class groups, such as those often found in nursing electives, afford the unique opportunity to bring the entire class into the laboratory together. Having a smaller group allows all students to participate in the care of the patient, where nametags define the various students' responsibilities, such as primary nurse, medication nurse, documentation nurse, and the nurse who calls the healthcare provider for orders. If the group is larger, half can provide care while the rest observe. At a predetermined point in the SCE, the groups can change roles. For example, students learning about high-risk obstetrical complications might attend four class sessions in the simulation laboratory. The students prepare for the experiences by learning risk factors, assessment data, interventions, diagnostic testing, and patient education needs for patients with conditions such as placenta previa and abruptio placentae. Each is then assigned a role, which changes with each SCE. The entire class period is spent in the simulation laboratory rather than in the classroom listening to a lecture on the material.

Perhaps the easiest method of scheduling simulation is at post-conference time following a clinical day. Experiences for a course may be spread out over an entire semester and should focus on a problem or situation common to that level of student. For example, medical–surgical nursing students would care for a patient with an anaphylactic reaction to a blood transfusion, as this is the course where they learn to administer blood. The students might arrive at the simulation laboratory every Friday afternoon and spend the time from 1:00 P.M. to 3:15 P.M. in their clinical group. Half of the students could participate in a 45-minute SCE while the other half completes clinical paperwork or another assigned activity. Following the completion of the first group's experience, they change places. When both groups' SCEs are complete, they are debriefed together. Any sensitive debriefing should occur in the small groups prior to combining them.

The simulation laboratory can also be used as a clinical site, with nursing students attending in their clinical group for an entire day. Nursing educators should critically consider each of their clinical sites to determine if they are providing beneficial experiences for the students. In many cases, clinical sites have been added to programs simply because student numbers have grown— not necessarily because they offer the best experiences. In this type of context, students should come to the simulation laboratory instead. For example, pediatric nursing students in their first course could attend the simulation laboratory from 7 A.M. to 3 P.M. one day per semester. During the course of the day, they would provide care for four pediatric patients with the following conditions: asthma, gastroenteritis with dehydration, septic appendix, and diabetic ketoacidosis. The instructor role-plays the patient's mother and has a different parental personality for each patient, an approach that allows students to provide care for the child within the context of the family. Debriefing would occur following each patient encounter. The same level of clinical preparation and paperwork would be expected for the SCEs as when students work at the traditional clinical site.

Table 18-1 provides an example of how simulation has been integrated throughout the curriculum at one nursing school.

Simulation in Nonclinical Courses

Many opportunities exist to use simulation in nonclinical courses, such as those dealing with physiology, pathophysiology, and pharmacology. The

Table 18-1 Simulated Experiences Integrated Throughout an Undergraduate Nursing Curriculum

Course	Simulated Clinical Experience (SCE)	Scheduling
Health Assessment Across the Life Span	Basic Assessment of the Adult Patient with Asthma Basic Assessment of the Cardiac Patient (with Murmur) Basic Assessment of Abdominal Complaints (Adult and Pediatric)	Station during assessment lab time
Nursing Care I (first medical–surgical course)	Basic Assessment of the Postoperative Gastrectomy Patient Asthma Attack in the Pediatric Patient (Basic) Diabetic Ketoacidosis and Pneumonia (Pediatric) Fluid and Electrolyte Imbalance (Pediatric) Septic Pediatric Patient Secondary to a Ruptured Appendix	Morning of first clinical day prior to going to hospital. One day of clinical spent in simulation lab: each SCE with debriefing is approximately 1.5 hours.
Nursing Care II (second medical–surgical course)	Renal Dysfunction Secondary to Acute Streptococcal Glomerulonephritis Anaphylactic Reaction to Blood Administration	In classroom post-conference scheduled one afternoon weekly over semester.
Nursing Care III (advanced medical–surgical and critical care)	Cardiopulmonary Arrest [without Advanced Cardiac Life Support (ACLS)] Asthma Attack in the Pediatric Patient (Advanced)	All groups completed over 3 days.
Family Health Nursing	Postpartum Hemorrhage 2 Hours Following Delivery	All groups completed over 3 days.
Psychiatric Nursing	Intentional Overdose of a Hypnotic	Two 4-hour sessions over 2 days.

Table 18-1   Simulated Experiences Integrated Throughout an Undergraduate Nursing Curriculum *(continued)*

Course	Simulated Clinical Experience (SCE)	Scheduling
Nursing Management	Managing Conflict and Delegation while Caring for Chronic Obstructive Pulmonary Disease (COPD) Patient	Broadcast to classroom via two-way interactive video; four students care for patient.
Level II Nursing Practicum (summer intensive)	Postoperative Care of the Patient with Complications: Pneumonia	Post-conference for each clinical group.
Level III Nursing Practicum (summer intensive)	Admission of Patient with Pneumonia	Post-conference for each clinical group.
Critical Care Nursing (Elective)	Adult Respiratory Distress Syndrome Leading to Death (on Ventilator) Cardiopulmonary Arrest (with ACLS)	4-hour session for each group of four students.
Caring in Times of Death, Dying, and Bereavement (Elective)	End-of-Life Care	Broadcast to classroom via two-way interactive video; two students care for patient.
Forensic Nursing (Elective)	Gunshot Wound Trauma (Deceased): Evidence Collection	Broadcast to classroom via two-way interactive video; four students care for patient.
Emergency Nursing (Elective)	Gunshot Wound Trauma Acetaminophen Poisoning (Pediatric) Motor Vehicle Collision with Abdominal Injury with Internal Bleeding and Hypovolemic Shock	Broadcast to classroom via two-way interactive video; three students care for each patient.

Table 18-1   Simulated Experiences Integrated Throughout an Undergraduate
Nursing Curriculum *(continued)*

Course	Simulated Clinical Experience (SCE)	Scheduling
Expanded Concepts in the Nursing Care of Infants and Children (Elective)	Traumatic Brain Injury (Pediatric)	Class takes place in simulation lab.
High Risk Obstetrics (Elective)	Pregnancy Induced Hypertension Abruptio Placentae Secondary to Cocaine Abuse Amniotic Emboli	Class takes place in simulation lab—3 weeks of course.
Pharmacology	Cardiac Medication and Dose Effects on Different Patient Types	During classroom time using computer software.

simulation software can be used alone or in conjunction with the simulators to teach concepts related to fluid volume, medication effects, hemodynamic status, and respiratory or cardiovascular abnormalities.

Effects of hypovolemia and hypervolemia can be demonstrated on the simulation software by having students observe hemodynamic parameters such as blood pressure, heart rate, mean arterial pressure, and cardiac output. Simulating blood loss through the software will lead to decreased blood pressure, tachycardia, and eventual decrease in cardiac output. Infusing too large a volume of crystalloids or colloids will lead to hypertension and decreased heart rate. The effects of altered fluid volume status can be simulated in a young healthy patient, an elderly patient, a pregnant patient, or any number of different patient types that can be programmed into the software.

Medications can also be administered through the software so that nursing students can see their effects. This experience is particularly valuable when the same dose of medication is administered to several different types of patients, as it allows students to understand that one dose is not appropriate for all patients. Additionally, after observing the immediate increase in heart rate and blood pressure associated with epinephrine, nursing students better understand the importance of educating the patient on the medication effects prior to medication administration.

Numerous hemodynamic changes happen when cardiac arrhythmias occur. The simulation software can be used to show changes associated with a variety of arrhythmias such as heart blocks, atrial fibrillation, ventricular tachycardia, and ventricular fibrillation. Additionally, critical hemodynamic changes that occur with pneumothorax, cardiac tamponade, or other life-threatening conditions can be simulated without risk to human life.

CONCLUSION

The Program for Nursing Curriculum Integration was created to assist nursing faculty in overcoming many of the barriers and challenges to integration of patient simulation throughout their curricula. This program offers SCEs designed for use with all levels of pre-licensure nursing students and occur in a variety of settings. The PNCI is designed to eliminate or decrease much of the time typically invested in scenario development so that nursing faculty can begin integration quickly.

One challenge for nursing faculty continues to be the logistics of how to integrate high-fidelity patient simulation fully across the curriculum. This chapter has outlined a variety of methods to facilitate use of simulation in clinical and nonclinical courses. Providing nursing students with repetitive learning experiences in an environment free of risk to human life allows them to increase their confidence and competence.

It is vital that nursing educators contribute to the body of knowledge related to simulation outcomes. Early research focused on student preference for learning with simulation and satisfaction with the methodology. Now, however, the literature needs to address the effectiveness of this teaching method and its ability to affect patient safety.

References

Alinier, G., Hunt, W. B., & Gordon, R. (2004). Determining the value of simulation in nurse education: Study design and initial results. *Nurse Education in Practice, 4*, 200–207.

American Association of Colleges of Nursing (AACN). (2002). Hallmarks of the professional nursing practice environment. Retrieved February 3, 2007, from http://www.aacn.nche.edu/Publications/positions/hallmarks.htm

American Association of Colleges of Nursing (AACN). (2005). Faculty shortages in baccalaureate and graduate nursing programs: Scope of the problem and strategies for expanding the supply. Retrieved February 2, 2007, from http://www.aacn.nche.edu/Publications/WhitePapers/FacultyShortages.htm

American Association of Colleges of Nursing (AACN). (2006). Student enrollment rises in US nursing colleges and universities for the 6th consecutive year. Retrieved January 18, 2006, from http://www.aacn.nche.edu/Media/NewsReleases/ 06Survey.htm

Baigis, J., & Caines, B. (2000). *Colleagues in caring.* The District of Columbia Consortium for Nursing Education and Practice. Retrieved September 4, 2006, from http://www.georgetown.edu/organizations/dccnep/Focus%20Group%20Report%202000.pdf

Bastable, S. (2003). *Nurse as educator: Principles of teaching and learning* (2nd ed.). Sudbury, MA: Jones and Bartlett.

Benner, P. (1984). *From novice to expert: Excellence and power in clinical nursing practice.* Menlo Park, CA: Addison-Wesley.

Berlin, L., Stennett, J., & Bednash, G. (2003). *2002–2003 enrollment and graduations in baccalaureate and graduate programs in nursing.* Washington, DC: American Association of Colleges of Nursing.

Billings, D., & Halstead, J. (1998). *Teaching in nursing: A guide for faculty.* Philadelphia: W. B. Saunders.

Bond, W., Kostenbader, M., & McCarthy, J. (2001). Prehospital and hospital-based healthcare providers' experience with a human patient simulator. *Prehospital Emergency Care, 5*(3), 284–287.

Casey, K., Fink, R., Krugman, M., & Propst, J. (2004). The graduate nurse experience. *Journal of Nursing Administration, 34*(6), 303–311.

Chopra, V., Gesink, B., DeJong, J., Bovill, J., Spierdijk, J., & Brand, R. (1994). Does training on an anesthesia simulator lead to improvement in performance? *British Journal of Anaesthesia, 73*(3), 293–297.

Clark, R., & Mayer, R. (2003). *E-learning and the science of instruction: Proven guidelines for consumers and designers of multimedia learning.* San Francisco: Jossey-Bass.

Dunn, W. (2004). Education theory: Does simulation really fit? In W. F. Dunn (Ed.), *Simulators in critical care education and beyond* (pp. 15–19). Des Plaines, IL: Society of Critical Care Medicine.

Fanaroff, A. (1999). Challenges for neonatology and neonatologists. *Journal of Perinatology, 19*(5), 329.

Feingold, C., Calaluce, M., & Kallen, M. (2004). Computerized patient model and simulated clinical experiences: Evaluation with baccalaureate nursing students. *Journal of Nursing Education, 43*(4), 156–163.

Gladwell, M. (2005). *Blink.* New York: Little, Brown.

Gordon, J., Wilkerson, W., Shaffer, D., & Armstrong, E. (2001). "Practicing" medicine without risk: Students' and educators' responses to high-fidelity patient simulation. *Academic Medicine, 76*(5), 469–472.

Hunt, E. (2004). *Simulation of pediatric cardiopulmonary arrests: A report of 34 mock codes performed over a 40-month period focused on assessing delays in important resuscitation maneuvers and types of errors.* Presented at the 2005 International Meeting on Medical Simulation, Miami, FL.

Institute of Medicine. (IOM). (2004). *Keeping patients safe: Transforming the work environment of nurses.* Washington, DC: National Academy of Science.

Kozmenko, V., Yang, T., Chauvin, S., DiCarlo, R., & Hilton, C. (2005). *Teaching clinical skills for undergraduate medical students through inquiry with the use of high fidelity human patient simulator.* Presented at the 2005 International Meeting on Medical Simulation, Miami, FL.

Larew, C., Lessans, S., Spunt, D., Foster, D., & Covington, B. (2006). Innovations in clinical simulation: Application of Benner's theory in an interactive patient care simulation. *Nursing Education Perspectives, 27*(1), 16–21.

Lupien, A. (1998). Simulation in nursing anesthesia education: Practical and conceptual perspectives. In L. C. Henson & A. C. Lee (Eds.), *Simulators in anesthesiology education* (pp. 29–38). New York: Plenum Press.

McLaughlin, S., Doezema, D., & Sklar, D. (2002). Human simulation in emergency medicine training: A model curriculum. *Academic Emergency Medicine, 9*(8), 786–794.

McMahon, G., Monaghan, C., Falchuk, K., Gordon, J., & Alexander, E. (2005). A simulator-based curriculum to promote comparative and reflective analysis in an internal medicine clerkship. *Academic Medicine, 80*(1), 84–89.

Morton, P., & Rauen, C. (2004). Using simulation in nursing education: The University of Maryland and Georgetown University experiences. In M. Oermann & K. Heinrich (Eds.), *Annual Review of Nursing Education* (Vol. 2, pp. 139–161). New York: Springer.

National League for Nursing (NLN). (2005). Despite encouraging trends suggested by the NLN's comprehensive survey of all nursing programs, large number of qualified applicants continue to be turned down. Retrieved September 14, 2008, from www.nln.org/newsreleases/nedsdec05.pdf

Nehring, W., & Lashley, F. (2004). Current uses and opinions regarding human patient simulators in nursing education: An international survey. *Nursing Education Perspectives, 25*(5), 244–248.

Peteani, L. A. (2004). Enhancing clinical practice and education with high-fidelity human patient simulators. *Nurse Educator, 29*(1), 25–30.

Pew Health Professions Commission. (1998). *Recreating health professional practice for a new century.* San Francisco: Author.

Prensky, M. (2001, October). Digital natives, digital immigrants. *On the Horizon* (NCB University Press), *9*(5). Retrieved May 18, 2008, from http://www.marcprensky.com/writing/Prensky%20-%20Digital%20Natives,%20Digital%20Immigrants%20-%20Part1.pdf

Rhodes, M., & Curran, C. (2005). Use of the human patient simulator to teach clinical judgment skills in a baccalaureate nursing program. *CIN: Computers, Informatics, Nursing, 23*(5), 256–262.

Robertson, B. (2006). An obstetric simulation experience in an undergraduate nursing curriculum. *Nurse Educator, 31*(2), 74–78.

CHAPTER 19

Evaluation

Pamela R. Jeffries and Angela M. McNelis

Healthcare professionals need to be prepared so that their work will ensure safe and efficient practice environments. Faced with the many challenges apparent today in healthcare education, nursing educators must explore innovative ways to teach nursing students real-world clinical practice in a cost-effective, productive, and high-quality manner. In recent years, developments in educational technology have made a wide array of options, such as sophisticated simulators, available to faculty to facilitate experiential learning. Such developments also create an environment conducive to systematic and substantial change. To create the most effective and efficient ways of teaching nursing students, educators need to employ a wide range of methods for engaging them in learning activities, including simulation. The traditional path of providing nursing students with limited clinical experiences and immersing them in lecture content and small-group work can impart technical knowledge, but is *inadequate* to prepare them for the complexities of the workplace. Clinical simulation, combined with actual clinical experience and experiential teaching methods, is a powerful tool to prepare nurses for competent clinical practice (Morton, 1999).

Incorporating clinical simulations into a curriculum is just one approach to preparing nurses for safe, efficient practice. Although more healthcare clinical simulations are being used to enhance learning, little is known about the outcomes of this educational approach, including which teaching practices contribute to positive learning outcomes, what the educator role needs to be for the students, or how the simulation design can contribute to the overall teaching and learning. This chapter focuses on the importance of the evaluation plan when developing and implementing simulation in a nursing course or program. Information is provided on developing a simulation evaluation plan, including high-fidelity patient simulation, specifically as it relates to four areas: (1) evaluating the quality of a simulation design; (2) evaluating the implementation of a simulation and the steps involved; (3) evaluating student learning outcomes designed for the simulation; and (4) using the simulation activity as an evaluation mechanism to document student behaviors and competencies.

A number of small studies (Bruce, Bridges, & Holcomb, 2003; Chau, Chang, Lee, Ip, Lee & Wotton, 2001; Jenkins & Turick-Gibson, 1999; Johnson, Zerwic, & Theis, 1999; Jones, Cason, & Mancini, 2002; Ost, DeRosiers, Britt, Fein, Lesser, & Mehta, 2001; Peterson & Bechtel, 2000; Rauen, 2001; Ravert, 2001; Weis & Guyton-Simmons, 1998) have assessed the use of simulations in nursing, medicine, and related disciplines. Many of these studies, however, have employed small sample sizes and measured various outcomes using instruments with questionable or unknown reliability or validity. Furthermore, the ways the simulations were designed and implemented were neither well documented nor empirically measured. Therefore, the emphasis in this chapter is on the process of developing and conducting an evaluation of the use of clinical simulations that are incorporated into the teaching–learning process or used as an evaluation measure for specific course competencies.

THE EVALUATION PLAN AND PROCESS

Identify the Purpose

As described in the introduction to this chapter, evaluation in relation to simulation must consider the relationship between the activities (the simulation) and the desired outcomes (knowledge, skills, critical thinking, learner satisfaction, self-confidence) as the relationship between a cause and its effects. Evaluation then becomes an activity that yields comprehensive information for analyzing, discussing, and judging a learner's performance relative to valued abilities and skills. In the context of simulation, focus on a learner-centered paradigm will guide both formative and summative evaluation approaches (as defined later in this chapter). According to Huba and Freed (2000), learner-centered evaluation can contribute to quality education in the following ways:

- Promoting high expectations
- Respecting diverse talents and learning styles
- Engaging students in meaningful intellectual work and helping them discover connections between what they learn in school and what they will use in their profession
- Synthesizing experiences, fostering ongoing practice of learned skills, and integrating education and experience
- Using knowledge to address issue and problems

- Actively involving students in learning and promoting adequate time on task
- Providing prompt feedback
- Fostering collaboration
- Increasing student–faculty contact

Consideration of these factors will help determine components of the evaluation.

Formative versus Summative Approaches

Scriven (1996) has separated evaluations into formative and summative approaches. Put simplistically, summative evaluation tells us what happened, whereas formative evaluation tells why or how it happened.

Formative evaluation is a method of judging the worth of a program while the program activities are forming or happening. This type of evaluation focuses on the *process* that occurs during the activity or effort. The intent is to improve or change the process by identifying progress toward goals, objectives, or outcomes. If the simulation fails to meet the course objectives, formative evaluation may tell us why. If the simulation is successful in meeting some of the objectives, formative evaluation also has the potential to tell us which activities or components worked well and which did not work well. The major advantage of this evaluation approach is that results can be used to improve the simulation before the course or semester has ended. Disadvantages include the potential for educators to make decisions based on preliminary data or to make judgments before the course is completed (Scriven, 1996).

Summative evaluation, by contrast, examines the effect of the activities or effort on the outcomes; in the case of simulation, the outcome may be assigning grades or certifying competency. An advantage of the summative evaluation is that all work has been completed and final results can be documented. The major disadvantage of this approach is that no changes can be made until the program or activity is concluded (Scriven, 1996).

Simulation as a Teaching–Learning Intervention versus Evaluation for a Grade

The educator decides if the evaluation will focus on the student's progress toward an outcome (formative) or on the attainment of the outcome (summative). Likewise, the simulation may be designed to focus on either the teaching–learning process or attainment of learning objectives.

When simulations are used as a teaching–learning activity, the idea is to improve student performance. Angelo (2007) identifies six purposes for formative evaluation:

- To focus learners' attention
- To illuminate and undermine misconceptions
- To increase motivation to learn
- To provide learners with feedback
- To promote self-assessment and monitoring
- To improve academic success

Thus, from this perspective, students receive feedback from the educator and from peers, and they reflect upon their knowledge, skills, and critical thinking relative to the simulation. Additionally, evaluation at this stage can involve examining the instructional design for purpose, clarity, timing, fidelity, cues, and learning activities of the simulation. Student satisfaction with learning and self-confidence in learning using simulations can also be evaluated.

When simulations are used to assign grades, learners receive feedback about attainment of learning objectives and/or final competency goals at the conclusion of the teaching–learning activity. Angelo (2007) describes five purposes for summative evaluation:

- To sort learners
- To compare learners with one another
- To compare learning against criteria
- To certify competence
- To award degrees and other qualifications

When used summatively, evaluation often becomes the basis for progression in a course or program.

SETTING UP AN EVALUATION PLAN

Purpose

One of the first steps in setting up an evaluation plan is to determine what the purpose of the simulation is and what the intended learning goals are for the activity. It is essential that the purpose of the evaluation is clear, as this factor determines the questions asked and the type and timing of those questions, guides the selection of evaluation instruments, and facilitates data collection, analysis, and interpretation. The plan needs to specify the procedure for data collection, including answers to the following questions: *Which data will be collected? How will the data be collected? Who will collect the data? Where will the data be collected? When will the data be collected?* A well-organized process for evaluation is essential to success.

If the purpose of the simulation is formative in nature, the questions are likely to focus on assessment of progress or performance of *selected* activities. If the simulation is summative in nature, the questions are more likely to focus on the *whole* of the experience and assess critical skills and behaviors of the student in achieving the desired outcomes.

Timeline

Once the purpose of the evaluation is determined, the time frame for the evaluation logically follows. If the simulation is designed to assess formative learning, the evaluation will occur during some point in the learning experience. Generally, evaluation occurs after the critical learning event or important teaching point has happened so that assessment of students' progress toward *selected activities* can be determined. Thus evaluation would take place after the students have completed the simulation activity, but while opportunities and time exist for them to use the feedback to improve their knowledge, skills, and/or performance.

When the simulation is summative in nature, the timing of the evaluation must occur at the conclusion of the course or module, when students would be expected to have acquired the intended knowledge, skills, critical thinking, confidence, and/or skill competence. The focus in this case is on the *whole* to assess attainment of learning objectives. As mentioned earlier, because it is a cumulative assessment, summative evaluation often affects student progression in a course or program.

Evaluation Instruments

Instruments to measure the constructs are selected according to the purpose and goals of the simulation. There are two major requirements of valid measures used in evaluation research: They must be valid and reliable for the population being studied and they must be adequately direct in measuring the construct of interest (Kerlinger, 2000; Ray, 2006). In addition, the instruments should be appropriate for the situation and level of participant. The educator needs to consider how much time is available for evaluation and make decisions about the breadth and depth of the measurements. Another consideration should be cost, as some instruments have a fee attached to their usage.

Evaluation instruments are simply the tools used to collect data. The type of instrument used to assess a simulation is determined by the data collection method and the variables of interest. As the researcher, you should select the most appropriate instrument or instruments for your study. Existing instruments should always be considered as a first choice, especially if they have documented reliability and validity. In addition, existing instruments can help connect findings from individual nursing programs to previous research, and they can usually be adapted to the specifics of individual simulation programs. Many types of data collection instruments are available for use in nursing research, including self-report questionnaires, attitude scales, observational methods, checklists, and journaling. Some studies use more than one method to improve confidence in the study findings. All of the instruments discussed here can be used in both formative and summative evaluations.

Questionnaires

Questionnaires are a frequently reported method of data collection in published nursing studies. Using questionnaires is generally advantageous because they are an inexpensive and rapid way to collect data from a large number of students. Also, because they can provide data anonymously if desired, students are more likely to provide honest answers on questionnaires. Moreover, existing questionnaires that have known validity and reliability can be used to increase the accuracy of data collected. Questionnaires should be short to maximize completion; forms that can be completed in 10 minutes or less are desirable. Individual questions should also be kept short, preferably containing fewer than 20 words. It is important that the evaluator keep questions clear and simple, so that knowledge is assessed rather than the students' reading ability or persistence (Polit & Beck, 2008). Disadvantages to questionnaires include the possibilities that students may answer questions in a socially acceptable direction, skip some questions, or answer questions incorrectly because the meaning is misunderstood.

Questions can be either open-ended or closed-ended. Open-ended questions ask students to respond to questions in their own words; closed-ended questions force students to choose from select answers. Closed-ended questions can take the form of dichotomous questions (yes/no, true/false), multiple choice, matching, or a checklist where students check all answers that are correct or apply to them. Questionnaires may combine both types of questions, as in the format in which, after the closed-ended item is presented, space is provided for students to answer in their own words if none of the choices seem to apply or to expand on an answer.

Attitude Scales

Attitude scales are a type of self-report questionnaire that asks students to indicate their attitudes or feelings about a concept. Attitude scales usually employ Likert scale responses composed of five or seven responses for each item, such as responses ranging from "strongly agree" to "strongly disagree." The researcher will need to decide if he or she wants to include a "neutral" response for students to select as their answer. Proponents of a neutral response suggest that respondents need this choice because the answers may not reflect their attitude, whereas opponents believe that respondents should be forced to either agree or disagree with the item. If five responses are used, scores on each item generally range from 1 ("strongly disagree") to 5 ("strongly agree") (Nieswiadomy, 2008).

Observations

Conducting evaluations by means of observation requires gathering data visually, with the data collection typically being performed by the instructor or another trained participant. The observation occurs during the simulation to assess critical skills or behaviors of the student participant. Observations can range along a continuum from structured to unstructured. Structured observations usually involve some kind of checklist; the observer records the frequency of occurrence of expected behaviors or activities of interest, resulting in quantitative data. Conversely, in unstructured observations, expected skills or behaviors are not predetermined; thus extensive amounts of descriptive data that are qualitative in nature are collected. Both types of observations require decisions about what will be observed, who will observe, which observational procedure will be used, and what type of relationship will exist between the observer and the subjects. A combination of both types of observations is often used in research (Cone & Foster, 2006).

Checklists

As discussed in the preceding paragraph on observations, checklists are often used to record observed phenomena. Not all behaviors are recorded—just those identified as important or necessary (Polit & Beck, 2008). The instructor or other observer uses the checklist to tally whether a behavior, event, or characteristic occurs. The checklist can employ a yes/no response scale, indicating that the phenomena of interest did or did not occur, or a weighted scale, in which more important items receive greater weight. Checklists are useful in simulations in which a skill has multiple steps that must be completed, especially when the steps must occur sequentially.

Journaling

Research on cognition indicates that reflection enhances student learning (Cross, 1996). Journaling is a type of self-reporting reflection in which students record their feelings, activities, and thoughts about their simulation experience. Journals can be a one-time activity or a continuous activity throughout the course. Students are encouraged to reflect on their overall simulation experience; their individual performance in the simulation, including strengths and areas needing improvement; and the effects that this experience will have on their practice. Both students and instructors can use the data in the journal to evaluate critical thinking as well as intellectual and professional growth over time.

Data Collection

Evaluation data are collected immediately after the simulation is completed by the student and should be gathered systematically and consistently. A plan for data collection should be developed before the study begins, and factors to consider include the answers to the following questions: *Which data will be collected? How will the data be collected? Who will collect the data? Where will the data be collected? When will the data be collected?* When the data collection plan is developed, pragmatic issues such as cost, time constraints, participant burden, and the number of variables being assessed always need to be taken into account.

Data Analysis

A plan for data analysis should be developed before the study is implemented. The first step after data collection is to organize those data for analysis. All data collection sources, but especially self-report forms, should be checked for completion; decisions must then be made about missing data. Preferably, a statistician will work with the evaluator from the conception of the study and will be particularly active in the data analysis phase. Plans for analyzing the data should be made before obtaining the data, however. The statistician can help you to determine the number of students you need in your study, identify the statistical procedures that will be appropriate to answer your research questions, and interpret the data.

Data Interpretation

After data are analyzed, responses are interpreted to answer the questions about the simulation. Data analyses and interpretation depend on the purpose of the simulation. At the student level, assessment and interpretation occur in an attempt to understand individual student progress or to determine which specific parts of the simulation worked and which did not work. At a curricular level, interpretation focuses on how well learning outcomes or objectives were met using the simulation. At the practice level, the center of interpretation is attainment of those knowledge and skills needed for safe and effective patient care. The results of the simulation evaluation should also be compared with results from previous studies to ensure that they contribute to the existing body of knowledge on the study topic.

Evaluating the Quality of the Simulation

When designing simulations, the educator wants to ensure a quality simulation for the learners that has objectives and focus appropriate to the learning experience. All too often, simulations are developed or run "on the fly" without sufficient consideration of what the simulation is actually about or what the student needs to learn from it. To help ensure quality simulations, a small group of researchers funded by the National League for Nursing developed a *Simulation Design Scale* (SDS) that proposes five design features to be included in a simulation to ensure it is of high quality (Jeffries, 2007). These design features assist educators to attend to all important components needed in a simulation. The five components of the SDS are described next, and the importance of each is discussed in depth.

OBJECTIVES/INFORMATION

When first deciding to develop a clinical simulation for students, the objectives of the simulation need to be considered so the activity can be mapped out to meet the needs of the course or activity. One simulation may serve many purposes—for example, enhancing therapeutic communication skills, patient safety competency, and care of an insulin-managed patient, all in one 20-minute scenario. The objectives should reflect the intent of the specific scenario, indicating a general direction for the student but not providing such specific objectives that the student is aware of how the entire scenario will unfold. Many educators are finding that the identification of three to five learning objectives for the simulation is sufficient to help inform students and to provide a quality learning experience for them (Jeffries, 2007).

In addition to objectives of the scenario, educators need to provide students with some basic information about the simulation as a preview of the learning experience. For example, the components of the simulation scenario need to be identified, so that students can anticipate what is expected and how much time they have within the simulation to achieve the objectives of the activity. Many educators also provide students with various types of pre-simulation information such as worksheets, Web-based modules, or simple reading assignments to review prior to the experience.

Fidelity (Realism)

Clinical simulations need to mimic clinical reality, be process-based, and have established validity (Cioffi, 2001). Clinical simulations must be authentic and include as many realistic environmental factors as possible to make the students' learning more relevant to the real world (Aronson, Rosa, Anfinson, & Light, 1997; Cioffi, 2001; Hample, Herbold, Schneider, & Sheeley, 1999; Hotchkins, Biddle, C., & Fallacaro, 2002; Jones et al., 2002; Peterson & Bechtel, 2000). Hotchkins et al. (2002) noted the lack of systematic study regarding the authenticity of simulation experiences, particularly in connection with anesthesia. Although high-fidelity patient simulation can rarely be a completely realistic situation, as close an approximation as possible should be attempted to promote better learning outcomes. Barrow and Feltovich (1987) have suggested the structure of a realistic simulated clinical situation requires three elements: (1) relatively little information should be available initially; (2) the clinician should be allowed to investigate freely, employing questions in any sequence; and (3) the clinician should be given the clinical information over time during the simulation.

Beaubien and Baker (2004), in a discussion of teaching teamwork and collaboration skills in health care, state that high-fidelity simulation is only one of many tools that may be effective. They describe three dimensions of fidelity: environmental, equipment, and psychological. Of these dimensions, they propose that psychological fidelity is the most important for team training. Depending on goals and objectives of a simulation, educators may need to focus on realism in the environment, for instance, but not necessarily just in relation to the patient mannequin.

What this means for nursing educators who are designing simulations is that educators have a responsibility beyond assuring realistic equipment. Clearly, learners can become quickly engaged in caring for a high-fidelity patient simulator that features heart sounds, running IV fluids, and real-life lung sounds, but there is more to the simulation than just the high-fidelity patient simulator. Consideration must be given to what learners are thinking and feeling during the experience.

Rudolph, Simon, Rivard, Dufresne, and Raemer (2007) describe four modes in which humans think about reality: physical, conceptual, emotional, and experiential. For example, the *physical* aspects of a simulation need to mimic reality, such that the environment should physically look like the setting that is implied in the scenario. With high-fidelity mannequins that can talk, have realistic heart sounds, and feature a chest that inflates with breathing, the physical realism is improved over what it used to be only a few years ago. An example of *conceptual* realism occurs when the patient is short of breath in the scenario: The student applies oxygen, and then the pulse biox increases, indicating that the patient's oxygenation status is improving. In this situation, the concept of oxygenation has been demonstrated, and the student's behavior indicates that he or she made the connection with the oxygenation concept. The *emotional* aspect of scenarios is also part of the realism and is created by the events, the real props, and all of the other factors that help to immerse students in the environment, such as alarms sounding, the patient deteriorating quickly as the blood pressure drops, and the moaning of the patient with chest pain. With these components built into the scenario, the emotional aspect is created so the student can experience factors that can influence quick assessments and interventions needed for the patient. Finally, the *experiential* realism of a simulation is that learners get to do hands-on care, assessment, and intervention.

PROBLEM SOLVING (COMPLEXITY)

Another design feature to consider when developing clinical simulations is the problem-solving feature, which requires some type of decision-making process or clinical decision by the nursing student. Developing the scenario around realistic events that could potentially happen with patients on a clinical unit provides nursing students with an opportunity to assess the patient and make a decision about what to do next. When designing the clinical simulation scenario, the nursing educator needs to set up the simulation so that the scenario gradually unfolds and a decision or decisions need to be made by the nursing student. Providing opportunities for nursing students to make decisions during this educational activity serves many purposes:

- It creates a safe, nonthreatening environment in which nursing students can make decisions and see the consequences and outcomes of their interventions and choices.
- It assists nurse educators in assessing how nursing students can critically think and problem-solve while being immersed in a realistic clinical setting.
- It constructs a hands-on learning experience for nursing students that approximates a real-life clinical situation.

STUDENT SUPPORT (CUEING)

Student support is a design feature that is discussed in the literature as an important component of simulations, although little evidence and few details about this component have been published to date. What is known is that students feel supported by instructors when a debriefing session after the simulation is facilitated by the instructor, rather than just having that instructor be present during the simulation.

Other support activities include providing cues or hints during the simulation to direct the student down a certain path or to evaluate his or her thinking and connection to the cue provided. For example, a nursing manager might bring in a lab report during a simulation showing that the patient has a potassium level of 2.8 mEq/L. On the patient monitor, the patient is shown to be experiencing sinus tachycardia with multifocal PVCs. With the lab report showing hypokalemia, the cue is the report, with the intent that the student will correlate or associate the hypokalemia with the multifocal PVCs and then treat the cause.

In Chickering and Gamson's (1987) *Best Practices in Undergraduate Education*, the authors propose that student–faculty interaction is one of the principles of best practices. Students want to be supported and have quality time with faculty members who facilitate their learning and achievement of course outcomes.

DEBRIEFING (GUIDED REFLECTION)

Guided reflection is defined as a process in which a facilitator promotes the learner's development of insight using semistructured cue questions. The act of debriefing consists of reviewing a real or simulated event by having participants explain, analyze, and synthesize information and reactions (emotions) related to the scenario, with the goal being to improve their performance in similar situations (Decker, 2007). Both guided reflection and debriefing are important activities to include once the simulation scenario is completed.

In the National League for Nursing study (2003–2006), simulation design features were evaluated in eight small outcome studies in addition to one large, multisite study testing selected outcomes on care of a postoperative patient (Jeffries, 2007). In these studies, the design feature consistently deemed to be most important to nursing students was the guided reflection/debriefing activity in which they could discuss their performance in the simulation, identify their feelings and emotions relative to the care of the simulated patient, have any of their mistakes corrected, and receive explanations about what should have been done.

According to Peters and Vissers (2004), learning occurs and is encouraged in debriefing. By allowing participants to discuss their perceptions, evaluate their performance, and give a rationale for their interventions, this activity provides high-level learning opportunity for students (Rhodes & Curran, 2005).

While reflecting, learners are able to examine what happened during the simulation and to verbalize what they learned from being immersed in the experience (Jeffries & Rogers, 2007; Lederman, 1992). For example, a study by Savoldelli et al. (2006) demonstrated how anesthesia residents who received either oral debriefing or debriefing using video had a significantly greater improvement ($P < .005$) in nontechnical skills from a pre-test to post-test simulated scenario than those participants who received no debriefing/guided reflection.

EVALUATION INSTRUMENT

To evaluate the quality of a simulation, the *Simulation Design Scale* (SDS; Jeffries, 2007) can be used to measure the five features recommended from the literature (Jeffries, 2005). The SDS is a 20-item instrument with five subscales: information/objectives, fidelity, student support, problem solving, and debriefing. These subscales are used to measure each design feature as rated by the participants. Table 19-1 lists the five design features and sample items from

Table 19-1   The Simulation Design Scale and Sample Items

Design Feature	Sample Items	5 Strongly Agree	4 Agree	3 Neutral	2 Disagree	1 Strongly Disagree
Objectives/ Information	I clearly understood the purpose and objectives of the simulation.					
Student Support	My need for help was recognized.					
Problem Solving	I was encouraged to explore all possibilities during the simulation.					
Fidelity	The scenario resembled a real-life situation.					
Guided Reflection	Feedback provided was constructive.					

the SDS. These features are postulated by Jeffries (2005) to be integral to positive learning outcomes in a simulation. The content validity of the SDS instrument was determined by a panel of eight nurse experts. The Cronbach's alpha coefficient reflecting reliability was 0.94 (Dobbs, Sweitzer, & Jeffries, 2006; Jeffries, 2007).

EVALUATING THE IMPLEMENTATION OF THE SIMULATION

Not only is the design and development important to the quality of simulations, but the way the simulation activity is implemented is also important to enhance learning outcomes. As part of the implementation phase, educators need to consider Chickering and Gamson's (1987) *Best Practices in Undergraduate Education*. According to these educational researchers, studying good teaching, incorporating specific evidence-based educational practices, and using them consistently are all measures that can improve student learning and satisfaction (Chickering & Gamson, 1987). The seven key principles in the context of simulations include active learning, prompt feedback, allowing diverse styles for learning, student–faculty interaction, time on task, collaborative learning, and high expectations. These principles can be used to guide simulation design and implementation.

An instrument called the *Educational Practices in Simulation Scale* (EPSS) was designed to measure these principles of best practice in simulation. The EPSS is based on a simulation framework (Jeffries, 2005) that incorporates these best practices (see Figure 19-1). This instrument, which consists of a 16-item scale that the participant completes after experiencing the simulation, measures the extent to which each principle of best practice is perceived to have been incorporated in the simulation itself and identifies how important that educational practice is to the student in his or her learning. Factor analysis on the scale resulted in collapsing the seven principles of best practice in education into four subscales (Cronbach's alpha = 0.92 on the overall scale). Content validity of the instrument was determined by a panel of nine nurse experts, and the Cronbach's alpha coefficients for the four subscales ranged from 0.78 to 0.92. Table 19-2 lists the four educational practices in simulation and gives a sample item for each.

EVALUATING STUDENT LEARNING OUTCOMES
WHEN IMPLEMENTING SIMULATIONS

Simulations also provide faculty with a way to more accurately assess each student's competency, in that they overcome the limitations associated with the variability and unpredictability of clinical experiences and supervision in

Figure 19-1   The Simulation Framework

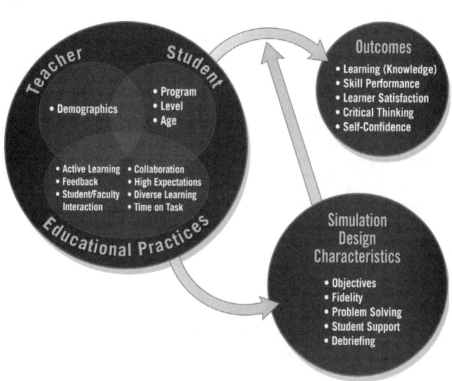

Source: Jeffries, P. R. (2007). *Simulation in nursing education: From conceptualization to evaluations.* New York: National League for Nursing.

actual healthcare settings (Becker, Rose, Berg, Park, & Shatzer, 2006). By constructing scenarios that test specific aspects of clinical practice (Comer, 2005), faculty can ascertain the adequacy of each student's performance related to specific competencies. Educators employing simulation technology can also assure that *every* student has experience in particular areas, including risky situations, by including threats to patient safety as part of the simulation experience. In this way, simulation can assist faculty to more clearly and reliably detect effective and ineffective student performance (Jeffries, 2005) and remediate students when particular skills are absent, inadequate, or not fully developed (Bremner, Aduddell, Bennett, & VanGeest, 2006).

Different types of simulations can be used to provide learners with opportunities to learn and practice in a controlled environment that closely mirrors the realities and complexities of practice without the risk of causing harm to

Table 19-2   Educational Practices in Simulation Scale (EPSS) and Sample Items for Each Subscale

Best Practice	Sample Instrument Item	5 Strongly Agree	4 Agree	3 Neutral	2 Disagree	1 Strongly Disagree
Active Learning	I received cues during the simulation activity in a timely manner.					
Diverse Ways of Learning	The simulation offered a variety of ways in which to learn the material.					
High Expectations	The objectives for the simulation experience were clear and easy to understand.					
Collaboration	I had the chance to work with my peers during the simulation.					

patients, in addition to providing a mechanism to evaluate student learning outcomes (Henneman & Cunningham, 2005; Jeffries, 2005). Although the literature often equates the term "simulation" with the use of high-tech equipment, such as high-fidelity patient simulators, faculty can use a variety of simulated experiences in their teaching and evaluation, including, but not limited to, the use of role-playing (Comer, 2005; Goldenberg, Andrusyszyn, & Iwasiw, 2005), standardized patients (Becker et al., 2006), interactive media (Jeffries, 2001; Jeffries, Woolf, & Linde, 2003), and mannequins and task trainers (Alinier, Hung, Gordon & Hardwood, 2006; Jeffries, 2005).

Good educators attempt to make learning meaningful so that students can make connections, solve problems, and critically think. Simulation appears to be effective in promoting problem solving, recall, and the connecting of information. When faculty decide whether to develop and incorporate simulation in the learning environments, the learning outcomes of the scenario need to be considered.

SUMMARY

As simulations become used more frequently in clinical teaching and learning in the health professions, it is essential that educators be well prepared to develop, implement, and evaluate those experiences. Experts in education (Chickering & Gamson, 1987; Huba & Freed, 2000) recommend that learning should be student-centered; simulations, when designed properly, meet this criterion. In simulations, students construct knowledge through gathering and synthesizing information and integrating it with general skills of inquiry, communication, critical thinking, and problem solving. Students are actively involved in their learning, with an emphasis on using and communicating knowledge effectively to address enduring and emerging issues and problems. Learning occurs in real-life contexts, and the instructor's role can be either to coach and facilitate or to judge. In this model, teaching and assessing are intertwined, and assessment is used to promote and measure learning by generating better questions and learning from errors. Moreover, desired learning is assessed directly through performance. Simulations also lend themselves to interdisciplinary collaboration, which helps to make the experience *real* in the context of practice.

Currently, clinical simulations incorporating high-fidelity simulators and other types of simulation scenarios are being used as part of clinical experiences for nursing students. Evaluation of these uses and clinical substitutions and enhancements are being studied to investigate the clinical judgment and the benefits of this type of clinical learning (Rhodes & Curran, 2005). To accomplish these lofty goals, evidence of best practices in simulation education must be generated. Utilizing the information presented in this chapter, educators can construct quality simulations that will result in data to guide future teaching and learning practices.

References

Alinier, G., Hunt, B., Gordon, R. & Harwood, C. (2006). Effectiveness of intermediate-fidelity simulation training technology in undergraduate nursing education. *Journal of Advanced Nursing, 54,* 359–369.

Angelo, T. A. (2007, November). *Doing assessment as if learning matters most.* Workshop presented at the meeting of the 2007 Assessment Institute, Indianapolis, IN.

Aronson, B., Rosa, J., Anfinson, J., & Light, N. (1997). A simulated clinical problem-solving experience. *Nurse Educator, 22*(6), 17–19.

Barrow, H. S., & Feltovich P. J. (1987). The clinical reasoning process. *Medical Education, 21*(2), 86–91.

Beaubien, J. M., & Baker, D. P. (2004). The use of simulation for training teamwork skills in health care: How low can you go? *Quality and Safety in Health Care, 13*(suppl 1), i51–i56.

Becker, K. L., Rose, L. E., Berg, J. B., Park, H., & Shatzer, J. H. (2006). The teaching effectiveness of standardized patients. *Journal of Nursing Education, 45*(4), 103–111.

Bremner, M. N., Aduddell. K., Bennett, D. N., & VanGeest, J. B. (2006). The use of human patient simulators: Best practices with novice nursing students. *Nurse Educator, 31*, 170–174.

Bruce, S., Bridges, E. J., & Holcomb, J. B. (2003). Preparing to respond: Joint Trauma Training Center and USAF Nursing Warskills Simulation Laboratory. *Critical Care Nurse Clinics of North America, 15*, 149–152.

Chau, J., Chang, A., Lee, I., Ip, W., Lee, D., & Wootton, Y. (2001). Effets of using videotaped vignettes on enhancing students' critical thinking ability in a baccalaureate nursing programme. *Journal of Advanced Nursing, 36*(1), 112–119.

Chickering, A. W., & Gamson, Z. F. (1987, March). Seven principles for good practice. *AAHE Bulletin*, 3–7.

Cioffi, J. (2001). Clinical simulations: Development and validation. *Nurse Education Today, 21*, 477–486.

Comer, S. K. (2005). Patient care simulations: Role playing to enhance clinical understanding. *Nursing Education Perspectives, 26*, 357–361.

Cone, J. D., & Foster, S. L. (2006). *Dissertations and theses from start to finish* (2nd ed.). Baltimore, MD: United Book Press.

Cross, K. P. (1996). New lenses on learning. *About Campus, 1*(4), 4–9.

Decker, S. (2007). Integrating guided reflection into simulated learning experiences. In P. R. Jeffries (Ed.), *Simulations in nursing education: From conceptualization to evaluation* (pp. 73–85). New York: National League for Nursing.

Dobbs, C., Sweitzer, V., & Jeffries, P. (2006). Testing simulation design features using an insulin management simulation in nursing education. *INACSL Online Journal, 2*(1), 1–9.

Engum, S., Jeffries, P. R., & Fisher, L. (2003). Intravenous catheter training system: Computer-based education vs. traditional learning methods. *The American Journal of Surgery, 186*(1), 67–74.

Goldenberg, D., Andrusyszyn, M. A., & Iwasiw, C. (2005). The effect of classroom simulation on nursing students' self-efficacy related to health teaching. *Journal of Nursing Education, 44*, 310–314.

Hample, J., Herbold, N., Schneider, M., & Sheeley, A. (1999). Using standardized patients to train and evaluate dietetics students. *Journal of the American Dietetic Association, 99*, 1094–1097.

Henneman, E. A., & Cunningham, H. (2005). Using clinical simulation to teach patient safety in an acute/critical care nursing course. *Nursing Education, 30*, 172–177.

Hotchkins, M., Biddle, C., & Fallacaro, M. (2002). Assessing the authenticity of the human simulation experience in anesthesiology. *AANA Journal, 70*, 470–473.

Huba, M. E., & Freed, J. E. (2000). *Learner-centered assessment on college campuses: Shifting the focus from teaching to learning*. Needham Heights, MA; Allyn & Bacon.

Jeffries, P. R. (2001). Computer versus lecture: A comparison of two methods of teaching oral medication administration in a nursing skills laboratory. *Journal of Nursing Education, 40*, 323–329

Jeffries, P. R. (2005). A framework for designing, implementing, and evaluation simulations used as teaching strategies in nursing. *Nursing Education Perspectives, 26*(2), 96–103.

Jeffries, P. R. (2007). *Simulation in nursing education: From conceptualization to evaluation.* New York: National League for Nursing.

Jeffries, P. R., & Rogers, K. J. (2007). Evaluating simulations. In P. R. Jeffries (Ed.). *Simulation in nursing education: From conceptualization to evaluation* (pp. 87–103). New York: National League for Nursing.

Jeffries, P. R., Woolf, S., & Linde, B. (2003). Technology-based vs. traditional instruction: A comparison of two teaching methods for teaching the skill of performing a 12 lead ECG. *Nursing Education, 24*(2), 70–74.

Jenkins, P., & Turick-Gibson, T. (1999). An exercise in critical thinking using role playing, *Nurse Educator, 24*(6), 11–14.

Johnson, J., Zerwic, J., & Theis, S. (1999). Clinical simulation laboratory: An adjunct to clinical teaching. *Nurse Educator, 24*(5), 37–41.

Jones, T., Cason, C., & Mancini, M. (2002). Evaluating nurse competency: Evidence of validity for a skills re-credentialing program. *Journal of Professional Nursing, 18*(1), 22–28.

Kerlinger, F. N. (2000). *Foundations of behavioral research* (4th ed.). New York: Harcourt Brace.

Lederman, L. C. (1992). Debriefing: Toward a systematic assessment of theory and practice. *Simulation and Gaming, 23*(2), 145–160.

Morton, P. (1999). Using a critical care simulation laboratory to teach students. *Critical Care Nurse, 17*(6), 66–68.

Nieswiadomy, R. M. (2008). *Foundations of nursing research* (5th ed.). Prentice Hall, NJ: Pearson Education.

Nicol, M., & Freeth, D. (1998). Assessment of clinical skills: A new approach to an old problem. *Nurse Education Today, 18*, 601–609.

Ost, D., DeRosiers, E., Britt, J., Fein, A., Lesser, M., & Mehta, A. (2001). Assessment of a bronchoscopy simulator. *American Journal of Respiratory Critical Care Medicine, 164*, 2248–2255.

Peters, V. A. M., & Vissers, G. A. N. (2004). A simple classification model for debriefing simulation games. *Simulations & Gaming, 35*(1), 70–84.

Peterson, M., & Bechtel, G. (2000). Combining the arts: An applied critical thinking approach in the skills laboratory. *Nursing Connections, 13*(2), 43–49.

Polit, D. E., & Beck, C. T. (2008). *Nursing research: Generating and assessing evidence for nursing practice* (8th ed.). Philadelphia: Wolters Kluwer/Lippincott Williams & Wilkins.

Rauen, C. (2001). Using simulation to teach critical thinking skills. *Critical Care Nursing Clinics of North America, 13*(1), 93–103.

Ravert, P. (2001). Critical thinking of nursing students: Pre and post use of human simulator. Retrieved November 10, 2004, from http://www.anestech.org/Publications/IMMS_2002/Ravert.html

Ray, W. J. (2006). *Methods: Toward a science of behavior and experience* (8th ed.). Pacific Grove, CA: Brooks/Cole.

Rhodes, M. L., & Curran, C. (2005). Use of the human patient simulator to teach clinical judgment skills in a baccalaureate nursing program. *Computers, Informatics, Nursing, 23*, 256–262.

Rudolph, J. W., Simon, R., Dufresne, R. L., & Raemer, D. B. (2006). There's no such thing as "nonjudgmental" debriefing: A theory and method for debriefing with good judgment. *Simulation in Healthcare, 1*(1), 49–55.

Savoldelli, G. L., Naik, V. N., Park, J., Joo, H. S., Chow, R., & Hamstra, S. J. (2006). Value of debriefing during simulated crisis management. *Anesthesiology, 105*(2), 279–285.

Scriven, M. (1996). Types of evaluation and types of evaluator. *Evaluation Practice, 17*(2), 151–161.

Weis, P., & Guyton-Simmons, J. (1998). A computer simulation for teaching critical thinking skills. *Nurse Educator, 23*(2), 30–33.

Unit 4

The Future

CHAPTER 20

Using High-Fidelity Patient Simulation: What Does the Future Hold?

Felissa R. Lashley

The use of high-fidelity simulators is growing quickly in the education of health professional students. It has been adopted for purposes such as new skill acquisition and other continuing education activities for already established professionals and for assessing skills for newly hired individuals in healthcare agencies. The contributors to this book have set forth the present context and past basis for using high-fidelity patient simulation in nursing and other health-related professions. Looking ahead, the following question can be asked: What does the future hold for the use of high-fidelity patient simulators in nursing and health professional education?

The evolution of this modality has occurred relatively quickly, as has its adoption by health professionals. The increased use has been spurred for reasons related to the equipment and its makers, and also for reasons not directly related to the product itself.

Product-related factors driving the use of high-fidelity patient simulation include the following issues:

- Advancement of elements of technology that make the equipment more and more realistic.
- Greater affordability of equipment.
- Greater awareness of the availability of these models among nursing educators and administrators through greater exposure to this modality. This has occurred because of presentations at professional conferences;, articles in professional journals and books, albeit to a lesser extent; and marketing initiatives by the manufacturers of these products so that potential users become cognizant of the range of products available.

The impetus to use high-fidelity patient simulation has also resulted because of reasons related to health professionals' education and to societal pressures, and because of the clear advantages to using patient simulation for training. Many of these reasons were highlighted in a report from the Institute of Medicine, entitled *To Err Is Human: Building a Safer Health System* (Kohn, Corrigan, & Donaldson, 2000). These factors are summarized here:

- Public demand for fewer patient complications (Ahlberg, Heikkinen, Iselius, Leijonmarck, Rutqvist, & Arvidsson, 2002).
- A decrease in accepting the use of animals or human cadavers for surgical or other types of practice or experimentation (Ahlberg et al., 2002).
- Need for improvement of health professionals' clinical competence.
- Need for improvement of health professionals' clinical expertise.
- Need for competency assessment before health professionals deliver actual patient care (Grenvik & Schaefer, 2004).
- Enhancement of the quality of patient care (Issenberg, 2006).
- Enhancement of the safety of patient care (Issenberg, 2006).
- Provision of a nonthreatening environment for students to practice without worry about harming the patient or concern about their own responsibility to the patient (Morgan, Cleave-Hogg, McIlroy, & Devitt, 2002).
- Ability for students to repeat procedures over and over without consequence or concern about the inconvenience, discomfort, or effect on the patient (Freeman, Thompson, Allely, Sobel, Stansfield, & Pugh, 2001; Issenberg, McGaghie, Petrusa, Lee Gordon, & Scalese, 2005; Treloar, Hawayek, Montgomery, Russell, & Medical Readiness Trainer Team, 2001).
- Ability for students to make errors and then follow them through to see what the ultimate effect will be without risk to the patient (Ziv et al., 2006).
- Capacity to allow inquisitive students to ask "What if?" questions and, for example, to administer different doses of various drugs to observe the physiologic and pharmacologic results. Thus students are active participants rather than passive learners (Issenberg et al., 2005).
- Exposure of the student to rarer conditions and illnesses that might not be typically encountered in the clinical situation (Lashley & Nehring, 2009).
- Ability to recreate specific patient encounters for multiple groups of learners (Vozenilek, Wang, Kharasch, Anderson, & Kalaria, 2006).
- Ability to teach both technical and nontechnical skills.
- Ability to practice communication, decision making, critical thinking, clinical reasoning, and leadership skills within a specific profession or across professions in a specific patient situation (Kuiper, Heinrich, Matthias, Graham, & Bell-Kotwall, 2008; Parr & Sweeney, 2006).
- Ability to assess individual performances as well as the performance of the entire team (Kozmenko, Paige, & Chauvin, 2008).

- A decrease in the acceptability of "practicing" skills for the first time on actual patients.
- Growing scarcity of clinical placements for health professional students.
- Restrictions on the types of clinical procedures that agencies will allow students to perform.
- The provision of the best possible education for students.

In addition, mistakes made while using simulation do not harm actual patients, so they are more easily exposed, discussed, and reviewed without concerns of liability, guilt, or blame. Making mistakes while using simulation allows for breaking the culture of silence as well as avoiding any denial about whether mistakes were made and questioning of competence (Ziv et al., 2006). The practice of debriefing as discussed in this book facilitates such discussion and review.

The various types of simulation used to educate nurses include standardized patients, computer-based patient case studies, and other types of educational models, virtual reality, haptic feedback trainers, partial task trainers, and high-fidelity patient simulators. Indeed, these technologies have found a clear—and valued—place in the educational system for most of the health professions. To a greater or lesser extent, more complex simulators are being used, or their use is being discussed, as a substitution for a percentage of required clinical time in the curriculum, and as part of licensure and certification examinations (Dillon, Boulet, Hawkins, & Swanson, 2007; Nehring, 2008).

Nevertheless, some concerns or barriers related to increased future use of high-fidelity patient simulators do exist:

- Equipment cost, which remains relatively high.
- Other instructional costs, such as for hiring additional knowledgeable faculty or a dedicated technician and providing instruction for faculty members.
- Perceived additional workload for faculty.
- Need for space for the necessary equipment.
- Inability of simulation to match the realistic nature of other methods such as standardized patients. For example, patient simulators do not provide spontaneous vocalization.
- Limited to a relatively small number of learners who are direct participants.
- Lack of a base of available data to demonstrate increased learning or skill acquisition, both immediate and across time, thereby providing the evidence base needed to advocate for using this method of instruction.

This is especially the case when high-fidelity patient simulation is compared to other methods of learning.

The obvious benefits of high-fidelity patient simulation for learning both technical and nontechnical skills in the health professions have been delineated earlier. These benefits, when coupled with the following factors, combine to make high-fidelity patient simulation an increasingly viable modality for teaching both technical and nontechnical skills:

- Increased awareness and interest of students, faculty, and clinicians
- The more affordable models available now and those that will be developed in the future
- Increasing realism and ease of use of the models and equipment
- The further development and dissemination of sample and standard scenarios
- Awareness of the place of simulation in undergraduate and graduate curricula with a theoretical base (such as in critical incident nursing management [Nehring, Lashley, & Ellis, 2002])
- The sharing of effective uses of this technology
- The drive to ascertain student mastery of skills in a standardized setting for licensing and certification processes
- The diminishing number of clinical practice sites
- The need for various professions to work in a collaborative manner
- The accelerated public demand for well-qualified, safety-conscious healthcare practitioners and optimal care

In summary, the availability of simulation centers that can be shared in various partnerships among the professions and between educational programs and healthcare agencies will result in greater opportunities for creative uses of simulation. We can expect to see an exponential growth in the use of high-fidelity patient simulation in nursing education, nursing licensure, advanced practice nursing credentialing, orientation programs, and continuing education in the future. This trend will be accompanied by further research and additional innovative uses of this exciting technology as advancements in technology, reduced costs, and increased demand will beget increased use.

References

Ahlberg, G., Heikkinen, T., Iselius, L., Leijonmarck, C. E., Rutqvist, J., & Arvidsson, D. (2002). Does training in a virtual reality simulator improve surgical performance. *Surgical Endoscopy*, *16*, 126–129.

Dillon, G. F., Boulet, J. R., Hawkins, R. E., & Swanson, D. B. (2007). Simulations in the United States Medical Licensing Examination™ (USMLE™). *Quality and Safety in Health Care*, *13*(suppl 1), i41–i45.

Freeman, K. M., Thompson, S. F., Allely, E. B., Sobel, A. L., Stansfield, S. A., & Pugh, W. M. (2001). A virtual reality patient simulation system for teaching emergency response skills to U. S. Navy medical providers. *Prehospital Disaster Medicine, 16*, 3–8.

Grenvik, A., & Schaefer, J. (2004). From Resusci-Anne to Sim-Man: The evolution of simulators in medicine. *Critical Care Medicine, 32*, S56–S57.

Issenberg, S. B. (2006). The scope of simulation-based healthcare education. *Simulation in Healthcare, 1*, 203–208.

Issenberg, S. B., McGaghie, W. C., Petrusa, E. R., Lee Gordon, D., & Scalese, R. J. (2005). Features and uses of high-fidelity medical simulations that lead to effective learning: A BEME systematic review. *Medical Teacher, 27*, 10–28.

Kohn, L. T., Corrigan, J. M., & Donaldson, M. S. (Eds.). (2000). *To err is human: Building a safer health system.* Washington, DC: National Academy of Sciences.

Kozmenko, V., Paige, J., & Chauvin, S. (2008). Initial implementation of mixed reality simulation targeting teamwork and patient safety. *Studies in Health Technology and Informatics Journal, 132*, 216–221.

Kuiper, R., Heinrich, C., Matthias, A., Graham, M. J., & Bell-Kotwall, L. (2008). Debriefing with the OPT model of clinical reasoning during high fidelity patient simulation. *International Journal of Nursing Education Scholarship, 5*, Article 17, e-pub April 3, 2008.

Lashley, F. R., & Nehring, W. (2009). Clinical simulation and the need for evidence-based policy. In G. L. Dickson & L. Flynn (Eds.), *Nursing policy research* (pp. 219–231). New York: Springer.

Morgan, P. J., Cleave-Hogg, D., McIlroy, J., & Devitt, J. H. (2002).Simulation technology: A comparison of experiential and visual learning for undergraduate medical students. *Anesthesiology, 96*, 10–16.

Nehring, W. M. (2008). U.S. Boards of Nursing and the use of high-fidelity patient simulation in nursing education. *Journal of Professional Nursing, 24*, 109–117.

Nehring, W. M., Lashley, F. R., & Ellis, W. E. (2002). Critical incident nursing management using human patient simulators. *Nursing Education Perspectives, 23*, 128–132.

Parr, M. B., & Sweeney, N. M. (2006). Use of human patient simulation in an undergraduate critical care course. *Critical Care Nursing Quarterly, 29*, 188–198.

Treloar, D., Hawayek, J., Montgomery, J. R., Russell, W., & Medical Readiness Trainer Team. (2001). On-site and distance education of emergency medicine personnel with a human patient simulator. *Military Medicine, 166*, 1003–1006.

Vozenilek, J., Wang, E., Kharasch, M., Anderson, B., & Kalaria, A. (2006). Simulation-based morbidity and mortality conference: New technologies augmenting traditional case-based presentations. *Academy of Emergency Medicine, 13*, 48–53.

Ziv, A., Erez, D., Munz, Y., et al. (2006). The Israel Center for Medical Simulation: A paradigm for cultural change in medical education. *Academic Medicine, 81*, 1091–1097.

Index

Locators annotated with *f* and *t* refer to figures and tables.